APPLIED PSYCHOLOGY

APPLIED PSYCHOLOGY

Research, Training and Practice

Second edition

Edited by Rowan Bayne and Gordon Jinks

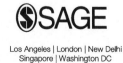

Los Angeles | London | New Delhi
Singapore | Washington DC

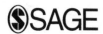

Los Angeles | London | New Delhi
Singapore | Washington DC

SAGE Publications Ltd
1 Oliver's Yard
55 City Road
London EC1Y 1SP

SAGE Publications Inc.
2455 Teller Road
Thousand Oaks, California 91320

SAGE Publications India Pvt Ltd
B 1/I 1 Mohan Cooperative Industrial Area
Mathura Road
New Delhi 110 044

SAGE Publications Asia-Pacific Pte Ltd
3 Church Street
#10-04 Samsung Hub
Singapore 049483

Editor: Michael Carmichael
Editorial assistant: Alana Clogan
Production editor: Imogen Roome
Marketing manager: Alison Borg
Typeset by: C&M Digitals (P) Ltd, Chennai, India
Printed by MPG Books Group, Bodmin, Cornwall

Editorial arrangement © Rowan Bayne and Gordon Jinks 2013

Chapter 1 and 18 © John Radford 2013
Chapter 2 and 9 © Brian R. Clifford 2013
Chapter 3 © David J. Harper, Kenneth Gannon and Mary Robinson 2013
Chapter 4 © Maria Castro, Christopher Whiteley and Mary Boyle 2013
Chapter 5 © Mark Fox 2013
Chapter 6 © Carla Gibbes, Mark Holloway and Donald Ridley 2013
Chapter 7 © Paula Nicolson 2013
Chapter 8 © Chris Hackley 2013
Chapter 10 © Ashok Jansari 2013
Chapter 11 © James Beale and Marcia Wilson 2013
Chapter 12 © Jill Mytton 2013
Chapter 13 © Kate Hefferon and Ilona Boniwell 2013
Chapter 14 © Volker Thoma 2013
Chapter 15 © Gordon Jinks 2013
Chapter 16 © Ho Law and Christian van Nieuwerburgh 2013
Chapter 17 © Jenny Bimrose, Rachel Mulvey and Nelica La Gro 2013
Chapter 19 Editorial arrangement and Personality theory © Rowan Bayne 2013
The humanitarian and third sectors © Sarah Davidson 2013
Green living © Nicky Hayes 2013
Community psychology © Carolyn Kagan 2013
Applying psychology to the layout of printed text © James Hartley 2013
Clinical psychology © Susan Llewelyn 2013
Educational psychology © Irvine Gersch 2013
Occupational and organisational psychology © Clive Fletcher 2013
Occupational psychology © Chris Lewis 2013
Investigative interviewing © Ray Bull 2013
Forensic psychology in the prison and probation services © Ruth E. Mann 2013
The use of virtual reality-based environmental enrichment for patients recovering from brain injury © Paul R. Penn and F. David Rose 2013
Strengths © P. Alex Linley 2013
Psychological ethics: the good, the defensive and the utilitarian © Richard Kwiatkowski 2013
Reflections on the place and usefulness of psychology © Colin Feltham 2013
Psychology today © Nicky Hayes 2013

First published 2013

Apart from any fair dealing for the purposes of research or private study, or criticism or review, as permitted under the Copyright, Designs and Patents Act, 1988, this publication may be reproduced, stored or transmitted in any form, or by any means, only with the prior permission in writing of the publishers, or in the case of reprographic reproduction, in accordance with the terms of licences issued by the Copyright Licensing Agency. Enquiries concerning reproduction outside those terms should be sent to the publishers.

Library of Congress Control Number: 2012939736

British Library Cataloguing in Publication data

A catalogue record for this book is available from the British Library

ISBN 978-0-85702-834-1
ISBN 978-0-85702-835-8 (pbk)

MIX
Paper from
responsible sources
FSC
www.fsc.org   FSC® C018575

CONTENTS

ABOUT THE EDITORS AND CONTRIBUTORS

Rowan Bayne is Emeritus Professor of Psychology and Counselling at the University of East London where he was a core tutor on counselling and psychotherapy courses for over thirty years. His books include *How to Survive Counsellor Training*: *An A–Z Guide* (with Gordon Jinks) (Palgrave Macmillan, 2010) and *The Counsellor's Guide to Personality: Understanding Preferences, Motives And Life Stories* (Palgrave Macmillan, 2013).

James Beale is a Senior Lecturer in Sport & Exercise Psychology in the School of Health, Sport and Biosciences at the University of East London. James specialises in the applied domain where he has over ten years' experience. James has worked in a number of sports including, but not limited to, Premier League Football, First Class County Cricket and Elite League Speedway.

Professor Jenny Bimrose is Deputy Director of the Institute for Employment Research, University of Warwick. She has over thirty years of experience teaching, researching and managing in higher education, acted as an expert on careers guidance to various government bodies and the Council of Europe and published extensively in the area of careers. Many recent research projects have focused on the theory, policy and practice of career counselling and guidance. She is co-editor of the *British Journal of Guidance and Counselling*.

Dr Ilona Boniwell is a Principal Lecturer, the Founder and Inaugural Programme Leader for the on-campus Master's Degree in Applied Positive Psychology (MAPP), currently leading international and distance learning MAPP developments. Her research interests include: subjective time use, time perspective and hedonic and eudaimonic well-being. Ilona is also interested in practical applications of positive psychology, being a qualified coach and a developer of educational programmes.

Mary Boyle is Professor Emeritus of Clinical Psychology at the University of East London where she was Director of the Clinical Psychology Doctorate until 2006. She was also an NHS psychologist initially in adult services and more recently in women's health. Her main interests are in critical analyses of the medical model and the development of alternatives, and in feminist approaches to women's health. She has published widely in these areas.

Ray Bull is Professor of Forensic Psychology at the University of Leicester. In 2010 he was 'elected by acclaim' an Honorary Fellow of the British Psychological Society 'for the contribution made to the discipline of psychology' and in 2008 he received from the European Association of Psychology and Law an 'Award for Life-time Contribution to Psychology and Law'. His books include Bull, R. (ed.) (2011) *Forensic Psychology – A Four Volume Set of Readings* (London: Sage and Wilcock) and R. Bull and R. Milne (2008) *Witness Identification in Criminal Cases* (Oxford: Oxford University Press).

Dr Maria Castro is Senior Lecturer and Academic Tutor for the Professional Doctorate in Clinical Psychology at the University of East London. Previously, she was an NHS Clinical Psychologist in Older People's Services. Maria's core interests are in creative and collaborative praxis, particularly with people and communities largely marginalised, and in teaching, learning and researching as dialogical processes.

Brian R. Clifford (PhD) is Emeritus Professor of Psychology at the University of East London and Honorary Research Professor at Aberdeen University. He has published over two hundred research papers, reports, chapters and monographs and four books, two in the area of forensic psychology (eyewitness psychology). His main research interests lie in the application of memory research in real-life situations, especially children's and adults' recall and recognition abilities. He has successfully supervised over 26 PhD candidates in these fields. He has taught high-level research methodology to postgraduates for many years. He has served as an expert witness in several cases within the UK where issues of testimony and identification have been in dispute. He has also written several chapters on the nature and scope of experimental psychologists as expert witnesses.

Dr Sarah Davidson is a Consultant Clinical Psychologist at the Tavistock and Portman Foundation NHS Trust and the Deputy Clinical Director on the Professional Doctorate in Clinical Psychology at the University of East London. She is the Psychosocial Advisor for the British Red Cross and leads the MSc in International Humanitarian Psychosocial Consultation at the University of East London.

Colin Feltham is Emeritus Professor of Critical Counselling Studies, Sheffield Hallam University. His most recent publications include *Critical Thinking in Counselling and Psychotherapy* (Sage, 2010), *The Sage Handbook of Counselling and Psychotherapy* (3rd edn, co-edited with Ian Horton, Sage, 2012) and *Failure* (Acumen, forthcoming).

Clive Fletcher is an Honorary Professor at Warwick Business School, Professor Emeritus at Goldsmiths' College, University of London, and Managing Director of Personnel Assessment Ltd. Clive is a Fellow of both the British Psychological Society and the Royal Society of Medicine. He has published nearly two hundred books, chapters, journal articles and conference papers in the field of occupational psychology, mainly in relation to leadership assessment and development in work settings. Clive has acted in a consultancy capacity to many organisations in both private and public sectors.

Dr Mark Fox is Programme Director for the Professional Doctorate in Educational and Child Psychology at the University of East London. He has worked as an educational psychologist for over thirty years both for local authorities and the voluntary sector where he was head of the Advisory and Assessment Services at SCOPE. He has written extensively on the training and evidence base for educational psychology. His professional interest is in children with severe and multiple disabilities and developing their quality of life.

Kenneth Gannon (PhD) is Research Director on the Doctorate in Clinical Psychology programme at the University of East London. Dr Gannon's research interests lie in the broad area of health psychology.

Irvine Gersch (PhD) is Professor of Educational Psychology at the University of East London. He has served as Chairperson of the British Psychological Society Training Committee for Educational Psychology and as a member of the DfES working group on the future role and training of educational psychologists. He has co-edited three books, and published chapters in books and articles in the fields of listening to children and pupil involvement, behaviour management, school leadership, systems analysis, management, educational psychology training, conciliation and mediation in special needs and teacher stress. In 2002, he received the British Psychological Society's annual award for Distinguished Contributions to Professional Psychology.

Dr Carla Gibbes is the Programme Director for the Doctorate in Occupational Psychology at the University of East London. A Chartered Occupational Psychologist, Carla is active as an external consultant to many public sector organisations. Her research interests include work–life balance, post-traumatic stress disorder and susceptibility to stress.

Chris Hackley is Professor of Marketing in the School of Management at Royal Holloway, University of London, teaching advertising and marketing. He has also taught social and introductory psychology as an Associate Lecturer for the Open University. Chris was already a management academic when he obtained his BSc Hons Social Science and Postgraduate Diploma in Psychology by distance learning. He learnt social psychological discourse analysis from Potter and Wetherell (1987) and he applied some of this knowledge to his qualitative PhD research into the creative development process in advertising agencies. His research interests focus on the linguistic and socio-cultural understanding of marketing and consumption. Recent projects have engaged with policy issues related to alcohol and young people and UK television product placement. His most recent book is the second edition of his text *Advertising and Promotion: An Integrated Marketing Communications Approach*, published by Sage in 2010.

David Harper (PhD) is Reader in Clinical Psychology at the University of East London. He is a co-author of *Deconstructing Psychopathology* (Sage, 1995), a co-editor of *Qualitative Research Methods in Mental Health and Psychotherapy* (Wiley, 2012) and co-author of *Psychology, Mental Health and Distress* (Palgrave MacMillan, 2013).

James Hartley is Research Professor of Psychology at the University of Keele, Staffordshire, UK. His main research interests are in written communication, but he is also well known for his research into teaching and learning in higher education. His publications include *Designing Instructional Text* (3rd edn, Kogan Page, 1994); *Learning and Studying: A Research Perspective* (Routledge, 1998); (with Alan Branthwaite) *The Applied Psychologist* (2nd edn, Open University Press, 2000); and *Academic Writing and Publishing* (Routledge, 2008).

Nicky Hayes is a Chartered Psychologist specialising in social and organisational issues. She is now semi-retired, but during her academic career she conducted research into subjects as varied as organisational cultures, team management, the psychology of interactive science exhibits and exam stress. She also had a varied teaching career, which involved teaching psychology in colleges and universities at levels ranging from GCE to postgraduate degree work. Her extensive knowledge of psychology, and ability to draw connections between different specialisms, meant that she was much in demand for her broad-ranging and informative guest lectures, both in the UK and abroad. In 1997 she was awarded the British Psychological Society's Award for Distinguished Contributions to the Teaching of Psychology, and she is a Fellow of the British Psychological Society and an Honorary Life Member of the Association for the Teaching of Psychology. She has published over 20 books, and her clear writing style opened up an interest in psychology for both new readers and struggling students.

Dr Kate Hefferon is a Chartered Psychologist, Senior Lecturer and Co-Programme Leader on the Msc in Applied Positive Psychology at the University of East London. Her research interests lie within the area of post-traumatic growth, physical activity, health and well-being.

Mark Holloway is the Programme Director for the MSc in Occupational & Business Psychology at the University of East London. A Chartered Occupational Psychologist, Mark is active as an external consultant and is currently working on specialist projects with the Department for Education and the Ministry of Defence. His research interests include impostors and deception in the workplace.

Dr Ashok Jansari got his degree in Experimental Psychology from King's College Cambridge and then his Doctorate at the University of Sussex where he conducted research on memory and amnesia. Following a two-year postdoctoral fellowship in the United States at the University of Iowa Hospitals & Clinics, he has created an extensive research programme looking at different aspects of memory loss including the development of rehabilitation regimes, the creation of a virtual reality assessment of brain damage, impairments in face-recognition (known as 'prosopagnosia' or face-blindness) and 'synaesthesia' or cross-sensory perception (in which an individual upon *hearing* the word 'Monday' will claim to *see* the colour red). In 2004, he was awarded the International Neuropsychological Society's Cermak Award for the best research in memory disorders and in 2011 he was awarded a Live Science residency at the Science Museum in London to run the largest ever study on face-recognition in the UK.

Gordon Jinks is Principal Lecturer in Counselling and Psychotherapy at the University of East London's School of Psychology, where he is programme leader for the MA/ Postgraduate Diploma in Counselling & Psychotherapy, and leader in collaborative provision, responsible for managing links with programmes at the Tavistock Centre for Couple Relationships, the Psychosynthesis Education Trust and East London NHS Trust among others. He has led the development of innovative undergraduate pro- grammes in counselling, counselling studies and counselling and mentoring at the University of East London and previously at York St. John. As a practitioner he has worked in university counselling services and in the mental health field (for the NHS and MIND) as well as in private practice. He is an integrative practitioner and has a particular interest in how clients learn from therapy and go on to apply that learning as new issues arise in their lives. Earlier in his career he worked for sixteen years as a psychiatric nurse and nurse tutor in Yorkshire and Lanarkshire. His first degree was in physics and he maintains a layman's interest in the ways the universe is not only stranger than we imagine, but stranger than we *can* imagine.

Carolyn Kagan is Professor of Community Social Psychology at Manchester Met- ropolitan University and Director of the Research Institute for Health and Social Change. She is also a qualified social worker and registered counselling psychologist. She has written widely about community psychology and has worked on local and international participative and collaborative research projects for over thirty years in fields including learning disability, poverty, women and community activism, migration, community participation, and university–community engagement. She is a founder editor of the international journal *Community, Work and Family*.

Richard Kwiatkowski (PhD) is a Senior Lecturer in Organizational Psychology at Cranfield Business School. He has been focused on developing people and organisations for over 25 years in a variety of contexts. He is both a Chartered and Registered Occupa- tional Psychologist and a Counselling Psychologist. He is a former Chair of the British Psychological Society's Division of Occupational Psychology and of the British Psychologi- cal Society's Ethics Committee and a former associate editor of *The Psychologist*.

Nelica La Gro is a Senior Lecturer in the School of Psychology, University of East London and has worked as programme leader for the p/g Diploma in Career Guidance (QCG). She is a fellow of the Higher Education Academy, on the ICG Research Committee and has recently qualified in mediation and conflict resolution. She has contributed to EU funded research projects over the last decade and has a keen interest in the develop- ment of innovative approaches to professional learning.

Dr Ho Law is an International Consultant and Practitioner Psychologist, Registered Occupational Psychologist, Chartered Scientist, Chartered Psychologist, Registered Applied Psychology Practice Supervisor, Fellow of the Chartered Management Institute, Fellow of the Higher Education Academy, Fellow of the Royal Society of Medicine, and Associate Fellow of the British Psychological Society. Ho has had over twenty-five years' experience in psychology and management consultancy. He delivered numerous workshops/conference seminars and carried out consultancy work in the UK and abroad (the East and West). Ho values diversity in people, and respects their cultures and believes in equal opportunities for all. He was one of the first equality advisors to the Assistant Permanent Under Secretary of State in the Home Office, and the Deputy Chair of the British Psychological Society Standing Committee for Promotion of Equal Opportunities. Ho is passionate about helping people to develop their talents and achieve their full potential through coaching and mentoring. Ho was the first Head of Profession in Coaching (Association for Coaching, 2004). He is a founding member and Chair (2010) of the British Psychological Society Special Group in Coaching Psychology and founding Director and member of the International Society for Coaching Psychology. He is the principal author of *The Psychology of Coaching, Mentoring & Learning* (Wiley, 2007), interviews editor of *Counselling Psychology Quarterly* and consulting editor of *The Coaching Psychologist*. He has published over forty papers and received numerous outstanding achievement awards including the Local Promoters for Cultural Diversity Project in 2003, the Positive Image (Business Category) in 2004 and Management Essentials Participating Company 2005. At the University of East London School of Psychology, Ho is a Senior Lecturer (0.5), Admissions Tutor and Leader in the MSc coaching/coaching psychology distance Learning programme and Leader in the coaching and mentoring BSc modules. He is also the Director of Studies, supervising PhD students: one is 'The Role of Space In Learning: Spatio-Educational Experiences of Female Students within Emirati Higher Education'; and another is 'The Impact Evaluation of Creating a Coaching Culture within a Third Level Educational Institution in the Gulf'.

Chris Lewis is a Registered Occupational Psychologist, an Associate Fellow of the British Psychological Society and a Fellow of the Royal Statistical Society. He is Principal of the consultancy Aver Psychology. He was Course Director of the MSc in Occupational Psychology at the University of East London for seventeen years and is a past chair of the British Psychological Society Division of Occupational Psychology. His main interests are assessment and the critical evaluation of current psychometric methodology. He has authored many widely used psychometric tests, over 100 papers and technical reports and a number of books and book chapters including *Employee Selection* (2nd edn, Stanley Thornes, 1992).

Dr P. Alex Linley is a Chartered Psychologist and Founding Director of Capp (www.cappeu.com). He works as an organisational consultant applying strengths psychology to organisational development and people practices, serving a range of major global clients. Alex has written, co-written or edited more than 150 research papers and book chapters, and seven books, including *Positive Psychology in Practice* (Wiley, 2004), *The Strengths Book* (CAPP Press, 2010) and the *Oxford Handbook of Positive Psychology and Work* (Oxford, 2010).

Professor Susan Llewelyn is Director of the Oxford Doctoral Course in Clinical Psychology, Professor of Clinical Psychology at Oxford University and Senior Research

Fellow at Harris Manchester College, Oxford. She trained at Sheffield and Leeds Universities and has worked in both the NHS and university sectors in Nottingham, Sheffield, Dorset, Southampton and Edinburgh. She has a particular interest in the psychological therapies, and her clinical work has concerned therapeutic interventions for adult survivors of childhood sexual abuse. Sue also has a specific interest in professional issues, leadership and teamwork and has written or co-authored six books and over one hundred academic and professional papers.

Ruth E. Mann (PhD) is a Chartered and Registered Forensic Psychologist employed by the National Offender Management Service. Her particular area of expertise is the assessment and treatment of sexual offending. In 2010, Ruth received the British Psychological Society Division of Forensic Psychology senior award for her contribution to forensic psychology in the UK.

Professor Rachel Mulvey is a Fellow and Past President of the Institute of Career Guidance; she is also a Fellow of the Higher Education Academy. Rachel was Vice-Chair of the Parliamentary task force on the career guidance profession that reported in October 2010. She is on the steering group for a pan-European research team looking at innovative training of career guidance. Her own research centres on public policy for career guidance and graduate employability. Rachel is Professor of Career Guidance.

Jill Mytton (MSc) is a Chartered Counselling Psychologist in private practice. She is also currently working part time as a research supervisor on the Doctorate in Existential Counselling Psychology and Psychotherapy at the New School of Psychotherapy and Counselling, London. Prior to this she was the Course Leader on the Counselling Psychology Doctoral Programme at London Metropolitan University. She has served on the Division of Counselling Psychology Committee as the Lead for conference for several years. In addition to contributing chapters to three books, she is the co-author with Windy Dryden of *Four Approaches to Counselling and Psychotherapy* (Routledge, 1999). As part of her own doctoral programme she is studying the relationship between mental health and being raised in fundamentalist sects/cults.

Paula Nicolson is Professor Emeritus of the University of London (Royal Holloway) in Critical Social Health Psychology, and an Organisational Consultant with Psychological Solutions London and Fitzrovia Organisational Consulting. Her research background includes health psychology issues in studies of domestic violence, sexuality, chronic illness, leadership in health care organisations and postnatal depression. She is a Chartered Psychologist, Fellow of the British Psychological Society, Academician of the Academy of Social Sciences, a member of the Tavistock Society of Psychotherapists (Allied Professions) and a Registered Practitioner Psychologist (Health Psychology). She is currently developing her private practice through further specialist training as a psychodynamic couple psychotherapist.

Paul R. Penn (PhD) is a Lecturer in Psychology at the University of East London and co-ordinator of the Virtual Reality Laboratory. He has research interests in the application of technology to the assessment and rehabilitation of brain damage and has published numerous works within this field. His other key interests centre around developing skills and employability provisions for psychology undergraduates. Paul is a Fellow of the Higher Education Academy, a Chartered Psychologist and a member of the British Psychological Society division for Teachers and Researchers in Psychology.

John Radford led the development of Psychology at West Ham College of Technology, a predecessor of the University of East London, from 1965, later becoming Dean of Science. He introduced Psychology as an A-level subject in 1970, and founded the Association for the Teaching of Psychology. He received the first awards of the British Psychological Society, of which he is a Fellow and Honorary Life Member, for Distinguished Contributions to the Teaching of Psychology and for Lifetime Achievement in Psychology Education. He has published eighteen books and numerous papers on many topics, including the teaching of psychology, higher education, child prodigies, the psychology of religion, gender differences, personality and individual differences, science fiction and Sherlock Holmes.

Donald Ridley is the Programme Director for the MSc in Applied Psychology at the University of East London. A Chartered Occupational Psychologist, Donald is expert in error prevention and safety critical systems. His research interests include the assessment of mental workload and the development of public sector organisations in the former Soviet Union.

Mary Robinson (PhD) is Associate Tutor/Senior Educational Psychologist at the University of East London.

F. David Rose (PhD) recently retired as the Dean of the School of Psychology and Pro Vice-Chancellor at the University of East London. He is now Emeritus Professor. For many years he has been involved in environmental enrichment research and has published extensively on brain damage rehabilitation and the possible applications of virtual reality in this area. He was responsible for establishing the first virtual reality laboratory in the UK.

Volker Thoma (PhD) is a Senior Lecturer at the University of East London. His research area is on dual processing in visual recognition of objects and in the area of decision-making, including the neuroscientific basis of cognition. He previously worked as a researcher in object recognition and visual attention at University College London and the University of California, Los Angeles. As a former human factors researcher at the Fraunhofer Institute of Industrial Science in Stuttgart he gained experience in the area of human-machine interaction, working on the design of interfaces such as ticket machines, computer software, as well as internet and virtual reality applications.

Dr Christian van Nieuwerburgh is Programme Leader for the MSc in Coaching and Coaching Psychology at the University of East London, Executive Coach for the West Midlands Coaching Pool and Chief Executive of the International Centre for Coaching in Education.

Christopher Whiteley (DClin Psy) is a Consultant Clinical Psychologist working in Specialist Addiction Services with East London NHS Trust. He is also an Honorary Clinical Tutor with the University of East London Professional Doctorate in Clinical Psychology. Christopher's clinical and research interests are in the associations between substance use and mental health.

Dr Marcia Wilson is a Principal lecturer in Sport Psychology and the Field Leader for Applied Sport and Exercise Sciences at the University of East London. Marcia's main area of research focuses on expectancy theory in sport. Marcia has extensive applied-sport psychology experience, mainly working with young elite female footballers.

INTRODUCTION

This book is a considerable revision and expansion of the first edition. It includes eleven new chapters and several substantial updates.

The book is intended for three groups of people:

1   psychology undergraduates who are considering a career in applied psychology and wondering which of the many possibilities is the most attractive and practical for them;

2   students on MSc psychology courses who want an overview of issues and new directions in applied psychology;

3   tutors on those MSc courses who, by definition, are shaping and developing applied psychology.

The book is organised into three parts. The first part is a general context for applied psychology including a critique of questions about evidence-based practice. The second part discusses research, practice and training in the traditional areas of applied psychology, eight relative newcomers and four areas not always regarded as applied psychology: counselling, coaching, careers guidance and lecturing. The latter group are examples of disciplines that are intrinsically psychological but do not require a psychology degree for a career in them, such as nursing, occupational therapy, social work, human resources (HR) and management. The third part is a roundtable of expert practitioners commenting on the new directions they would like to see in their areas of applied psychology.

There is no definitive answer to the question 'What is applied psychology?' but the British Psychological Society's (BPS) *Directory of Chartered Psychologists and the Directory of Expert Witnesses* (2002 version), now an online publication at www.bps. org, made a detailed, brave, though probably quixotic, attempt. It distinguished fourteen broad areas in which chartered psychologists offer services and one hundred and eight specialist services within those areas. The fourteen broad areas are all represented in this book.

Training and practice in applied psychology has been firmly structured around such specialisms as clinical, educational, etc. for many years. In an incisive and radical critique of this situation, Peter Kinderman (2005) noted the anomaly of different approaches to training, pay and conditions in some of the specialisms when the psychologists in many of them work in 'very similar ways', and he argued that the resulting problems include both a general public who are confused about applied psychology and students who are deterred from a career in applied psychology. He proposed a revolution, to a three-year doctoral programme in applied psychology with specialisms in the third year only, and a unified career structure with five levels: undergraduate, associate psychologist, applied psychologist in doctoral training, applied psychologist with a particular specialism, and consultant. Thus, there would be a single route of training and a single career path. So far, any such revolution is happening slowly at best.

For authoritative and up-to-date information on becoming a chartered psychologist and on other aspects of careers and training in applied psychology, contact the BPS (www.bps.org.uk; phone: 0116 254 9568). The BPS will also give details of conversion courses for people who want to be eligible for postgraduate training in psychology but who do not have a psychology degree that is recognised by the BPS.

ACKNOWLEDGEMENTS

A warm thank-you to our authors and to our editors, Michael Carmichael, Sophie Hine and Alana Clogan, especially in uncertain and demanding times for universities and publishers.

PART ONE

Context

1

APPLYING PSYCHOLOGY

John Radford

This chapter discusses:

- the nature of Psychology as a discipline, subject and profession;

- the application of Psychology to the psychological professions, and to other special-isms and professions;

- the fallacy of distinguishing between 'pure' and 'applied' Psychology;

- the public understanding of Psychology, and why it is often poor;

- critical views of Psychology;

- how Psychology can achieve wider acceptance, and why it should.

INTRODUCTION

A distinction is made between Psychology, a scientific enquiry, and psychology, the subject matter of that enquiry. It is suggested that Psychology, like other such labels, refers to three distinct entities which should be distinguished. The *discipline* is a group of related problems, focused on the human individual, and the methods and findings resulting from investigating these problems. This gives unity to Psychology. The *subject* is organization of material and resources for practical applications includ-ing teaching. The *profession* is a body of people practising in various contexts but based on the discipline. Professional psychologists are only a small number of those who obtain the Graduate Basis for Registration of the British Psychological Society (BPS). Some difficulties arising from this are discussed. Psychology can be and is applied in many contexts, and while there are some criticisms of this, it is suggested that a better understanding of human behaviour is fundamental to solving the many problems we face as a species.

In studying this subject we must be content if we attain as high a degree of accuracy as the matter of it admits. (Aristotle, c. 385–322 BCE, *Ethics*)

A science is said to be useful if its development tends to accentuate the existing inequalities in the distribution of wealth, or more directly promotes the destruction of human life. (G.H. Hardy, 1877–1947, mathematician)

We can tell nothing of our fellow men except by seeing what they do or say in particular circumstances ... If we refuse to use observation and experiment on other human beings, we start to regard them as wicked or foolish. I think this is a serious danger, and I have no doubt that the methods of empirical psychology are socially more hygienic, or to use the older and more robust phrase, morally better. (Donald Broadbent, *In Defence of Empirical Psychology*, 1973)

In another memorable quotation, reported by Joshua Reynolds, Dr Johnson remarked:

There are two things which I am confident I can do very well: one is an introduction to any literary work, stating what it is to contain, and how it should be executed in the most perfect manner; the other is a conclusion, shewing from various causes why the execution has not been equal to what the author promised to himself and to the public.

This chapter is not an introduction in Johnson's sense. Those that follow will speak for themselves, and whether his conclusion is necessary can be left to the reader. Rather, I raise some larger issues about what psychology is, and how it is or can be applied.

THE NATURE OF PSYCHOLOGY

I have in front of me a copy of *The Times* for today, 2 March 2011. I can find no mention of the word 'Psychology'. But there is a great deal of psychology. There are items about gender (as it is now called, previously sex) equality, racial prejudice, problem-solving and creativity, crime, aggression and murder, war and conflict, child development, education, mass media, propaganda and persuasion, leadership and, of course, sport. All of absorbing interest to psychologists, and not only professionally.

Psychology and psychology

The useful distinction between Psychology as a discipline or enquiry, and psychology as the subject matter of that enquiry, is due to Graham Richards (1987). This can be applied to any discipline, but it is particularly apt for some. The subject matter of Chemistry is chemistry, processes that can be studied at chemical level, so to say. But those processes are not themselves part of the investigation, only its object. With disciplines concerned with human behaviour the case is different. If the task of History is to understand the past, the whole of it, then what historians have said is part of that past, and has often helped to shape it. Psychology is more extreme still, for it is itself human behaviour, which is its subject matter. Psychologists themselves, and their theory and practice, are necessarily something that requires a psychological explanation. In other words, Psychology is by its nature reflexive. So too are other disciplines dealing with human beings, Anthropology, History, Sociology and so on. But the issue is most pertinent to Psychology because it focuses (I argue) on the individual human being. The argument can be taken further. Richards (1996) suggests that the language that Psychology uses itself constitutes psychology: 'Nobody before Freud had an Oedipus complex … nobody before c. 1914 had a high IQ … To put it bluntly, Psychology is produced by, produces, and is an instance of, its own subject matter.' This is not, as I understand it, a social constructivist view. *H. sapiens* must always have had intellectual capabilities, if not an IQ.

Medical examples

Consider two medical examples (not from Richards). In former times people often suffered from 'ague'. Today it is sometimes said that this was malaria (or influenza, or rheumatic fever). It was not. It was ague. The symptoms were real, but they were classified differently, and without knowledge of the disease entities. Malaria existed as a disease, but not as a medical or psychological reality. Similarly with schizophrenia, which did not exist until Eugene Bleuler invented it, or identified it as he would have said, in 1911 (Boyle, 1988). Since then there has been a long history of seeking to find the causes of schizophrenia by studying 'schizophrenics', that is, samples of persons diagnosed as such. Considerable progress has been made, though the process risks being circular. A leaflet on schizophrenia produced by the Royal College of Psychiatrists states that schizophrenia is 'a disorder of the mind which affects how you think, feel and behave' (para 3). The word 'schizophrenia' is used 'because there is not yet a better one for the pattern of symptoms and behaviours described' (para 2). But those symptoms and behaviours are so varied and inconsistent as hardly to merit the word 'pattern'. For example, they may or may not include hearing voices, and hearing voices may or may not indicate a disorder. This is even more the case if one considers different cultures and periods, in some of which hallucinations of various kinds can be normal or signs of exceptional gifts, such as receiving messages from the gods. Of course, it is not that there are no such things as hallucinations, or mental disorders, rather that Psychology and its subject matter are in a constant state of interaction and creation. And much of it depends on probabilities and reasonable estimates, just as Aristotle said. There are very real consequences for treatment and for public attitudes.

DISCIPLINE, SUBJECT AND PROFESSION

Discipline

An implicit assumption is perhaps that because there is a word 'schizophrenia', there must be a disease entity corresponding to it. But that is just what has to be found out. A similar fallacy has often underlain attempts to say what psychological concepts 'really' mean, for example intelligence (Radford, 1995), and indeed what 'Psychology' itself is, and particularly whether or not it is a unity (Radford, 2004). 'Psychology' is one word, and thus there must be one thing to which it refers. I have argued, I think first in Radford and Rose (1989), that words such as Chemistry, History or Psychology commonly refer to at least three distinguishable entities, which it is desirable not to confuse. I label them discipline, subject and profession. By a *discipline* I mean a set of problems that appear to be related, and the methods, theories and bodies of knowledge that are created in investigating them. A discipline is not defined by a list of subject matter, but by a focus; what the problems appear to have in common. The focus is not fixed but may change over time. It may be relatively wide or narrow. The focus of History can be either. A limited focus is the recorded past; a very wide one is all that has occurred. Obviously the first is a subset of the second. The focus of Psychology could be the individual human being, or *H. sapiens*, or living things, but a better label for that is Biology. I prefer 'individual', but that can only be understood as being at the centre of the other two – three concentric circles. Every discipline is more or less closely related to others. Psychology is close to Anthropology, Biology, Sociology and History. The individual might be seen as where all of these 'circles' intersect. Slightly more distant might appear Geography, Economics, Statistics, while Geology seems quite a long way off, but you never know. The 'circles' are imaginary. Disciplines are not static, and they do not have boundaries. New disciplines constantly emerge, and it is a matter of opinion and convenience when they should be regarded as independent. They are not territories. It is impossible to say in advance where new knowledge relevant to a problem will emerge. And it is absurd to reject it on the grounds that it is not part of a particular discipline. Anything at all may, in principle, be grist for the psychologist's mill. At the same time the focus on related problems and methods does, in my view, give unity to a discipline, however varied its practitioners may be.

Subject

I use the word '*subject*' to refer to the use of disciplinary material for purposes of dissemination and application. Unlike a discipline, a subject is legitimately territorial.

In education or in practice, it must have space, specialized accommodation, equipment, staff, support services and so on. All these depend in the last resort on attracting students, clients or other sources of finance. Psychology has often had to fight to be considered a 'science' subject, or a legitimate speciality, and this is not merely for prestige but because they relate directly to funding. One has to deal with the mundane needs of a subject as much as the vaulting ambitions of a discipline. Discipline content must also be ordered if it is to be conveyed to others. This is part of applying Psychology. A library is little use without a catalogue, but any classification system must be a partly arbitrary fitting of overlapping and inter-related material into boxes. Any educational course must be a selection from what its title might suggest (and usually more than that). An honours degree in Psychology cannot cover anything like all that is available, and should also include something from related disciplines. A syllabus must be strictly defined, if only because it is a licence to examine. A student may be asked about what is in it, and must not be penalized for not knowing what is not. Books and journals must have some limits. The question then is, how to make the selection. In the case of a book, it is up to the author to defend the choice – or an editor to impose one. A practitioner similarly draws on one or more disciplines. The criterion must surely be relevance to the purposes of the education, dissemination or practice.

In education, there are three general cases. In one, Psychology is a component of training for something other than professional psychology. Teaching, social work, nursing, medicine, police work, management are obvious examples and there are many others. A second case is general, non-vocational education, such as most GCE A-levels. The third case is courses, specifically first degrees, that are preparation for a psychological career. The second and third cases overlap, due to the well-known fact that of those who graduate (major) in Psychology, only some 15 to 20% will go on to a professional psychological career. The majority have careers that may or may not involve Psychology directly or indirectly. (Former students of mine have taken up jewellery making, journalism, picture-framing, market gardening, managing pop groups, working the stock market, menswear retailing and many other trades. Some at least have said they value their degree.)

Profession

By a *profession* I mean a body of people who are usually but not always formally qualified, but who conform more or less to the characteristics I discuss in more detail elsewhere in this volume (Chapter 18), including a commitment to the best interests of the client, a shared basis of knowledge both theoretical and practical, accountability for what is achieved rather than for specific procedures, responsibility of the individual practitioner and autonomy of the professional group. Like a subject, a profession is legitimately territorial. It is right for medical practitioners to try to ensure that quacks are seen for what they are, and prevented from doing harm. This is, however, a double-edged weapon. It can result in rejecting new advances merely because they are not accepted practice, or have arisen through unconventional routes. Professionals must not seek to extend their control beyond their competence, and must respect the role of other professionals (which does not mean necessarily deferring to it). Protection of the public can lapse into concealment of malpractice. There must be robust monitoring systems with external input. Professions are usually linked to one main discipline, but often draw on several others. Medicine is a profession based on the discipline of Medicine, focused on the treatment of disorders, but which also draws on many others that exist in their own right, including Psychology.

Professions may be defined both informally, as above, and formally. The formal criteria for psychological professions normally include academic qualifications, Chartered status granted by the BPS and, since 2009, for seven domains of psychological practice, registration with the Health Professions Council (HPC)[1]. This last is the outcome of a prolonged campaign for legal establishment, which has ended, by governmental insistence, in a more or less shot-gun wedding, inasmuch as many professional psychologists have little or nothing to do with health as such. The domains are occupational, clinical, forensic, counselling, health, educational, and sport and exercise.

---

[1] Also known as the Health and Care Professions Council (HCPC).

The effect is that no one may legally describe themselves as any of these varieties of psychologist without being registered. The generic term 'psychologist' is not protected, and anyone may describe themselves as one. The argument is that it would be impossible to set standards that would apply to all varieties. In addition, it was felt that psychologists in research or teaching should be able to describe themselves as such, but should not have to be registered.

APPLIED PSYCHOLOGY

'Psychology', then, can refer to all these things. As I have tried to show, they are not aspects of the same thing. This is relevant, I think when considering how Psychology can be or should be 'applied', for example to the training of other specialists. One approach to this is essentially to give a potted version of 'Psychology', the discipline, and then try to show its relevance. Another method is to ask what a lawyer or a medical general practitioner (GP) has to do, and then what, if anything, there is in the psychological cupboard, so to say, that could be of use to him or her. These are not absolute opposites, rather a matter of emphasis. One example of the first, to my mind, is *Psychology and the Teacher*, by Dennis Child (2007), and of the other, *The Psychology of Behaviour at Work*, by Adrian Furnham (2005). The titles themselves suggest the difference. To the question of what is relevant, we should not be afraid to say, nothing. It does not follow from the all-embracing aims of the *discipline*, that there is anything valuable for a particular *subject* or *profession*. Increasingly, there is, but there is still an obligation to prove it.

Applied psychologists

'Applied Psychology' usually refers, as it does in this volume, mainly to psychologists who work in particular specialisms. In the past, it has sometimes been used in particular for work concerned with occupations and organizations, but now is extended to many other areas. The BPS uses the term 'Types of Psychologist' on its website (BPS, n.d.). I think this is misleading. All psychologists share, in principle, a common background in their first degrees. Further qualifications are more specialized for different fields, but, as Hartley and Branthwaite (1989) put it, 'the work which psychologists actually do in these various areas has more similarities than differences'. (I would say that the discipline is the same also.) 'It is the subject matter of their jobs that differs, rather than the roles, skills and ways of working.' Hartley and Branthwaite describe seven overlapping roles that psychologists may need to fill, regardless of specialism: counsellor, colleague, expert, toolmaker, detached investigator, theoretician and change agent. Bekerian and Levey (2005) rather similarly express this as psychologists working in different 'rooms': crime, court, work, war, treatment, sport. It is true that some specialists feel strongly that they should be clearly distinguished from others, and hence agree with the present system of Chartered status as specifically Clinical, Occupational and so on. My guess is that this means rather little to the general public, who would more readily understand a generic title of Chartered Psychologist. I have not seen any investigation of this hypothesis.

Professionals also like to distinguish themselves sharply from the unqualified, as I discuss elsewhere in this volume. This distinction runs more widely in higher education (Radford, 2003a; Radford et al., 1997). There is a long tradition, going back at least two hundred years now, of upholding a dichotomy between the 'pure' and the 'applied'. Warnock (1988), for example, in *A Common Policy for Education*, referred to the distinction, 'the most important there is' between 'the *practical* and the *theoretical*'. A reviewer in *The Times Higher Education Supplement*, on 27 May 1988, commented:

> ... teaching the English language as part of a national curriculum is practical, and therefore right; but teaching English literature is theoretical and not 'user-oriented'. So its separation from language becomes 'a matter of urgency'. Yet it is difficult to imagine how an effective teacher of language, seeking a creative response, could fail to draw on examples from literature.

Pure and applied

Even more strongly may it be questioned whether there is a useful distinction between pure and applied Psychology. In the first place, a great deal of Psychology originated in practical problems. To give just one familiar example, one of the roots of the investigation, indeed discovery, of systematic individual differences was the famous occasion in 1796 when the Astronomer Royal, Nevil Maskelyne, a meticulous observer, dismissed his assistant, named Kinnebrook, because the latter's recordings of a particular event, stellar transits, were consistently slower than his own. Much later, in 1820, another astronomer, Bessel, guessed correctly that this might have been due not to carelessness but to differences in what we now call reaction times. This was really a fundamentally new and important concept, upsetting the notions that thought was effectively instantaneous, and that all human minds worked in the same way. It is not too much to say that individual differences are fundamental to all psychological work. A later stage in the same story was the development of psychometric measurements; again, partly from a practical problem, occasioned by the introduction of education for all children. It soon appeared that some seemed incapable of benefiting from it, and Alfred Binet, a medical doctor in France, was asked to devise a way of picking them out. He came up with a test of 'mental age', based essentially on what an average child might be expected to do at each year of life. This was the beginning of what became intelligence tests, which took off in a big way from yet another practical problem. This arose when the USA entered the First World War in 1917, and was faced with handling large numbers of new army recruits, some unable to read English. A group of psychologists developed the Army Alpha (for English readers) and Army Beta (for others) tests of intelligence. Between September 1917 and January 1919, 1,750,000 men were tested with Alpha. For the full stories see Boring (1957) and Tuddenham (1966) among others. Intelligence tests, and psychometrics generally, have been used, misused and abused for alleged harm they have done, but they remain a prime example of applied Psychology.

Secondly, it can be argued from the reflexive nature of Psychology that it cannot be other than applied. Psychologists, as part of our own subject matter, cannot stand completely apart from it, as a mathematician or a chemist could reasonably be said to do. Sigmund Freud discovered one example of this when he found that he had to deal not only with a patient's reactions to him, but with his own to the patient, the counter-transference as it came to be called. More generally, nearly all, if not all, the matters to which Psychology is applied, directly involve people, and frequently decisions that affect them. The psychologist's own attitudes, opinions and beliefs must come into this. I will return to this, but my view would be that one can be aware of it, and try to balance objectivity with human concern.

Thirdly, Psychology often exemplifies the 'blue skies' problem. There is constant pressure on scientists, from funding bodies and politicians, to make their work 'relevant'. One answer to this is that it is never possible to say exactly what work will turn out to have practical applications. A tiny psychological example is perhaps short-term memory for digits. This was investigated for years in the hope of understanding memory itself. It suddenly turned out to be very relevant when all-digit telephone numbers were introduced.

PREPARATION FOR APPLIED PSYCHOLOGY

Professional training

Applied psychologists normally have some specialized training, as described elsewhere. But all (in the UK) are expected to have a first degree (or equivalent) approved by the BPS as the Graduate Basis for Registration (GBR). I and others have suggested previously two main criticisms of this (e.g. Gale, 2002; Radford, 2008). One is that it is too narrow, and too focused on content at the expense of skills and experience. The aim is to ensure that graduates have covered the 'core areas' of Psychology discipline knowledge. Gale pointed out that several years may pass between graduating and even starting professional training, let alone entering a career, while psychological content can change rapidly. And as I suggested above, a Psychology graduate really ought to know at least something of various other approaches to human behaviour. My preference, for what it is worth, would be to start not from lists of content, but from the methodology and context of Psychology. To put it simply, how and why we (and others) go about investigating behaviour. The second criticism is that the whole concept of GBR is misconceived. If the purpose is to maintain and enhance professional standards, the way to do this is to ensure, first, that on qualifying, an individual is equipped to do what she or he has to do. A professional qualification is like a driving test, an assurance of minimum competence. Second, that the individual understands and accepts the principles of professional work, as I discuss elsewhere. The GBR at present seeks to ensure *professional* standards by defining the *subject,* i.e. of the first degree, and hence, since students will take only one such degree, the *discipline*.

General education

We are left with the large body of students with GBR qualification, but for whom Psychology is not clearly vocational, which includes the majority of first degrees and effectively all pre-degrees. Some may be doing it simply out of interest, or to make up a timetable. But we must surely hope that it will be of some value to them. I suggest two ways in which Psychology may apply, though they are not sharply distinct. One is relevance to what students will do, now and later. To make an obvious point, all students study (at least in principle), and they may want to, or have to, go on doing so in later life. Psychology tells us how to study better. All or virtually all students will enter a job, perhaps cope with unemployment or change of career, marry and rear children, manage a household, deal with retirement, old age, illness and bereavement of themselves and family, have a social and recreational life and so on and so forth. To all of this, psychological knowledge is relevant. The second way is more generally educational, for want of a better word. What this means has varied widely across human societies. But it is generally seen to involve both some form of personal, individual development, and some form of service or contribution to other individuals and wider society. And it would be odd to urge one of these without the other. Both are intimately related to Psychology. They are hardly possible without an attempt to understand why we and others behave as we do. For most of history such attempts have rested on tradition, folk wisdom, religion, superstition, personal preferences and prejudices, and so on. Psychology offers the hope of a more systematic and empirically based attempt, one which has made worthwhile progress and promises more. Many others have developed this theme at length, e.g. Miller (1969), Broadbent (1973), Zimbardo (2004), MacKay (2008).

OTHER PERSPECTIVES

The popular view

There are at least two other ways of looking at Applied Psychology. One is that of the non-psychologist, the general public. They are the main consumers of Psychology, and they pay for it either directly as clients or indirectly, through government agencies or organizations that employ psychologists and pass on the costs to customers. The other perspective is that of a number of varying views grouped together as 'critical' or 'radical' Psychology, to the effect that much of the discipline is not beneficial, or even positively harmful, and that it ought to be much more pro-active in changing society in various ways.

In the first case, it might seem that a reflexive science would be particularly interested in understanding how it is seen by others. Published research on this is somewhat scanty, but overall gives a fairly consistent picture. Psychology is regarded reasonably favourably, but is not well understood, particularly as regards its scientific nature and wide range of activities. Anderson (2006) reported a study done in the mid-1990s in the USA, in which 1087 adults were interviewed by telephone. Asked what psychologists do, 45% said 'help with problems, counselling' and 30% 'study behaviour, analyse people'. Multiple responses were allowed, but there were no other major ones. Respondents were asked which of psychologist, psychiatrist or social worker they would be most likely go to for help with various problems. Psychologists were favoured for stress, marriage, children, bereavement, work or illness related. Psychiatrists were chosen for mental illness, suicidal tendencies, severe depression and anxiety. Social workers were apparently not first choice for anything. Other questions were not really relevant to the UK; for example 80% said psychologists work in private practice.

Howard and Bauer (2001) drew on references in the press to 'psychology' which the BPS has collected since the 1980s, in particular those from the *Daily Telegraph*, *Guardian*, *Daily Mail* and *Daily Mirror*, 1988 to 1999. The most notable finding was that coverage increased fourfold in that period, which contrasts with a twofold increase in that for science. They also found that treatment of Psychology became more serious and less ironic or facetious, with 85% of references considered serious by 1999. A closer analysis suggested, however, that Psychology has to some extent become assimilated to the supernatural; it is more accepted, but partly because 'it is affiliated to the religious desire for an explanation of evil'. Bailey (2010 and personal communication), using focus groups and an online survey, found attitudes generally favourable to Psychology, but accurate knowledge somewhat deficient. Mills (2009) reports a survey of 1,000 randomly sampled adults in the USA, with 82% regarding Psychology very or fairly favourably. Psychology was not however considered a 'hard science' comparable with Biology, Chemistry, Physics or Medicine. It was concerned with treating individuals, like medicine, but was more akin to psychiatry and social work.

An unusual approach was taken by Hartwig (2002) who asked respondents (Australian, seventy-one female, forty-eight male) to draw 'a psychologist'. While the results were variegated, it appeared that a sort of 'typical' psychologist was a male in a suit and tie, bald or balding, with glasses. This is surprising, because perhaps the most robust finding about how psychology appears to the general public is that it is more appropriate for females than males, both as an occupation and as a subject to study. Data support this from the USA, various European countries including the UK, and China (Radford and Holdstock, 1995; Radford and Holdstock with Wu Rongxian, 1999). It is of course borne out by the fact that recruitment to degree and pre-degree courses is invariably around 75–80% female. It appears that this relates to attitudes towards both disciplines and occupations varying along a masculinity/femininity dimension, which in turn relates broadly to interests in things versus people. Psychology is seen as concerned with people, and thus tends to attract the more 'feminine' oriented students, who naturally tend to be female. It does seem a cause for concern that a discipline that, by definition applies to all people, should attract such a biased sample, and should not be generally better understood. (For a further detailed discussion see Lilienfeld, 2012.)

Critical Psychology

The second perspective has been variously explored at least since the early 1970s, e.g. Brown (1973). It is by no means a unified view, but there are some frequently expressed themes (Fox et al., 2009). One is that Psychology puts too much stress on the individual and individualism, which hinders the development of mutuality and strengthens social injustice. 'Mainstream' Psychology accepts uncritically the values of Western, capitalist society, which depend on an 'individualistic world view that sees economic class as a natural rather than a constructed state of affairs'. The underlying assumptions and allegiances of mainstream Psychology disproportionately hurt the powerless and marginalized by facilitating inequality and oppression. This occurs regardless of psychologists' individual or collective intentions to the contrary. Some psychologists contribute directly to oppression, for example by advising on methods of torture. The majority however seek to help individuals, but tend to do so by, as it were, fitting them back into the social and economic settings that caused the problems in the first place. Mainstream Psychology seeks to provide impartial scientific knowledge, but unlike Anthropology, Sociology, History and even Law, has not fully embraced reflexivity, and realized that 'social science is neither neutral nor value-free' (Fox, 2009).

The essence of critical Psychology, according to Prilleltensky and Nelson (2002), is 'standing with disadvantaged people, speaking out against social injustice, and acting for social change. Psychology needs to get more political'. Fox (n.d.: para 3) asserts that 'social justice is central'. A problem with this is that what counts as social justice is not a given but is itself culturally variable. Critical psychologists feel that the mainstream view is restricted to one ethos, that of Western capitalism, but a similar charge might be made against them. 'Social justice' might seem obviously to entail abolition of slavery and of rigid hierarchical structures. But many societies have felt, on the contrary, that social justice depends on them. Slavery was a normal condition of society in antiquity, while the feudal system of mediaeval Europe, the caste system in India and the 'four categories' of people in China were all seen as essential to a stable and ordered society. Individual psychologists should certainly be politically aware, as all citizens ideally should. We should also realize that dominant theories and methods may not be as objective as we would wish, and may have arisen from, or be biased by, unquestioned assumptions that have little to do with scientific enquiry. Psychology, as a reflexive discipline, does not comprise completely objective observations of neutral matter. Perhaps in the last resort no science does. It is possible, nevertheless, to be more objective or less, to acknowledge our own involvement and yet pursue a scientific enquiry. It is another matter to urge that 'Psychology' should take a political stand and seek to change society in a particular direction, and not only because Psychology is not an agent for deliberate change or anything else. Only individuals can be such agents.

But individual psychologists, like everyone else, will vary in their views of what is right and wrong. For example, Seligman and Fowler (2011) mount a robust defence of the work of psychologists in the armed forces. As they point out, not all will agree. They argue that the (American) military carry out policies determined by a democratically elected government. Further, that those policies are aimed at preserving democratic government from forces seeking to overthrow it. It is the duty of psychologists to assist in this. This takes us back to the previous point, in that it assumes the inherent rightness of democratic over other forms of government. Ultimately this is a matter of values, and thus of debate, not facts. Psychological science can contribute, it may be suggested, in various ways. One is by helping to keep it a matter of debate rather than open conflict, through the study of decision-making, conflict resolution and so on. Another is by showing what conditions lead to what effects, for example what treatment tends to reduce criminal recidivism. More widely, Wilkinson and Pickett (2009) present much evidence that more equal societies tend to score more highly on almost all 'good' criteria, such as low rates of crime, suicide, etc. A third way involves seeking an empirical basis for values, such as human rights. Warnock (2010), taking her cue from Aristotle, has argued that rights can only exist as general agreements, often enshrined in law. They cannot be absolute. They are not inherent in human beings, nor are they divinely granted. Slaves (not her example) do not have a right to be free; indeed it is precisely the lack of such a right that constitutes being a slave. It is a question rather of whether there is a general consensus that all people ought to be free. Here, although Warnock does not say so, social or psychological science comes in. Seligman (e.g. Seligman et al., 2005) and Hauser (2006) report just such widespread consensus on ethical and moral issues across many cultures, races and religions.

CONCLUSION

'My mind's made up, don't confuse me with facts' is attributed to Samuel Goldwyn the film producer. Whether authentic or not, it points to two problems of Applied Psychology. One is that the nature of any applied work is that it often has to be done in the absence of conclusive evidence. Physicians and psychologists must treat patients, film producers must commit resources or not, and so on. In the case of the first two, and similar occupations, we must rely on clinical judgement, which in turn rests on professional training, experience and commitment to standards. The other problem is that even when we have convincing evidence, it may not be accepted by its intended recipients. Munro (2011) discusses how prior beliefs may cause rejection of evidence that runs counter to them. This may be a particular problem for psychology, for various reasons. Psychology often does not carry the prestige of 'hard' science, of which it lacks some of the trappings such as white coats and laboratories. There is a general (usually correct) assumption that human behaviour is less predictable than are inanimate objects.

Psychological findings are nearly always in terms of probabilities rather than absolutes, and are thus harder to grasp. Some people feel that psychological findings are derived from and possibly influenced by the ideology of the researcher (as 'critical psychologists' aver). Then too, we are all perforce experts in human behaviour, or at least have experience of it and generally firm ideas about it. Nevertheless, there are ways of increasing acceptance of scientific findings about ourselves, in the longer term, Munro suggests, by better education (see also Tan and Halpern, 2006).

Human problems

In the longer term too, one more quotation: 'If the world is to be saved at all, it will be saved by Psychology'. This was quoted by Professor C.A. Mace when he greeted new students including me over fifty years ago. He attributed it to Abraham Maslow but I have been unable to find a specific reference. In the short term, Psychology has done and is doing an ever-increasing amount of valuable applied work, as this volume I hope illustrates (in contrast to the pessimistic view of G.H. Hardy). In the longer term, or even in the medium, it hardly needs repeating that the problems we humans face – conflict of all kinds, ignorance and prejudice, disease and starvation, failure to deal with natural disasters and all the rest – are the result of human behaviour. We must understand ourselves better. That is Applied Psychology.

QUESTIONS FOR REFLECTION AND DISCUSSION

1   Is the overwhelmingly feminine intake to Psychology courses a problem for Applied Psychology?

2   Should Psychology be more political?

3   How can the public image of Psychology be improved?

4   Are there too many Psychology graduates?

5   What has Applied Psychology done for us?

SUGGESTIONS FOR FURTHER READING

Donaldson, S.I., Berger, D.E. and Pezdek, K. (eds) (2006) *Applied Psychology: New Frontiers and Rewarding Careers.* Mahwah, NJ: Lawrence Erlbaum Associates. Discussions of the growth of Applied Psychology particularly in the USA, and new approaches and applications, by different authors.

Fagan, T.K. and VandenBos, G.R. (1993) *Exploring Applied Psychology: Origins and Critical Analysis.* Washington, DC: American Psychological Association. Chapters by different authors on various branches and how they developed, mainly from an American point of view.

Hearnshaw, L.S. (1964) *A Short History of British Psychology 1840–1940.* London: Methuen. For recent graduates this constitutes more or less pre-history, but it is still valuable in showing where British Psychology came from and how.

Prilleltensky, I. and Nelson, G. (2002) *Doing Psychology Critically: Making a Difference in Diverse Settings.* Basingstoke: Palgrave Macmillan. Applications of a 'radical' approach to areas such as teaching, counselling, health and community work, seeing psychologists as agents of change.

Radford, J. (2008) 'Psychology in its place', *Psychology Teaching Review,* 14 (1): 38–50, and various responses to this in the subsequent issue – 14 (2): 3–61. Although mainly from a teaching point of view, these articles raise many general issues relevant to applied work.

Richards, G. (1996) *Putting Psychology in its Place: An Introduction from a Critical Historical Perspective.* London: Routledge. This is a more argumentative account seeking to show some of the pressures, attitudes and assumptions that have shaped the discipline.

2

RESEARCH: THE UBIQUITOUS HANDMAIDEN OF PROFESSIONALISM

Brian R. Clifford

This chapter discusses:

- the nature of research;

- several fundamental considerations when humans are the subject matter of investigation;

- numerous specific research methods;

- a major research methodology debate;

- the promises and pitfalls of a major new research tool;

- the availability of 'canned' statistical packages to help move from data to information (the end-point – knowledge – requires the researcher's reasoning capacity).

INTRODUCTION

This chapter makes the case that <u>research</u> underpins all professional activity because change is ever-present, both in the discipline and in the level of professional expertise exhibited by the exponent of the service provided. It makes the case that although research execution is as much art as science, nonetheless certain basic considerations are present in all exploration of <u>human behaviour</u> and experience. Having established these basic considerations, the various research approaches are presented and their strengths and weaknesses detailed. A major debate within research methodology, qualitative versus quantitative approaches, is then presented and the core elements of the dispute are laid bare and their implications for the research approach adopted spelt out. The chapter closes by arguing that whatever the pre-theoretical assumptions are that one adopts, there are certain principles of operation in research that cannot be ignored and that must be adhered to if the research product is to have validity, reliability, replicability and applicability.

RESEARCH: THE FOUNDATIONAL BASIS OF ALL PROFESSIONS

Irrespective of which profession you seek to enter there is one component of your education that will always appear in whatever course you undertake: research. This is necessarily the case because no discipline or practice is static: new frontiers are always being opened; the envelope is always being extended; and past and present work must always be evaluated for usefulness for incorporation into new mechanisms, practices and policies in your profession of choice. Evidence-based – or at least, evidence-guided – practice is becoming the watch-word of all professions. Thus, research becomes seminal in all professional induction.

RESEARCH

So what is research? Research means different things to different people and in different professions. Broadly, it extends all the way from *re-searching* extant knowledge, practice or theory, to the *creation* of new knowledge, practice or theory. Its focus can thus be retrospective or prospective; it can be empirical or rational; it can be creative or it can be algorithmic.

Scholarship is concerned with fully understanding what someone else has said and possibly reformulating the accounts given. Research on the other hand is concerned with the production of new knowledge, new insights, new laws, mechanisms, procedures or processes. The distinction may be formulated as the ability to wonder (scholarship) versus the ability to know (research). The former is essentially open ended whereas the latter is essentially closed. Research is closed because to conduct research that is meaningful requires adherence to a number of methodological 'rules' and 'tactics' that are generally accepted by the research community as rigorous, meaningful and productive of knowledge or understanding (Figure 2.1).

The various research methods found across the professions of clinical, occupational, educational, health and forensic psychology are many and varied. Often this variety is forced by the topic of enquiry; often variation is forced by compromise and research becomes as much art as science in its execution. However, underlying the myriad varieties of research that exist can be detected the strain towards the canons of research. Whatever the topic of research, whatever the field of enquiry, nonetheless there is the strain to maintain the principles of research design, implemented within a framework of ethical acceptability. To paraphrase Medawar (1972), research begins as a speculative adventure, an imaginative preconception of what might be – a thought

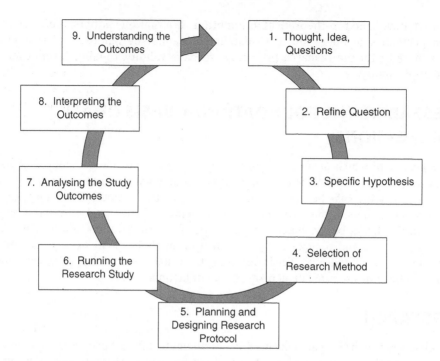

Figure 2.1   The ideal research cycle/spiral

that goes beyond anything you have logical or factual authority to believe. It is the power to wonder, the invention of a possible world. You then expose your thought, idea or conjecture to critical scrutiny – by way of a critical literature review or practice audit. Having established a prima facie case for your idea, you are then set to take the next research steps. This involves clarifying your concepts, identifying the variables of interest and then setting about exploring the hypotheses you feel justified in holding.

Now this appears so clear-cut and ordered to the beginning researcher: you start with a desire to understand better some phenomenon; by the application of some selected systematic means you obtain meaningful data; then following careful reflection and interpretation, you end up with conclusions concerning your initial phenomenon of interest. However, unlike this 'reconstructed logic of science' (Kaplan, 1964) that you will meet in the published literature, real research is often messy, intensely frustrating and fundamentally non-linear. As stated above, it is as much art as science, as much compromise as design, especially in the applied, real-world context.

BACKGROUND CONSIDERATIONS

Despite the above-acknowledged gulf between the rhetoric and the reality of research, once you are clear on the question(s) you wish to address then the next question is how to proceed. This is a difficult question because the available methods are numerous. However, certain guidelines are available to render the task of selection manageable.

⌐The basic aim of research is to gather objective data to support (verify) or challenge (falsify) or clarify (understand) your idea⌐ this emphasis on data is what differentiates psychology from, for example, philosophy. Thus, cognitive psychology emphasises experimental data; occupational psychology, psychometric data; developmental psychology, longitudinal data; and social psychology now emphasises qualitative data. Applied psychology in general, because of the difficulty of conducting 'true experiments', emphasises interviews, observational methods, field research and quasi-experimental designs. So where do you begin?

If truth be told, the professional area you enter, and the department within which you study, may have a 'preferred method' and you will be dragooned into utilising this approach. Allowing for this pragmatic solution to research design selection, you should nonetheless be aware of the various approaches available, and the overall problems that attach to any and all approaches by virtue of psychology's unique subject matter – human beings. These overall problems emanate from the fact that neither the respondents nor the researchers are inert beings.

PARTICIPANT EFFECTS

Coolican (1998) argues that human participants exhibit a number of biases (Box 2.1).

Box 2.1   Participant effects in research

- Hawthorne effect

- Social desirability responding

- Evaluation apprehension

- Placebo effect

- Response acquiescence set

The well-known *Hawthorne effect* exhibits participants' reactivity. The Hawthorne effect showed that whatever was done to workers in an electrical factory (positively or negatively) their productivity went up. This indicates clearly that humans are not inert – rather they are thinking, feeling, sentient beings who will react in different ways if they 'know' or think they are being evaluated. As Coolican indicates, in real-life research, naturalistic or participant observation methods are means of getting over this.

Social desirability responding is another human reactive phenomenon whereby participants attempt to present a public image of social respectability. Clearly all self-report measures run the risk of eliciting this response, as do any questions in questionnaires that request views on socially sensitive matters. Related to this aspect of reactivity, but different from it, is *demand characteristics*. Because partici-pants are active, sense-making beings they will pick up cues as to what the research is about, and the usual norms of social interaction will come into play, for example, co-operation.

The *placebo effect* serves to demonstrate that humans who 'know' they have received a treatment, intervention or a manipulation, will behave as they believe they are expected to behave. This is related to but distinct from *evaluation apprehension*, which refers to research participants' eagerness to do well, which may not pertain in real-life situations.

Lastly, *response acquiescence set* refers to the tendency of participants to respond in one direction rather than another, and usually positively. This response set can be detected and controlled for by inserting 'opposite' questions and including a lie scale (e.g. as in Eysenck's Personality Inventory (EPI)).

RESEARCHER EFFECTS

Complementary to participant bias in human research is bias in researchers and research designs (Box 2.2).

Box 2.2   Researcher effects in research

- Self-fulfilling prophecy
- Pygmalion effect
- Halo effect
- Data mining
- Omission of non-confirmatory data
- Falsification of results

The *self-fulfilling prophecy* is the clearest demonstration of this bias. Labelled people will actually begin to demonstrate the labelled behaviour. This is also referred to as the *Pygmalion effect* – researcher's expectations or hopes have actual effects upon participants. The standard control procedure for this effect is the single, or better still, double-blind technique whereby neither the participant (single blind) nor the data gatherer (double blind) know which condition(s) the participants are in.

Another well-known research effect is the *Halo effect* whereby an examiner or assessor's overall positive or negative evaluation affects their evaluation of a specific trait, ability or response.

The above biases are unconscious influences on the researcher. There are also more pernicious, conscious, biases such as *data mining* for any congenial findings, omission, ignoring or burying of uncongenial or *non-confirmatory data*, and lastly, *falsification of results*. All these latter biases are reprehensible and should not be countenanced under any circumstances.

For the moment, suffice to say that in *any* research there are a multitude of possible confounding effects, and a great deal of effort and thought must be devoted to either eliminating or statistically controlling these possible confounding variables as explanation.

These *participant*, *experimenter* and *structural* biases are potentially present in all research, so although they act as a backdrop to considerations of specific method selection they do not serve to make that selection. As has been said, tradition, local predilection and sheer necessity frequently force the choice of method. So what methods are available?

RESEARCH METHODS: SPECIFIC TECHNIQUES

Box 2.3 presents a list of the various research techniques that are used across the board by the various psychological subdisciplines.

Box 2.3   Categories of research methods

- True experiments

- Quasi-experiments

- Correlational methods

- Interview-based research

- Questionnaires and survey-based research

- Observational methods of research

- Case studies

- Diary methods of research

- Archival research

Experiments

At the positivist end of research the true experiment is the method of choice. Here participants are allocated at random to either the control or the experimental group. These two groups are treated identically except that the experimental group under-goes a treatment whereas the control group does not. Both groups are then measured on the same variable. The manipulated variable is referred to as the independent variable and the measured variable is called the dependent variable. With all other variables controlled, the manipulation of the one variable is assumed to be the cause of any observed consequent change in the dependent variable. This is Mill's (1874) 'method of difference'. Note, what has been described is the archetypal experimental design. In reality several independent variables can be manipulated simultaneously (e.g. a multifactorial design) and several dependent variables can be measured (e.g. multivariate designs). However, the logic of causation remains the same.

Within the experimental method, further decisions will have to be made between repeated measures (within-subject) designs, matched-subject designs, and factorial (between-subject) designs. The deciding factors here will be economy of time and/or respondents and control of variance (variability). Finally, it is possible to conduct designs where some variables are manipulated within-subjects, while others appear as between-subject factors or variables. This gives rise to the so-called split-plot or mixed design.

The experimental method is not without its detractors. A frequent criticism is its artificiality and lack of ecological validity or mundane realism, or, in forensic psychology, its legal verisimilitude. In short, it is frequently argued that although the experiment has good internal validity it has poor external validity. As we will see later the ontology, epistemology and model of the human that underpins the experimental method is currently under attack.

Quasi-experiments

Quasi-experimental methods are available for research purposes when conditions pertain that exclude the conducting of 'true' experimentation. A great deal of research in the professional literature is of this type. The interested reader is directed to Campbell and Stanley (1963) for what still remains the best account of the many quasi-experimental designs available.

Broadly, quasi-experimental methodology is employed when either you cannot randomly allocate participants to conditions, or you have less than perfect control over the independent variable, or both. Thus, a great many experimental studies con-ducted *in situ* are quasi-experiments where either intact groups have to be used under different conditions, or variables cannot be manipulated but either happen infre-quently, by chance or not at all. In addition, although a study may begin as a true experiment, reality may intrude and the researcher has to be creative in salvaging his or her research and engage in damage limitation.

So what are quasi-experimental designs and how valuable are they? Fundamen-tally, their value resides in how well or badly they retain internal and external validity. Internal validity is the basic minimum without which any experiment is un-interpretable. Essentially, did the treatment(s)/manipulation(s) make a difference? External validity refers to the result's generalisability – to other populations, settings, treatment and measurement variables.

With respect to internal validity in quasi-experimental designs, eight different threats have to be guarded against. (1) *History* – uncontrolled specific events outside the experiment can happen at the same time as the experimental manipulations or interventions are being undertaken. (2) *Maturation* – changes in the respondents can occur co-terminously with the manipulation. (3) *Testing* – an initial test (to establish a baseline) can have an unintentional effect upon the scores of a second testing. (4) *Instrumentation* – unnoticed changes in the measuring instrument, the scorers, or the participants over time. (5) *Regression to the mean* – a statistical phenomenon whereby extreme groups move closer to the overall mean on second testing, irrespective of what was done to them. (6) *Selection artefacts* – these are caused by differential selection methods being used for the different groups or treatments. (7) *Experimental mortality* – across time a differential rate of loss of participants can occur in comparison groups. This would not be a major problem if it had been possible to allocate participants to groups randomly. (8) *Selection–maturation interaction* – here different intact groups may be undergoing different changes unrelated to the experimental manipulations.

All these threats are threats of confounding. The researcher can mistakenly assume that observed change or difference is due to the manipulation whereas such change or difference may, in reality, be due to these various extraneous factors.

External validity or representativeness of quasi-experimental designs is jeopardised by four main threats. (1) Reactive or interactive effects of testing. For example pre-testing may influence eventual responsiveness, which would not vary if pre-testing had not been undertaken. (2) Interaction effects of selection bias and the experimental variable. (3) Reactive effects of the experimental arrangements. For example, non-reinforced or control groups may become resentful (resentful demoralisation, or more prosaically, the 'screw you' effect). (4) Multiple-treatment interference. Prior treatments/manipulations are usually not erasable. In the true experiment this can be controlled for by counter-balancing: in quasi-experimental designs it cannot.

The researcher seeking qualifications in professional psychology will rarely be capable of running true experimental designs, though the research psychologist (experimentally based M Phil or PhD postgraduate) should have more scope for executing the true experiment.

It is when the true experiment is not possible that students begin to realise that research methodology is as much an art as a science. Research is not carried out in a vacuum: rather it is frequently the outcome of compromise, creative construction and plausible recoverability.

Correlational methods

Apart from the practical impossibility of running a true experiment or even a quasi-experiment, ethics may not allow the conducting of such a study. However, we can still explore the relationship between variables of interest. This is achieved by selecting a correlational rather than an experimental methodology. Correlation methodology explores the co-variation between two or more variables (via linear and multiple regression techniques). Although correlation can never disclose causation, modern techniques can certainly approach it. Several correlations compared across time, known as a cross-lagged design, can tease out the directionality of association, and path analysis can indicate the magnitude of different associations.

In the developmental, forensic, occupational, health and clinical fields, correlational studies are frequently based on longitudinal or cross-sectional group comparisons. Both these group comparison methods have their problems, but all other things being equal, the longitudinal design is to be preferred to the cross-sectional. In terms of practicalities, master's and doctoral theses usually allow only of cross-sectional designs, the more time-consuming longitudinal studies being reserved for well-funded post Master's or post Doctoral studies.

Interview methods

Another major research methodology is that of the interview. The interview can be face to face, over the telephone, by email or over the internet. Additionally, the interview can range from structured to unstructured. The structured interview will be characterised by containing exactly the same questions for all respondents and a closed – probably Likert scale – response format. The semi-structured interview uses more open-ended questions, but is still designed to obtain similar types of information from each interviewee. The semi-structured interview is more respondent-led and is designed to allow the interviewee's unique perspective to emerge clearly and comprehensively.

The non-directive interview is designed to allow the respondent as much freedom as possible when addressing the research topic of interest, and to ensure a rich and 'thick' response to emerge. Despite being interviewee-led the researcher must retain some degree of specifiable focus if meaningful data are to be captured.

Clearly the costs and benefits of these different types of interview method must be weighed carefully. The more structured the interview, the more reliability there will be, the easier will data be to compare across individuals or groups and the greater will control be. The more unstructured the interview, the richer the data but the less comparable will any two respondents' data be. Depending upon your meta-theoretical assumptions and research orientation, quantification possibilities may not be an issue. However, some framework of understanding will have to be 'imposed' on the accumulated responses if sense is to be made of the data. Thus, as in most research, a compromise has to be made.

In the case of interview data, that decision will be between obtaining rich, full and comprehensive accounts, and obtaining data that can be organised and understood within a well-prescribed, and communicated, research topic. Discourse analysis, content analysis, thematic analysis, grounded theory and conversational analysis are likely research techniques that will be brought to bear upon these interview data. As we will see below, statistical and software packages now exist to aid 'sense-making' and to ensure tractability of the data that can arise.

Questionnaires and surveys

These research methods form a large part of postgraduate research output. Basically this research method can range from simply asking (research related) open, exploratory, believed-to-be relevant questions, to administering tests that have a theoretical and normed underpinning, such as aptitude, ability, personality, intelligence and attitude tests and questionnaires.

It is unfortunately the case that postgraduate students frequently perceive research based upon questionnaires as an 'easy option'. Nothing could be further from the truth. Major problems of reliability and validity must be addressed if constructed measuring instruments are to be of any value. Reliability is a question of consistency: external reliability asks whether the same results will pertain with the same participant at a later date; internal reliability asks whether the test is internally consistent. This in turn can be assessed by split-half reliability, item analysis and Cronbach's alpha. Validity refers to how well the test or questionnaire tests what it purports to test. Validity can be checked by face validity considerations, content validity, criterion validity and construct validity. A consideration that is rarely if ever met in postgraduate work with new scales, questionnaires or tests is standardisation. Without standardisation of a measurement instrument we can never be fully confident in its reliability and validity. As has been said, this research choice is not an easy option.

Observational methods

Observational research methods exist and are exploited fully most noticeably in educational, occupational and developmental research. As Coolican (1998) indicates, observational studies can be ranged along four dimensions: structure (whether data are recorded within a predetermined framework and scoring system, or are open-ended); setting (whether contrived or naturalistic); level of observer's participation (uninvolved, participant observer or observing participant); and lastly, disclosure (participants are aware or not of being observed). Clearly such studies involve major considerations of what to measure, where to measure, how to measure, when to measure and whom to measure. In addition, in such open-ended flexible research, problems of interpretation and reliability loom large.

Case studies

Case studies have been an enduring research method within psychology and yet their status is somewhat ambiguous. While Bromley (1986) points out that they are the 'bedrock of scientific investigation', they seem to contravene the canons of experimental psychology (random allocation to groups) and by definition they lack external validity (because unique). Case studies involve the intensive study of one individual, group or organisation, usually *in situ*.

Within experimental psychology, and especially cognitive neuropsychology, they are frequently referred to as '$n=1$' studies. For example, a person exhibiting a rare cognitive deficit is examined intensively and an independent variable of interest is manipulated. By utilising such an *n*=1, or case study, an existence proof can be established of some process or mechanism as being of importance in normal functioning. In applied psychology research generally, case studies can provide extremely rich data but they do lack generalisability and replicability, by definition. McLeod (2010) reviews case study research's historical development and the specific methods and issues involved in carrying out systematic and rigorous case studies, distinguishing among five models that are available.

Diary methodology

Diary studies require participants to keep more or less detailed and comprehensive records of their thoughts, behaviour or emotional reactions to people, events or happenings. These types of study are frequently used in clinical (e.g. panic attacks), cognitive (e.g. autobiographical memory), health (e.g. smoking cessation) and forensic psychology (e.g. post-traumatic stress disorders). Again, rich and fully meaningful data can be produced, but again the dangers are human frailty in terms of forgetfulness, reliability, and, it must be said, honesty, together with a lack of research control and objectivity.

Archival studies

A last approach to be detailed is archival research. This can be conceptualised as a secondary form of observation. Objectively, however, the data are 'frozen' and no manipulations can be applied, although the extant data-set can be re-partitioned and re-analysed in a number of interesting and research-directed ways. Research can be conducted on other people's research data (secondary analyses); on official or unofficial public and private documents (e.g. court cases or medical records); and finally on any published or unpublished source material whatever.

A MAJOR RESEARCH METHODS DEBATE

The perspicacious reader of this chapter will have noted that I have studiously avoided the use of the term 'scientific'. The scientific method emphasises understanding, explanation, prediction and control and the scientific approach, experimentation, which allowed these four aims of science to be achieved. Today, a deep philosophical disputation, frequently obscured by highly charged emotion, threatens to polarise the discipline of psychology, cause schisms within schools or departments of psychology and alienate colleagues within subdisciplines.

The headline dispute is between qualitative versus quantitative methodology as the better way to proceed in coming to understand human behaviour. Broadly, the debate rests on four pillars – ontology, epistemology, concepts of human nature and methodology. Fundamentally, two views exist of social science generally and psychology specifically. On the one hand, we have the view that social sciences are essentially the same as the natural sciences and are therefore concerned with discovering lawful relations regulating and 'determining' individual and social behaviours. On the other hand, the opposing view, although still concerned to describe and explain human behaviour, emphasises how people differ both from inanimate objects, and from each other. These two views eventuate in very different ways of viewing social reality and of how to interpret it.

The first issue is how to conceptualise the essence of social phenomena – is social reality external to the individual or group, or is it the product of individual thought and action? This is the ontological debate – found in philosophy as the nominalist–realist debate. The realist position argues that objects have an independent existence and are not dependent for their existence on a knower. The nominalist position argues the opposite.

The epistemological debate centres on the question of how we gain knowledge, and its nature and form. Are the objects of knowledge real, objective and 'out there' and capable of being apprehended, or is knowledge subjective, based on experience, and of a unique personal nature? Is knowledge extant or is it emergent? Depending upon one's stance on this epistemological question, so one will stress the researcher as an objective observer, with a dedication to the methods of science, or if knowledge is seen as subjective, personal and constructed, then the researcher should be a participant, and highly involved with their respondents.

The third pillar of the dispute is the conception held of the respondent or participant – are they 'determined' and responding almost 'mechanically' to outside forces, or are they initiators of their own actions and thoughts? This debate is most clearly focused in forensic psychology (but in other professions as well) where a key issue at trial can be whether the defendant is a product of their environment and conditioned by it (or their genes, or their psychological structure) or if the defendant is capable of free-will, and thus master of his or her own destiny. This is the long-standing debate between determinism and voluntarism: determinism and free-will.

The fourth pillar is a product of the foregoing three: different research methods are called for, depending upon the choice one makes between the contrasting ontologies, epistemologies and models of human beings available. Most generally, one will adopt a positivist stance or an anti-positivist stance. If one adopts the positivist stance then one adopts the view that the social world is similar to the natural world and exists independent of the experiencing individual, and will thus adopt but also adapt the existing methods, tactics and procedures of the natural sciences. The aim will be to establish regularities and relationships between factors of interest, and the approach to analysis will be predominantly quantitative. In a nutshell, this choice will be for the normative stance and for a nomothetic approach, selecting from among the plethora of research methods that fall within the scientific method.

However, if one adopts the alternative ontology, epistemology and model of the human being, then different consequences flow. If subjective experience in creating the social world is held to be important, the methods of science will be eschewed for other techniques or approaches already available in sociology and currently being developed in social psychology and cultural studies. These methods will be geared to understanding how individuals create, modify and negotiate meaning in the world. As such the methods will be qualitative rather than quantitative, and designed to document what is unique and particular to the individual (or group) rather than what is universal and general. Because of its stress on the individual and the particular, this approach will adopt the interpretive stance and the ideographic approach in research, selecting from among the numerous qualitative approaches now available. Wherever possible the imposition of external form and structure will be avoided since this would reflect the viewpoint of the observer as opposed to that of the actor directly involved. Theory and meaning extraction will be grounded in data generated by the research act, and theory will follow, not precede, the research.

Researchers of this persuasion point out that positivism failed to notice key differences between human beings and inert 'things' or objects. 'Social science, unlike natural science, stands in a subject–subject relation to its field of study, not a subject–object relation; it deals with a pre-interpreted world in which the meanings developed by active subjects enter the actual constitution or product of the world' (Giddens, 1976: 120).

Social science is thus a subjective undertaking rather than an objective one. But more than this, because of our self-awareness and power of language we must view social interaction as a different order of complexity from any other and thus no other system is capable of providing a sufficiently powerful model to advance our understanding of ourselves.

At base, this debate reflects the distinction between the mechanistic non-intentional causality inherent in natural science and the causality inherent in biological systems that have inbuilt goals, intentions and plans: that is, non-intentional versus intentional explanations. As Oatley (1992) points out, psychology is unique among academic disciplines in including both approaches. Some have questioned whether there are not dangers in giving up the methods of science for methods more akin to literature, biography and journalism, and Coolican (1998: 727) points out that skills of analysis must rise above common sense or more-or-less well-executed journalism. Others have asked, 'is it possible to move from the interpretation of one specific action or event ... to a theoretical explanation of behaviour' (Dixon 1973: 4–5). Only time will tell, as this is an ongoing and yet-to-be-concluded debate.

A MAJOR NEW RESEARCH TOOL?

A major new facility that can be used in both qualitative and quantitative research, and is increasing in frequency, is the internet. This tool, it is argued, can offer low-cost, high-quality, fast data collection. However, as with all chosen methodologies, there are both advantages and disadvantages that the researcher should be aware of (Box 2.4).

Box 2.4   Advantages and disadvantages of using the internet as a methodological tool

Advantages

1   You can collect large samples and thus increase power.

2   Collect data seven days a week, twenty-four hours a day.

3   Obtain a more diverse sample than in a localised study.

4   Obtain a faster turnaround time.

---

5   Data can be automatically coded and entered.

6   You can create cross-cultural studies more easily.

7   Experimenter demand and expectancy effects are avoided.

8   Respondents can often feel more at ease and anonymous than with live interviewers or experimenters.

9   This methodology can reduce financial costs.

10 Side-by-side studies have resulted in conclusions similar to those of more traditional methods (e.g. Birnbaum, 2004).

Disadvantages

1   Can be time consuming to set up initially.

2   Non-representative samples can be obtained.

3   Data may be 'noisier'.

4   Lack of control over some variables.

5   Participants may participate more than once.

6   Drop-out rates can be unpredictable (usually 10–20%).

7   Participants may perform the tasks in undesirable ways (e.g. continually stop-starting, rushing without due care and attention).

8   Frivolous responses are fairly frequent.

9   Internet-based research is still less acceptable than 'mainstream' methods.

10 'Flames' and 'letter bombs' can result from disgruntled recipients.

Despite these various disadvantages, and given the commercialisation of internet-based research, with the attendant development of sophisticated interactive surveys (via Java applets, JavaScript, VBScript and ActiveX technologies) there can be little doubt that this method of conducting research is here to stay and to increase in popularity and acceptability. Those students who are likely to explore this avenue of research methods should consult the BPS (2007) guidelines for ethical practice in psychological research online.

COMMONALITIES IN THE RESEARCH REPORT

If the most distinctive feature of psychological research is its data gathering, its second most noticeable feature is its set of procedures that serve not only to indicate what was done but also to allow replication by other researchers in the field. As we have seen, there is no one scientific method – no single invariant approach to problem-solving. Rather, 'What is important is the overall idea of scientific research as a controlled rational process of reflective enquiry, the interdependent nature of the parts of the process, and the paramount importance of the problem and its statement' (Kerlinger, 1970: 17).

All research, of whatever persuasion, must cohere with canons that stand as criteria against which a study can, and will be, evaluated. These canons are, according to Lincoln and Guba (1985) 'truthfulness', applicability, consistency and neutrality. Within the experimental, quantitative tradition, these canons are met by considerations of internal validity, external validity, reliability and objectivity respectively. Within the qualitative approach the equivalent considerations are credibility, transferability, dependability and confirmability respectively. Within the latter tradition, personal and functional reflexivity and triangulation of data, method, investigator and theory are important considerations in assessing the achievement of the canons of 'good research' (see Banister et al., 1994).

AND SO TO ANALYSIS

Assuming that the researcher has selected his or her preferred stance and consequent method, and executed the research programme efficiently and effectively, eventually they arrive at the data handling, analysing and interpretation stage.

For those researchers who capture their data via the experimental mode, statistical packages of great scope and power are now available (e.g. SPSS), together with a blizzard of 'idiot guide' handbooks. In addition bespoke meta-analysis, power analysis, structural equation modelling (SEM), path analysis (PA) and R packages exist and these techniques will have to become an essential part of the researcher's armoury.

Those of a qualitative persuasion will also have to become acquainted with PCQ3, PQMethod, NUDIST, ETHNIGRAPH and QUALPRO. The richness of qualitative data can be given precision by the application of these computer-based techniques.

Increasingly, then, for all researchers, of whatever persuasion, computer-based data handling will become important and a necessary skill that has to be acquired in order to be counted as a competent professional.

CONCLUSION

The argument has been advanced that research underpins all psychology professionalism. However, it has also been asserted that the actual research undertaken will be of a diverse nature depending upon the context of the research, the persons of interest in the research, the researcher's theoretical stance and numerous practical considerations. Notwithstanding the complexity of this initial decision matrix, any research method chosen should conform to canons of 'truthfulness', applicability, consistency and neutrality, based upon an approach characterisable as a controlled rational process of reflective enquiry. Only when the research conducted conforms to those canons can the resulting findings ensure warranted true belief and possibly carry policy confirmation or change implications.

QUESTIONS FOR REFLECTION AND DISCUSSION

1   Are there any **fundamental** differences in the research that are likely to be carried out under the rubric of clinical, organisational, educational, health, guidance, counselling, sport, coaching or forensic psychology?

2   Has the qualitative versus quantitative debate generated more heat than light?

3   Research methodology has a number of criteria by which its value is evaluated. What are they and can they be prioritised, or are the criteria context dependent?

4   Is research **really** necessary for the development of your chosen profession? Give reasons for your answer.

SUGGESTIONS FOR FURTHER READING

Campbell, D. and Stanley, J. (1963) 'Experimental and quasi-experimental designs for research in teaching', in N. Gage (ed.), *Handbook of Research on Teaching*. Chicago: Rand McNally. Given that most real-life research does not conform to the true experiment or its conditions, this book on quasi-experimental designs is essential reading for any professional concerned to conduct research that is designed to have maximum impact on knowledge accumulation or policy development.

Cryer, P. (2006) *The Research Student's Guide to Success*. Buckingham: Open University Press. Designed for the PhD student this book nevertheless is a mine of helpful hints for all researchers. In the Open University style, the book is replete with self-test questions and tasks that ease the learning and development of research skills and tactics.

Forrester, M.A. (ed.) (2010) *Doing Qualitative Research in Psychology: A Practical Guide*. London: Sage. This book provides a complete introduction to qualitative methods. Essentially a 'how to do it' manual, the book is linked with a specifically designed set of digitised video recordings and transcripts. Usefully, the book describes how to write up qualitative research.

Kinnear, P.R. and Gray, C.D. (2010) *PASW Statistics Made Simple 17*. Hove: Psychology Press. An absolute must for any researcher who has to analyse quantitative data and requires computational assistance. This replaces SPSS Statistics 17, the industrial standard for parametric and non-parametric analysis, and this book really does live up to its title, 'Made Simple'.

Robson, C. (2011) *Real World Research* (3rd edn). Oxford: Blackwell. The generalist's best introduction to types of research that any professional person is likely to need to know about. It covers models of the research process and deciding upon research questions. Methods of data gathering are discussed for a variety of research designs and approaches, and it takes you gently into data analysis and report writing.

3

BEYOND EVIDENCE-BASED PRACTICE: RETHINKING THE RELATIONSHIP BETWEEN RESEARCH, THEORY AND PRACTICE

David J. Harper, Kenneth Gannon and Mary Robinson

This chapter discusses:

- how applied psychologists attempt to ground their practice in research;

- the history of the evidence-based practice movement;

- problems with the scientist-practitioner model;

- alternative conceptualisations of the link between research evidence and practice;

- some of the problems with randomised controlled research trials;

- the social context of research;

- the need for a different approach, focusing on the views of participants and utilising a broader range of research methods.

INTRODUCTION

One of the distinctive things about applied psychology is that its practitioners are engaged in intervening in the world in a variety of ways, providing: psychotherapy, health psychology programmes, educational support interventions and so on. However, on what basis are these interventions designed? How can we tell whether an intervention has 'worked'? How might our interventions be improved? The applied psychologist needs to be able to draw on theory, research and practice in order to address such questions but how do these three domains relate to each other? It is on this question that this chapter is focused.

A range of policy initiatives now explicitly stress the importance of basing professional practice on firm evidence, what has become known as 'evidence-based practice'. The notion of the applied psychologist as a scientist-practitioner is one model of relating practice to evidence. However, such models present a number of dilemmas for the applied psychologist. If we only ever do what is deemed effective how do we develop innovative approaches? If 'absence of evidence is not evidence of ineffectiveness' (Department of Health, 2001: 40) how should psychologists work when dealing with issues where there is no firm evidence base? How can knowledge of groups help us in deciding how to approach an individual case? Do practitioners really base what they do on the research literature? There are often tensions in this debate between practitioners and academic researchers, for example about what kind of knowledge counts as evidence.

In this chapter, we begin with a review of the history of the evidence-based practice movement before examining the scientist-practitioner model and alternative approaches like the reflective practitioner. Then we consider some of the methodological problems faced in conducting randomised controlled trials (RCTs) in applied psychology, using trials of psychological therapy as an example. Of course, judgements about research evidence take place within a social and political context and so we investigate this in relation to the work of the UK's National Institute for Health and Clinical Excellence (NICE) before looking at how the perspectives of the recipients of interventions have been neglected. We make a case for a more pluralistic approach to gathering evidence before discussing examples of applied psychologists making use of evidence.

THE RISE OF THE EVIDENCE-BASED PRACTICE MOVEMENT

The phrase 'evidence-based practice' is now so commonly used it has become a cliché but it may surprise some readers how brief a history this concept has had. Originally the term 'evidence-based medicine' was employed and the focus was on the individual 'patient' (e.g. Sackett et al., 1996). However, increasingly the philosophy and methodology underpinning the approach have been applied to decisions on funding for treatments and in areas beyond clinical medicine. Many commentators trace its emergence to the work of epidemiologist Professor Archie Cochrane in Cardiff in the 1970s. During the 1970s and 1980s, however, his ideas were taken up by others and, in 1992, the National Health Service (NHS) set up the Cochrane Centre, which aimed to develop systematic reviews of clinical trials. In 1993 we saw the emergence of an international Cochrane Collaboration, and in 1999 the National Institute for Health and Clinical Excellence (NICE) was established. Similar aims were identified by the Social Science Research Unit based at the Institute of Education in London and, more directly, in the Evidence for Policy and Practice Information and Co-ordinating Centre established in 2003.

For private health insurance companies, especially in the USA, evidence-based practice provided a means of controlling their costs. For countries like the UK with a publicly funded health service, evidence-based medicine also offers a way of controlling costs to the taxpayer. Bodies like NICE offer the possibility of providing a rational and transparent process for making decisions about interventions, one freed from quackery or the influence of lobby groups like the pharmaceutical industry. However, as we discuss later in the chapter, these decisions still occur within a particular socio-political context.

It would be a mistake to assume that, before these policy developments, practice was not informed by research. Indeed, the scientist-practitioner model has been a dominant identity since the beginnings of applied psychology, and so it is to this that we turn first.

THE SCIENTIST-PRACTITIONER MODEL AND ITS CRITICS

This model was developed originally for clinical psychology graduate training programmes in the USA at a conference in Boulder, Colorado in 1949 but it has become a dominant model both in other fields of applied psychology (Hagstrom et al., 2007) and in other countries, including the UK. One of the motivations in developing the model was to train practitioners to apply the scientific method to understanding and aiding diagnosis and treatment, although in the UK clinical psychology became involved in treatment much later than in the USA (Pilgrim and Treacher, 1992). It was clear even at the time that this model was essentially a compromise position to prevent a split in the young profession between courses that emphasised either the scientist or practitioner side of the model (Pilgrim and Treacher, 1992). Clinical health psychology emerged as a distinct subdiscipline later than clinical psychology, but Murray (2010) has suggested that it too follows the scientist-practitioner model. Even sixty years on there is a lively debate in clinical psychology about this model (e.g. Clegg, 1998; John, 1998; Lane and Corrie, 2006; Long and Hollin, 1997; and Milne and Paxton, 1998).

Does the scientist-practitioner model accurately represent applied psychology? If by this we mean 'Do practitioners conduct research which is published in peer-reviewed journals?' then the answer appears to be largely 'no'. For example, Norcross et al. (1992) noted that the modal number of publications for UK clinical psychologists was zero – a well-replicated finding over the years in the UK and USA – with 8% of clinical psychologists producing approximately half of published work although 76% had published at least once in their careers. A similar result has been found in the USA (Norcross et al., 2005).

There are, of course, many valid reasons why applied psychologists may not be research active (Holttum and Goble, 2006) – many employers may prefer psychologists to be involved in direct interventions rather than research or consultancy. Thus Kennedy and Llewelyn (2001: 77) have suggested that the model represents 'an attitude to practice rather than a commitment to participation in the academic community', whereas Milne (1999) differentiates between scientist-practitioners and evidence-based practitioners. However, even here there are problems as few applied psychologists appear to read peer-reviewed research on a regular basis. For example, Milne et al. (1990) reported that only 20% of their sample of UK clinical psychologists had read an academic journal each week (although 45% did monthly); only 14% attended national scientific conferences; and only 16% thought published research had 'a lot' of influence on their work. Milne et al.'s (2000) more recent sample of UK psychological therapists had 'used guidelines and protocols on 56% of occasions, had on average drawn on research, CPD [continuing professional development] and audit approximately half of the time, but had been only minimally influenced by research, CPD or audit' (p. 8). It is, perhaps, not surprising that some commentators have argued that identifying oneself with the scientist-practitioner model may serve the rhetorical function of claiming the authority of science while, in practice, research has much less impact (Pilgrim and Treacher, 1992).

One could resolve some of the problems with the scientist-practitioner model by having a much broader and inclusive notion of 'science' and 'evidence', stepping away from simplistically modernist and naively realist views (Lane and Corrie, 2006). Larner (2001), advocating a critical practitioner model, has argued that 'the choice is not between psychological science and non-science, but between an exclusively logical-positivist and a critical science' (p. 40).

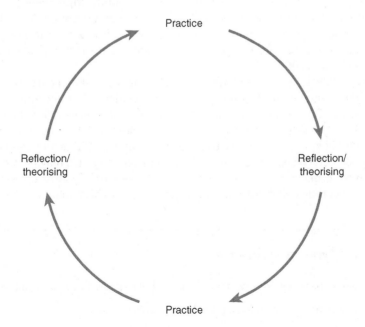

Figure 3.1

In recent years, the scientist-practitioner model has had competition from Schön's (1987) *reflective practitioner.* This approach was developed following studies where expert practitioners were identified by peers and then a consensual understanding developed of key elements of their practice. Interestingly, peers often focused on personal qualities such as wisdom, integrity and intuition. Although research-based knowledge was accessed by experts they combined it with knowledge of other cases that bore some similarity and with subjective, emotional perceptions about the particular therapeutic relationship or context (Clegg, 1998). Here then there is an emphasis on an integration of theory, research and practice at a more personal level and it also appears to draw on an active philosophy of learning that is consistent with previous work on philosophies of learning (e.g. Kolb et al., 1974) – see Figure 3.1.

Although in the USA, the scientist-practitioner model seems as strong as ever – in clinical psychology at least (Norcross et al., 2005) – there are signs in the UK that things may be changing as reflective practice has become an increasing influence (e.g. Stedmon and Dallos, 2009). For example, an examination in August 2011 of the programme descriptions on the website of the UK Clearing House for Postgraduate Courses in Clinical Psychology revealed that only five out of thirty programmes specifically noted that they followed the scientist-practitioner model whereas twice that number mentioned both scientist-practitioner and reflective-practitioner models (http://www.leeds.ac.uk/chpccp/Courses.html). In a similar vein some health psychology programmes in the UK align themselves with a reflective-scientist-practitioner approach (e.g. the University of Surrey). There are also challenges to the scientist-practitioner approach to health psychology from critical and community approaches (e.g. Murray, 2010). Within educational psychology the drive to incorporate evidence has been twofold: the search for interventions that have proven efficacy, and the need to assure quality of provision through the provision of outcome measures (Dunsmuir et al., 2009; Frederickson, 2002).

One of the differences between the applied scientist of old and current practitioners is that the evaluation of the quality of research evidence has become increasingly institutionalised. Bodies such as NICE now recommend interventions for particular diagnoses. Paradoxically, applied psychologists may now be discouraged from evaluating the quality of studies for themselves, instead taking a NICE recommendation as a proxy of quality. However, as we will see later in the chapter, this may be problematic. Bodies like NICE make certain assumptions about research quality, drawing on the work of the Cochrane Collaboration, viewing it in a hierarchical manner – see Box 3.1.

⊿ Box 3.1   Types of evidence

Type I evidence: at least one good systematic review and at least one randomised controlled trial.

Type II evidence: at least one good randomised controlled trial.

Type III evidence: at least one well-designed intervention study without randomisation.

Type IV evidence: at least one well-designed observational study.

Type V evidence: expert opinion, including the opinion of service users and carers.

Source: Department of Health (1999: 6)

Randomised controlled trials (RCTs) are at the top of this hierarchy. In these trials, research participants are allocated to different interventions – including a control group – in a randomised fashion. However, they suffer from a number of methodological problems and so the next section examines these in more detail, using RCTs of psychological therapies as an example.

THE TROUBLE WITH TRIALS – PROBLEMS ASSOCIATED WITH THE USE OF RCTs

A strong form of RCT is the double-blind procedure where neither the research participant nor the staff involved in their care should be able to tell what experimental condition they are in. This is because staff knowledge of the condition can introduce bias. However, participants in drug trials can often work out which condition they are in from the side-effect profile (Moncrieff, 2013) and it is possible that many participants in psychotherapy RCTs do too, introducing another form of bias. In a psychotherapy RCT the therapist certainly knows which condition the participant is in and thus there are no double-blind RCTs of psychological therapy. In drugs research there is increasing use of the triple-blind procedure, where the researcher does not know the condition, since even this has been shown to have an effect. There are no triple-blind RCTs of psychological therapy.

Moncrieff (2013) notes that other common problems with RCTs include: biases in the selection of participants (e.g. research samples are highly selected); high numbers of participants dropping out of a study over time (sometimes in quite high numbers); how findings and analyses are presented; and publication bias (i.e. positive findings are more likely both to be submitted for publication and published by journals). Kelly and Moloney (2013) note some more specific problems for psychotherapy RCTs including: the difficulty of achieving 'pure' randomisation; the impact of therapist allegiance effects (the well-replicated finding that therapists have better outcomes when giving a therapy with which they have an allegiance); the difficulties in achieving fidelity with a therapy; what kind of control group is selected (e.g. treatment as usual – a weak comparison – or a potentially powerful alternative therapy); and the length of follow-up. Guy et al. (2011) point out that RCTs tend to be very expensive to run and thus this limits who can conduct trials (often large university-based collaborations). Davey et al. (2012) note that many RCTs focus on symptomatic change in individuals rather than the second-order change – change within the system (e.g. a family, group or organisation) – on which, for example, systemic family therapists focus in their practice.

Over twenty years ago, Stiles and Stiles (1989) critiqued the drug metaphor underlying psychotherapy RCTs – the idea that an RCT can help determine the 'active ingredient' in a therapy in the same way as determining the active chemical in a drug. In psychotherapy RCTs the relational context in which therapeutic conversations take place is not considered. Moreover, there is a focus on comparing different 'brand name' therapies like cognitive–behavioural therapy (CBT) or psychodynamic therapy. One could argue that many RCTs obscure research progress since they tend to focus on the relatively small differences between, say, CBT and supportive counselling for people with psychotic experiences, rather than examining the larger common factors shared between these different therapeutic approaches (Paley and Shapiro, 2002; Shapiro and Paley, 2002) but proponents argue that equivalence between therapies may be a methodological artefact (Tarrier et al., 2002). However, whichever is the case, there are still some quite fundamental questions that have not been fully addressed – for example are cognitive strategies the active ingredient in CBT? Longmore and Worrell (2007), in their review, argue that the cognitive components of CBT do not appear to add anything to the behavioural components and thus are not necessary components of CBT.

There are also problems of generalisability. Randomised controlled trials tend to focus on the narrow issue of efficacy (whether an intervention 'works' in a highly controlled setting with a highly selected research population) rather than effectiveness (whether an intervention 'works' in the real world, making a real difference in a person's everyday life). In fact there are vastly more studies of efficacy conducted than of effectiveness (Cahill et al., 2010). Since RCTs are based on group means they tell us very little about individuals but, in practice, applied psychologists need to be able to work out what will help them in a particular situation. A related problem is the number of combinations of treatment that can be compared within an RCT. In routine clinical practice, interventions are frequently combined but trials rarely evaluate more than two (Marks, 2009), and it is easy to see why. If one wished to evaluate five different techniques in combination, for example, one hundred and twenty different combinations would be required. The issue of the clinical or practical significance of trial findings is an increasingly important topic – see the March 2010 issue of *Clinical Psychology: Science and Practice*. Roth (1999) has suggested the introduction of clinically meaningful analyses like the number needed to treat (NNT) criterion – that is, how many people would need to receive the experimental condition for one person to gain a benefit they would not have obtained from receiving the control condition. However, Shearer-Underhill and Marker's (2010) analysis of one hundred randomly selected papers published in the American Psychological Association's (APA's) *Journal of Consulting and Clinical Psychology* between 2000 and 2008 revealed that only four reported this statistic. Nevertheless, although analyses such as NNT are more helpful to clinicians making decisions about individuals than groups means they do not resolve some of the fundamental limitations of RCTs.

The dependence of bodies like NICE on RCTs is thus problematic but, of course, bodies like these do not evaluate evidence in a social and political vacuum. Indeed, as policymakers and public sector employers have increasingly sought to ensure that guidelines are followed by practitioners, judgements about evidence have become increasingly politicised and so it is to this issue that we turn next.

THE SOCIAL CONTEXT OF EVIDENCE-BASED PRACTICE: A *NICE* EXAMPLE

One of the problems with evidence-based policymaking is that the social context within which evidence gets produced can be obscured. Marks (2009) has argued that '[i]n truth, evidence consists of negotiable, value-laden and contextually dependent items of information. The evidence (= knowledge) base in science, medicine and health care is not an accident, but the outcome of a heuristic set of "gates" or "filters"' (p. 476). Research evidence does not just appear – researchers need to decide to research a particular topic and this will be dependent on the topics research funders are prepared to fund. Research funders may be influenced by issues other than the epidemiological importance of a problem. For example, in one of his Reith lectures Lord Martin Rees criticised the fact that health and pharmaceutical research expenditures were 'much, much higher' than the 'five trillion dollars a year' spent on research into energy which, he argued, was arguably a more pressing need because of climate change (Rees, 2010). This contrast is heightened because much pharmaceutical research is focused on products likely to be profitable and so, although malaria is a massive international problem, pharmaceutical companies were initially unwilling to develop cheap anti-malarial medication until extensive campaigning forced them to do otherwise (Crawford, 2007). Much health research is funded by charities, and the ability of a charity to generate money may depend a lot on the emotional appeal of a particular issue.

A great deal of research is funded by governments. Governments have a range of priorities – for example, worldwide military spending in 2010 was $1.6 trillion (Stockholm International Peace Research Institute, 2011). Government funding will be related to policy priorities and because politicians tend to work on electoral timescales of four to five years, policy initiatives may move ahead of the research evidence. Thus, for example, the UK government spent £200m setting up new cognitive–behavioural treatment services for people with a diagnosis of personality disorder who were also considered dangerous potential offenders (so-called DSPD) in advance of research demonstrating their efficacy. Subsequently, the researchers involved with the DSPD programme have noted that it 'has been less effective in managing those whom it was primarily targeting and may not have been cost-effective' (Tyrer et al., 2010: 95).

NICE provides a good example of the social context of evidence-based practice. For a start, it doesn't choose the topics on which it will develop guidelines – these are decided by ministers (though obviously with input from advisers).[1] Moreover, the topics

---

[1]Limitations of space prohibit a fuller discussion of the way in which evidence is utilised by policymakers – see Stevens (2011) for a fascinating account of one academic researcher's experience of being seconded to work in a UK government department.

are 'conditions' and thus the process is based on a medical diagnostic framework even though the guidelines for many of the mental health problems specifically note that the reliability and validity of many of these diagnoses are contested (e.g. the guidelines on borderline personality disorder and depression). The Midlands Psychology Group (2010) note that the 2006 NICE guideline on attention-deficit hyperactivity disorder (ADHD) includes the developers' response to a submission by the Critical Psychiatry Network:

> Thank you very much for your comprehensive and detailed critique of the concept, diagnosis, classification and treatment of ADHD and related categories. Unfortunately, we are unable to dismiss the diagnosis as we would be left without a guideline to undertake. (NICE, 2006: 34)

Once a topic has been selected, NICE then sets up Guideline Development Groups (GDGs). Guy et al. (2011) has criticised the composition of these groups, noting that the membership of the GDGs for the 2004 guidelines for anxiety and the 2009 guidelines for depression and schizophrenia were composed of: 6.7% psychological therapists; 10.7% service users or carers; 33% representatives of the medical profession; and 36% staff from the National Collaborating Centre for Mental Health (NCCMH) led by a partnership between the Royal College of Psychiatrists and the BPS's Centre for Outcomes Research and Effectiveness. Winter (2010) notes that, of the psychological therapy professionals included on mental health-related GDGs, the 'majority were cognitive behavioural in their therapeutic orientation' (2010: 6). He argues that allegiance effects are evident in the work of research reviewers like the GDGs. Citing examples of alleged bias in their work he comments:

> It is difficult not to conclude that such recommendations are based less on a balanced review of the evidence base than on the allegiances of members of the Guideline Development Group or political considerations, such as support of current NHS policies and initiatives. (Winter, 2010:.6)

Moreover, not all perspectives are given equal weight in GDG deliberations. Milewa reports – based on his interviews with NICE participants – that non-professional members 'were more likely to have their credibility or legitimacy questioned openly' (2006: 3108). Indeed, the two service user representatives on the self-harm GDG resigned because they felt the group was unwilling to question aspects of assessment and treatment (Midlands Psychology Group, 2010; Pembroke, n.d.).

Reviews of the research evidence are based on the hierarchical framework described earlier. However, Milewa and Barry (2005) note that NICE committees take into account a wide variety of considerations. For example, the GDG for antisocial personality disorder, finding that there was little RCT evidence in the area, instead drew on research into offending behaviour programmes.

Once the guidelines have been agreed they are published in four different versions. Learmonth (2006: 2) notes that there are important differences between these versions:

The Quick Reference Guide and shortened Guidelines are essentially synopses of the full Guidelines, but with all caveats and ambiguities removed. The effect of this is to make them read as hugely more 'authoritative' statements of fact, whereas the full Guidelines allow for far more questioning of both process and outcome.

The Department of Health then seeks to ensure, through managerial and policy directives, that only recommended interventions are utilised, and NHS managers often simply carry this out, rather than refer to the full, and more nuanced, versions of the guidelines. Typically, for the mental health guidelines, only interventions with RCTs are recommended. Roth (1999) has warned of the dangers of going down the US path of identifying 'empirically supported therapies' because of the way this has been used to restrict practice, especially by managed-care organisations. In the NHS there has been more of an emphasis on the development of clinical guidelines that involve both evidence and professional opinion (e.g. Roth and Fonagy, 2004) but, increasingly, room for discretion and for tailoring interventions for particular users of services have been removed.

WHOSE EVIDENCE? THE NEED TO INCLUDE THE PERSPECTIVES OF PARTICIPANTS

It is noteworthy that the views of those who receive interventions are placed at the bottom of the Cochrane Collaboration's hierarchy of evidence. Indeed, Marks (2009) has argued that '[i]n medicine and health care there is a large and increasing gap between what gets measured and what matters most to clients and patients' (p. 476). Perkins (2001), a mental health professional and mental health service user, has noted that one of the problems with the way the outcomes of mental health interventions are usually measured is that they tend to focus only on the reduction of psychiatric symptoms. She argues that a narrow focus on symptoms alone is a professional perspective and that this may not be the only or even the most important criterion of success from a service user's point of view – often they are more interested in issues relating to quality of life. She suggests that services need to systematically ascertain the goals of service users (as they define them) and accord them the status currently enjoyed by the views of professionals, and she questions whether many interventions would look effective if outcome was measured by service users' scores on scales like Rogers et al.'s (1997) measurement of empowerment. Rose et al. (2006: 110) concur, asking, 'Who decides what is evidence, or more precisely, whose versions of evidence are given priority?' They argue that the evidence gathered in relation to interventions is contestable from the viewpoint of different stakeholders (e.g. service users and carers, professionals, policymakers etc) and that researchers thus need to incorporate multiple perspectives. They noted that service users often had important views that were at variance with those of professionals, citing as an example Rose et al.'s (2003) study of service user perspectives on electroconvulsive therapy (ECT). This had found that service users gave much lower ratings of satisfaction for ECT compared with ratings collected in ECT trials, and that about a third of those who had signed consent forms for

ECT felt their consent had not been willingly given. Moreover, the measures of outcome were defined by what professionals considered important, not necessarily what service users did. The importance of attending to the views and experiences of service users is given additional emphasis by the recent focus in the UK on the importance of shared decision-making in relation to testing and interventions of various sorts (e.g. Coulter and Collins, 2011). This is a process in which clinicians and service users/patients work together to determine a course of action. Although it is generally conceptualised as occurring in the context of a consultation it clearly entails a central role for the 'consumer' of the intervention and thus has implications for research as well as good clinical practice. It is thus important in any study for applied psychologists to consider the perspectives of a range of stakeholders, especially those who receive our interventions.

A PLURALISTIC APPROACH TO GATHERING EVIDENCE

So far we have argued that a reliance on RCTs, studies of efficacy rather than effectiveness, statistical rather than clinical or practical significance, and professional- rather than participant-derived views and measures of outcome is problematic. Cornish and Gillespie (2009) have argued that the traditional hierarchy of evidence, with meta-analyses and RCTs at the top, reflects the prioritisation of a particular set of interests. Despite their limitations, RCTs are helpful to policymakers and purchasers of health care. They are less helpful, as we have seen, to practitioners making decisions about particular clients and to those wishing to understand the views of service users or the role of social and cultural factors in health and illness. There is a need both for researchers and independent gatekeepers like NICE to adopt a more pluralistic approach to evidence, and a number of suggestions have been made in the literature. Indeed, in a report on evidence-based practice Marks (2002a) concluded, among other things, that it was necessary to 'broaden the epistemological approach and evidence-base, and create more inclusive methods for synthesis of evidence' (p. 45). Hoshmand and Polkinghorne (1992) have talked of the need for new forms of knowledge and enquiry – a 'knowledge of practice' (p. 60) and, indeed, practice-based research has become increasingly popular, as have effectiveness studies (e.g. Cahill et al., 2010). Roth (1999) has noted that much psychotherapy research continues to focus on comparisons between 'brand name' therapies, and he has called for the further development of pan-theoretical research focusing on factors like the importance of the therapeutic alliance and the skilfulness with which interventions are implemented (see Norcross and Goldfried, 2005, and Prochaska and Norcross, 2009 for introductions to this kind of approach).

A number of commentators have argued for a greater role for qualitative research in applied psychology. For example, within the realm of psychotherapy, qualitative methods can provide an insight into change processes (Elliott, 2012; McLeod, 2011) or how people's engagement with services changes across time (McKenna and Todd, 1997) or how theoretical propositions are enacted in therapy (Roy-Chowdhury, 2003). There are some challenges, however. For example, a range of interventions are not based on modernist realist premises. Here, however, new forms of evaluation like the *Most Significant Change* technique[2] (Dart and Davies, 2003) can be useful. In this approach a range of stakeholders identify key domains within which change is desired from an intervention programme and there is then a consensual search for specific stories identifying change within these domains. This has proven to be a popular method for evaluating a variety of programmes, particularly in community development as it explicitly includes a range of stakeholders and is sensitive to social impacts.

There is a danger though in leaving evaluation just up to researchers and bodies like NICE. Practitioners too have a role both in consuming research (see Falzon et al., 2010 for an example of how practitioners can search the evidence base themselves) and also in evaluating their own work. Many organisations employing applied psychologists may gather data useful for evaluation but, as practitioners, we have an ethical duty to evaluate our own practice in a manner consistent with our approach. Here single case designs can be helpful but 'quick and dirty' approaches can also be enlightening and some practitioners have conducted simple audits of their work (e.g. Holmes, 2003). A quantitative approach can be useful for evaluating change over time but this need not be dependent on a modernist realist epistemology. For example, within mental health settings, simple ecologically valid scaling measures can be used that are not dependent on psychiatric diagnostic categories. For example in Shapiro's personal questionnaire technique (Shapiro, 1961) the client is asked to describe, in their own words, a particular problematic experience or 'complaint' (or 'symptom' within a diagnostic framework). Each complaint is then given a simple rating scale and so the client can be asked to give a rating over the course of an intervention (e.g. Barkham et al., 1989). A similar approach is adopted within solution-focused work, where scaling questions can be used to evaluate progress towards desired goals, confidence in maintaining progress and so on (e.g. George et al., 1999). These can complement anecdotal observations of the practitioner where 'very concrete stories are provided from multiple sources and for a period spanning weeks or months' (Kazdin, 2006: 47).

Box 3.2   An example of the use of evidence in practice: using CBT with a pupil in danger of exclusion from school

Kevin is a fourteen-year-old boy in secondary school, nearing the end of year nine. He has struggled to accept school rules throughout the current year and the advent of GCSE subject choice has brought the issues regarding 'rules' to the fore. Despite parental commitment to the school and a focus on academic success within the family, Kevin sees the solution to his current unhappiness as a change of school. At times when this has not been supported by parents or school, Kevin has withdrawn his co-operation in both settings and his challenging behaviour has resulted in a number of fixed-term exclusions.

(Continued)

---

[2]We are indebted to Angela Byrne for alerting us to this technique.

(Continued)

Kevin was raised as a priority concern during consultation with the educational psychologist working with the school. At a joint school and family meeting Kevin's parents reported their incomprehension regarding the change in Kevin's behaviour over the past year, the constant arguments and his apparent unreasonable resistance to all school rules. A period of direct involvement was agreed and CBT was proposed as the intervention most suited to bringing about a change in Kevin's relationships with adults at home and in school. CBT had been used with a number of pupils in the school following a review of its effectiveness (Pugh, 2010). A number of factors indicated that it might be an appropriate intervention here. For example, it was important for any intervention to be short term and CBT offered this. Moreover, it seemed to be important for Kevin to have an opportunity to identify links between his thoughts, feelings and behaviour so that he could then develop alternative strategies and so avoid further exclusions from school and CBT appeared to promise this.

Over a period of seven weeks, Kevin met with the educational psychologist on five occasions and together they explored his perception of how decisions were made regarding expectations of behaviour and his role in the process. It transpired that Kevin saw all adults as having the freedom to make choices whereas he saw them withholding a similar right from children. He saw this control by adults as insulting to his developing maturity and thus tended to rebel against rules. The sessions with Kevin focused on inviting him to notice rules across society and not just in school. For example, he was encouraged to take note of the rules governing the behaviour of respected role models in the community and the media. He also identified the personal rules he would apply if given the opportunity. He also examined the long-term consequences of taking an oppositional approach to rules in both school and home.

Part of the awareness that governed change in Kevin's approach was the realisation that, both at home and in school, all activities included both choices and rules (either self- or other-imposed). Moreover, an important element of freedom was the ability to choose to abide by certain rules. Of course, not all rules are of equal status and Kevin began to identify those that were negotiable and those that needed to be adhered to for practical and pragmatic reasons. Now in year ten, Kevin has moved to the upper area of the school and is engaged in his GCSE studies. He continues to work on negotiating his choices with parents and school but has accommodated to the notion of negotiation rather than resistance as an indicator of maturity and respect.

CONCLUSION

One of the important issues that appears to get lost in the debate about evidence-based practice is the reason why we need to gather evidence on our interventions. Rather than fetishise 'evidence' we see the major issue here as about *accountability*. Applied psychologists need to be accountable to a wide variety of stakeholders (including the recipients of their services) for what they do and so we need to be able to justify and give a theoretically reasoned rationale for why we have used one intervention rather than another. If we keep this notion in mind it means that we need to move beyond narrow modernist conceptions of science in evaluating our work.

In evaluating our theories we also need to draw on ethical principles and criteria to orient us to what count as better theories and practices. Some have argued that we need to debate the values that underpin much research and have called for 'ethics before effectiveness' (Bracken and Thomas, 2000: 22). The American social constructionist psychologist Ken Gergen has suggested that we need to focus more on the *usefulness* of our theories (Misra, 1993) and Cornish and Gillespie (2009) have proposed a pragmatic approach within health psychology. Of course, we also need to examine other ways of commissioning research, and increasingly researchers are looking at partnerships with users of services rather than only with the traditional commissioners and purchasers of services (e.g. Faulkner, 2012; Faulkner and Thomas, 2002; Lindow, 2001; Patel, 1999). We have argued here that we need to move away from simplistic conceptions of evidence-based practice and to seek a more dynamic and reflective conceptualisation of the relationship between theory, research and practice. This entails developing not only real-world criteria for evaluating research evidence but also different ways of going about the research enterprise itself, embracing a pluralistic approach to the selection of methodologies and the kinds of evidence gathered. Only then are we likely to find not just a more effective relationship between theory, research and practice, but also a more ethical one.

QUESTIONS FOR REFLECTION AND DISCUSSION

1   What is 'evidence-based practice' and what are its implications for applied psychology?

2   What kinds of evidence could psychologists gather apart from that found in RCTs?

3   As well as effectiveness, what additional factors might psychologists need to bear in mind in making judgements about the appropriateness of particular interventions? How might they go about investigating these factors?

4   What other stakeholders should be considered in carrying out research in applied psychology and how might they be involved?

SUGGESTIONS FOR FURTHER READING

Clegg, J. (1998) *Critical Issues in Clinical Practice*. London: Sage. A critical examination of different approaches to thinking about theory, research and practice. Written by a clinical psychologist but easily applicable to other areas of applied psychology.

David, T. (ed.) (2001) *Promoting Evidence-based Practice in Early Childhood Education: Research and its Implications, Volume 1*. Greenwich, CT: JAI Press. A good overview of current research in this area.

Marks, D.F., Murray, M.P., Evans, B. and Estacio, E.V. (2011) *Health Psychology: Theory, Research and Practice* (3rd edn). London: Sage. An introductory-level text to health psychology but with good discussions of epistemology, evidence-based practice and critical approaches.

Roth, A. and Fonagy, P. (2006) *What Works for Whom? A Critical Review of Psychotherapy Research* (2nd revised edn). London: Guilford Press. A thorough overview of psychotherapy research but also includes a sophisticated model outlining how practitioners might draw on evidence in exercising their professional judgement – written by two clinical psychologists but, again, applicable to other areas.

Sackett, D.L., Richardson, W.S., Rosenberg, W. and Haynes, R.B. (1997) *Evidence-Based Medicine: How to Practice and Teach EBM*. London: Churchill Livingstone. The classic text on evidence-based medicine. Written very much from a medical perspective but has lots that will be of interest to any clinician, such as information about NNT.

Schön, D.A. (1987) *Educating the Reflective Practitioner*. San Francisco: Jossey Bass. A good introduction to the reflective-practitioner model.

Web resources

A useful website on evidence-based practice can be found at: http://www.medicine.ox.ac.uk/bandolier/

PART TWO

Training and Practice

4

CLINICAL PSYCHOLOGY

Maria Castro, Christopher Whiteley and Mary Boyle

This chapter discusses:

- the structure and content of clinical psychology training;

- examples of the main settings in which clinical psychologists work and types of work they do;

- some of the major current issues relevant to training and practice, including challenges arising out of changes to the NHS and key contributions of clinical psychology to national health and social priorities;

- the context of recent government policies, such as NICE guidelines, New Ways of Working for Applied Psychologists, and the Improving Access to Psychological Therapies initiative;

- changes in statutory registration;

- models for training and the relationship between the personal and professional;

- uncertainty for training programmes at times of financial and political upheaval.

INTRODUCTION

What is clinical psychology?

There is still often confusion about the roles of clinical psychologists and other health professionals such as psychiatrists, counselling psychologists (see Chapter 12), and counsellors and psychotherapists (see Chapter 15), despite attempts to answer this question for the past two decades (Management Advisory Service (MAS), 1989; *The Psychologist*, October 1989). This may be due to the diversity of each role, posing difficulty in communicating succinctly its key elements. Furthermore, the British Psychological Society (BPS) Division of Clinical Psychology (DCP) estimates that there are just over 9500 clinical psychologists currently practising in the UK (some outside the NHS or working part time), the relatively small size of the profession also plays a part in the lack of a clear external profile. Nonetheless, in comparison with other health professionals, clinical psychology has done little to promote itself and enhance understanding among members of the public and colleagues alike.

The most stereotyped perception of a clinical psychologist is in a psychotherapy role with individual clients in an outpatient setting, where clients attend appointments for an hour a week over a period of time. Indeed, the *Core Purpose and Philosophy of the Profession* (BPS/DCP, 2010a: 2–3) defines the purpose and aims of the profession as:

> to reduce psychological distress and to enhance and promote psychological well-being by the systematic application of knowledge derived from psychological theory and data.

and

> to enable individual service users and carers to have the necessary skills and abilities to cope with their emotional needs and daily lives ... to make informed choices in order to enhance and maximise independence and autonomy; to have a sense of self-understanding, self-respect and self-worth; to be able to enjoy good social and personal relationships; and to share commonly valued social and environmental facilities.

Although many clinical psychologists would not disagree with these statements, they certainly do not capture the variety and breadth of what they do, such as working more exclusively with physical health problems, at the level of organisations and service planning, and focused on community or preventative work. Another complex factor is the idea that clinical psychology promotes well-being by 'the systematic application of knowledge derived from psychological theory and data', which may be desirable but is not without its problems, as we discuss in the section on training. Crucially, the *Core Purpose and Philosophy*, with its strong emphasis on the autonomous individual, can also be seen as de-emphasising the relational nature of people's lives (and problems) and the necessity of changing environments and contexts in order to reduce distress. Indeed, implicit in the language used is a particular epistemology, as exemplified by the constructs of 'sense of self', 'self-respect' and 'self-worth'. Additionally, the work of clinical psychologists is also relational and contextual, as clinical psychologists rarely work in isolation – at the very least relating to particular theoretical approaches. Thus, describing how the DCP statements translate into professional practice is further complicated by the wide diversity of models, settings and groups with which clinical psychologists work. Nevertheless, the importance of these statements lies in their move away from a medical language of diagnosing and treating illness or psychopathology, highlighting the necessity of integration between theory, research and practice.

In the late 1980s, the NHS/Department of Health commissioned a review tackling questions such as: 'What is clinical psychology?' and 'What do clinical psychologists do that others cannot?' (MAS, 1989). This concluded that clinical psychology operated on three levels (see Box 4.1); while Levels 1 and 2 were shared with other health professionals, only psychologists routinely operated at Level 3, which is to 'Formulate and respond to complex problems in terms of broadly based psychological knowledge'. Perhaps a sign of the quality of this piece of research is that it continues to be a relevant conceptualisation today; subsequent publications on the part of the profession have not so much sought to change the basic ideas from the report but, rather, elaborate on organisational and leadership roles for clinical psychologists (see New Ways of Working in Mental Health, 2007) and to address issues of access to psychologically based interventions (see *Good Practice Guide on the Contribution of Applied Psychologists to Improving Access for Psychological Therapies*, BPS, Care Services Improvement Partnership (CSIP) and National Institute for Mental Health in England, 2007).

Box 4.1   Levels of psychological skill derived from job analysis

Level 1: Skills in establishing and maintaining relationships; simple and often intuitive techniques of counselling and stress management.

Level 2: Undertaking circumscribed psychological activities (e.g. behaviour modification) – may be defined by protocol.

Level 3: Thorough understanding of varied and complex psychological theories and the ability to apply these to new problems to generate interventions.

Source: Management Advisory Service (1989)

The unique contribution of clinical psychology

The rather abstract statement of 'Level 3' activities could be thought of in terms of a process with four elements: *assessment, formulation, intervention* and *evaluation*. Without making the gross oversimplification to suggest that the process of trying to understand individuals', groups' (such as organisations) or communities' problems and engaging with the people who 'bring' these to enhance their well-being can be divided artificially into 'tasks' (which are neither discrete nor consecutive), the brief description of these aspects in Table 4.1 can help convey how these elements may be used to capture some of the complexity of people's lives and predicaments.

Clinical psychologists approach this process drawing on their in-depth knowledge of psychological theories, with a judgement-free interest and respect for the knowledge people have about themselves and their predicaments. Clinical psychologists

Table 4.1   Brief description of clinical psychologists' Level 3 skills

Assessment	Depending on theoretical orientation, *assessment* involves collecting information about the specific problem/s or exceptions to the problem (i.e. areas the problem has not entered), immediate and wider context, as well as some ideas about desired changes, goals, hopes or preferred ways of living. This may involve interviews, self-monitoring, observation, psychometric tests and questionnaires. It is crucial to side with and reach a full description from the person/s who bring the problem and, often, other significant people around them (e.g. relatives, partners or carers), since people who complain of 'anxiety' or 'depression' are using culturally available language to convey what may be very varied forms of distress with very different meanings for them. The *assessment* may also aim to clarify the circumstances at onset of the problem, its present occurrence and impact on the life of the person/s and those around; alternatively, it may focus on describing life before or outside of the problem.
Formulation	The *formulation* brings into relation information gathered during the assessment, using relevant psychological theory, to have working hypotheses or shared understandings about the factors contributing to and maintaining problems and/or exceptions to problems. To give an individual example, from what could be called a 'problem-centred' hypothesis, it may be that a person's auditory hallucinations are an understandable response to past sexual abuse, that the negative content of the voices relates to the person's thoughts about him or herself following abuse, and the voices are more likely to happen in situations where negative thoughts about the self are activated. A 'person-centred' hypothesis would focus on the person's ability to hold onto goals for their life, in the face of hallucinations and traumatic life events (e.g. past sexual abuse, forced admissions to hospital), because of resilience or determination, which can be tracked back through time and across relationships and are likely to continue to serve the person well in the future if made explicit and enriched.
Intervention	These hypotheses guide the *intervention* or may be *interventions* in themselves, aimed at reaching the person's stated aspirations. Therapeutic interventions are intended to move towards collaboratively developed goals. Depending on the psychological model guiding the intervention, the therapist/therapist's ideas or the person's own knowledge and skills will be more at the centre of the therapy. Interventions may be direct (with individuals, couples, families, communities or organisations) or indirect (e.g. working with care home staff when a person in their care has been referred due to problems such as aggression or, more broadly, influencing the home's practices and policies).
Evaluation	Another part of this process, which can be a final stage or an ongoing parallel element, is *evaluation*: a more or less systematic attempt to assess whether or how the desired changes have been achieved – the understanding being that this is a result of the process; but, clearly, life is complex and other aspects may come into play, beneficially or not. Clinical psychologists may employ the therapeutic conversation, self-monitoring or self-rating with a simple ten-point Likert scale, observation, psychometric tests or questionnaires in this part of the process.

have to remain open and curiously engaged with the person/s seeking help in this process since, as stated above, we consider that these elements are not linear: further important information available later is incorporated (*re-formulation*), as the utility of initial thinking is continually tested out (*evaluation*); similarly, questions aimed at gathering information during initial conversations (*assessment*) may be equally promoting of change (*intervention*).

These kinds of understandings and engagements are very different from those traditionally encountered in mental health settings – compare the very brief formulations of auditory hallucinations in Table 4.1 with the claim that these are a symptom of schizophrenia. Within this general framework, the nature of the work done by individual clinical psychologists is likely to be influenced by three broad factors: setting, client group and theoretical orientation.

The majority of clinical psychologists work in the NHS, including primary care, community multidisciplinary teams, general hospitals, specialist hospitals and clinics; others work with communities, in social services, prisons, charitable or private sectors. In addition to working directly with people across the lifespan and range of ability, clinical psychologists also undertake indirect work with staff, relatives and/or carers, and utilise their knowledge to bring a psychological perspective to service planning and policy development, consultation and supervision to colleagues, teaching and training, research and audit. Finally, clinical psychologists may adopt a particular theoretical model, or integration of models, which will influence the type of service offered. For example, those who adopt a cognitive–behavioural model will tend to work on a one-to-one or possibly group basis, whereas for those who use a systemic model, much of the work will be with families or organisations.

The diverse ways of working to achieve the core purpose of the profession is a substantial part of the attraction to training and working as a clinical psychologist. Table 4.2 provides some examples of the kinds of work carried out by clinical psychologists in various settings; some of the work would be done in collaboration with other professionals, but the illustrations are typical of those presenting to clinical psychologists.

CURRENT ISSUES AND THE FUTURE OF CLINICAL PSYCHOLOGY

Is clinical psychology acceptable to the diverse population it serves?

To date, despite a proportion of psychology undergraduates from minority ethnic groups similar to national demographics, clinical psychology is not demographically representative of the population it serves. Moreover, psychology has traditionally neglected the role in the development and maintenance of distress of those very experiences of disadvantage and disempowerment that people so often bring to consultations. Therefore, clinical psychology has never fully represented those to whom it aims to provide services and this has become much more apparent for three reasons. First, developments in the human sciences have both highlighted psychology's androcentric and Eurocentric traditions, and provided analytical tools for examining the implications of this and for constructing alternatives. Second, the UK population has become more diverse (particularly because of immigration and asylum seeking), and 'race' has been constructed as a primary marker, so that the differences between clinical psychologists and the people they work with are increasingly difficult to overlook. Third, social changes have increased the visibility and recognition of entitlement of

Table 4.2 Some examples of the day-to-day activities of clinical psychologists in various specialities

Child and family	Adults	Primary care	Learning disabilities	Older adults	Forensic
Design and facilitate a group for children who have lived through difficult parental divorce and separation	Assessment and intervention with a man who is threatened with loss of his job because of poor time-keeping due to prolonged checking rituals at home	Supervise a research project on the training needs of general practitioners (GPs) on screening for domestic violence, particularly looking at why they find it difficult to ask screening questions in consultations with patients	Devise and run a training course for people with learning disabilities working for an advocacy organisation involved in quality monitoring of services	Work with man and family where he has been given the label of Alzheimer's disease, to devise strategies to minimise impact of memory problems on day-to-day functioning	Assessment with a 19-year-old man from Bosnia on remand in a young offender institution, where staff report daily attempts to hang himself; potential admission to medium secure unit
Cognitive assessment of a girl who has been referred for school avoidance and who may have a specific learning disability	Teaching session to staff from accident-and-emergency departments on psychological analysis of self-harm and implications for clinical practice	Make a presentation to European visitors on psychologists' involvement with primary care services	Carry out assessment and intervention with a man with mild learning disabilities who is afraid to go out, following an attack	As part of a referral asking whether psychological intervention could be an alternative to electroconvulsive therapy, provide an assessment of a 75-year-old, recently bereaved woman who is refusing food	Weekly consultation session to probation staff, on risk assessment and risk management for people with psychological problems
Work with a boy and family where a diagnosis of attention-deficit hyperactivity disorder has been suggested	Assessment of suicide risk of a woman with long-standing intrusive thoughts of suicide, and who hears voices telling her to kill herself	Devise and deliver a training and education course for health visitors on supporting new parents when there are postnatal difficulties	Undertake an assessment of a woman with moderate learning disabilities who reports sexual abuse by male staff, as part of official investigations	Devise and deliver a training programme to staff on a unit for people with dementia aimed at helping them assess possible meanings and functions of residents' behaviour that staff find difficult to manage (so-called 'challenging behaviour')	Assessment of motivation to engage in psychological therapy for a man with long-standing sexual offending against women, to be presented at his Mental Health Act review tribunal hearing

Table 4.2 (Continued)

Child and family	Adults	Primary care	Learning disabilities	Older adults	Forensic
Teaching sessions on the development of sexuality and sexual identity for staff of the local adolescent inpatient unit	Participate in a support group for staff in a unit for people with a diagnosis of borderline personality disorder	Provide weekly clinic at GP surgery, including, e.g. assessment and intervention for a man referred for 'depression' and who is very ambivalent about seeing a psychologist	Work with the family of an adolescent boy with mild learning disabilities who is reported to be increasingly aggressive	Work with older people in local day centres to think with them how they maintain mental well-being and how they build on their resources to deal with any difficulties	Assessment and intervention with a woman with a history of serious interpersonal violence who has beliefs that agents from the Vatican wish to harm her
Form part of the team for a regular family therapy clinic	Assessment and intervention with a woman with a severe fear of driving	Meet with senior health visitors to discuss request to set up a support group for newly qualified health visitors	Carry out assessment of organisational and other aspects of hostel accommodation for six adults where there are a high number of reports of so-called 'challenging behaviour'	Help develop policy guidelines to ensure the inclusion of older people in decisions about their care needs	Family work with a man, father and sister in preparation for his moving from a medium secure ward to a community hostel, the main theme being relapse prevention
Intervention with a toddler and mother using behavioural management because the girl has severe 'tantrums'	Supervision of research project on effectiveness of referral practices in multidisciplinary team	Provide management supervision to counselling psychologists, including appraisal and planning of continuing professional development	Devise an education and support programme for a pregnant woman with moderate learning disabilities	Couple work where the man reports sexual problems following recent coronary by-pass surgery	Work with ward staff in designing and implementing a graded programme for a man who feels too anxious to come out of his room on the ward
Provide group supervision for a team of community psychiatric nurses working in a child and adolescent mental health service	Long-term intervention with a woman who was sexually abused as a child, has recurrent suicidal thoughts and who self-harms	Evaluate local population needs, such as those of a minority ethnic group and in consultation with them, help plan and deliver a service that they will feel able and willing to access to meet their needs	Run workshops for care staff on the provision of sex education to people with learning disabilities	Form part of a joint NHS and social services steering group to develop a new service for people with severe memory problems	Risk assessment with a man previously convicted of sexually abusing his step-child, requested by the local authority to contribute to discussions of his request to be allowed to live with his new partner and their young child

groups such as gay men, lesbians and people with disabilities, who are not willing to occupy the marginal social status previously assigned to them. Although there has been much discussion about clinical psychology becoming more representative, with an assumption that this would lead to increased service 'accessibility', a more persuasive argument would propose that examining the biases and assumptions of the theories the profession draws on, and the practices these lead to, is a better way to ensure 'acceptability' to the wide diversity of the population. Indeed, diversity in the workforce should not be assumed to automatically lead to, or be a substitute for, universal competence in working with people from diverse backgrounds. This has particular relevance in the NHS, where there is little or no choice or selection in assigning clinical psychologist and client. Furthermore, what would an appropriately diverse profession look like, given the potentially vast array of difference that might be considered: gender, age, sexuality, physical ability, ethnicity, class, faith and so on? It is not just a question of recruitment into the profession; the fact that women are over-represented within psychology has not changed its androcentricity. In order not to run the risk of colonising people's experiences with concepts and understandings dominant in clinical psychology today, changes are called for from its core in terms of the theory–practice taught in training programmes and promoted within services and wider contexts.

Clinical psychology in relation to current NHS developments

Arguably, the most substantive recent change to the field of psychological therapies has been the rapid expansion of services focused on providing 'evidence-based' interventions for 'common mental health problems'. These are known as IAPT services, after the strategic programme 'Improving Access to Psychological Therapies' (MHChoice, 2007). This initiative adopts a stepped-care model for service delivery, providing psychological interventions for a range of psychological difficulties with an accompanying growth in workforce; seeing the arrival of almost entirely new groups of practitioners – high-intensity psychological therapists and psychological well-being practitioners – in a structure interestingly reflecting elements of the MAS (1989) review referred to earlier. This nationally driven development has necessitated a shift in the roles of many clinical psychologists and to some extent added to further refinements to the role of clinical psychologists, for example, *The Clinical Psychology Leadership Development Framework* (BPS/DCP, 2010b).

Although clinical psychologists have made a central contribution to the programme, both at a national strategic level and in local service leadership, they have also levelled criticism at the initiative, particularly for its narrow focus on symptom reduction within diagnostic categories and the dominance of CBT models of psychological interventions. Furthermore, as stated above, it is not simply a matter of expanding or offering services in a wider variety of settings, i.e. attending to accessibility, but of more fundamentally examining the nature of these services and the theories that inform them, i.e. focusing on acceptability (a point we shall return to in the section on training). In this way, we can hope to avoid the traps of continuing to locate 'difference' in people seeking help, rather than in relationships or contexts, and of replicating in services the experiences of disadvantage and injustice that may have contributed to people's problems in the first place.

Statutory registration

The BPS's goal for the profession to be subject to statutory registration (i.e. registration as a legal requirement to practise) has only recently been achieved. This is a major shift for qualified clinical psychologists, who since 2009 are required to register with the Health Professionals Council (HPC) under the umbrella term of applied psychologists. Statutory registration has achieved some of the desired goals of the profession with regard to ensuring protection of the public, like preventing re-employment of a clinical psychologist in the NHS once removed from the register (it remains to be seen how far it will prevent the offering of private practice). Also prior to HPC registration, there was nothing to stop anyone offering their services under the 'clinical psychologist' title, whereas now this is a legally protected professional title, with the HPC setting the criteria for who can legitimately provide services under this title. However, with the introduction of HPC registration, requirements for continuing professional development (CPD) have changed, as have processes for the validation of training and qualifications, failing to secure the nature of statutory registration that many clinical and other applied psychologists aspired to; the UK Council for Psychotherapy has already challenged the HPC at the High Court for not meeting the required standards to regulate their members. Now the role of the BPS in regard to applied psychologists is in transition, with many calling for the organisation to establish its role, autonomy and utility.

Relationships with the public

In a recent paper, the author of the MAS review expressed his concern that this had been lost, as it had been 'a "big picture" review: it spoke to those who could see the wider landscape; [but] it was interpreted by those who couldn't or wouldn't' (Mowbray, 2010: 1). And, therefore, twenty years later clinical psychology is still defining its role and what it can offer. In recent years, the guidance published by NICE on the effectiveness of psychological interventions in a range of mental health problems – although heavily critiqued (see, for example, *NICE Under Scrutiny*, Guy et al., 2011) – has raised the status and potential visibility of psychology, publicly, professionally and politically. Arguably, the profession has made proactive attempts to contribute psychological theory, specifically, in areas where it had not been very visible (e.g. the publication and wide dissemination of the report *Recent Advances in Understanding Mental Illness and Psychotic Experiences,* BPS/DCP, 2000). Nevertheless, there remains a need for much wider engagement with the public on topics such as conceptualising and responding to psychological distress, evaluating psychological interventions and ensuring the people who use services contribute to their design and implementation. The alternative to such debates may be a defensive oversimplification of the issues in an attempt to 'educate' the public, rather than real engagement reflecting the complexity of what we do and trying to convey assertively how it is different from what is offered by others.

The political context

The intentions of the coalition government with regard to the future of the NHS as a whole, as well as mental health services in particular, are stated in the *White Paper: Equity and Excellence – Liberating the NHS* (Department of Health, 2010), and were finalised in legislation passed by Parliament in March 2012. With the legislation only recently passed, the specific implications of the major changes to the NHS are uncertain. Attention has focused around key strategic initiatives, such as commissioning led by groups of GP practices, and debates around the provision of services by private and charitable organisations. Concerns about the quality and effectiveness of services, including psychological services, have focused on the statement within the white paper 'any willing provider', raising concern about the competence of any such providers and quality of services.

As we see in the next section, training places have been increasing year on year in response to the growing demand for clinical psychologists; however, the current financial and political climate has led to a nationwide reduction in places for 2011–2012. The resulting growth in the profession presents opportunities for using our skills in creative and innovative ways within new and existing services, for example with the expanding role for 'talking therapies', although these are not the exclusive remit of clinical psychology. Some proposals have given rise to concerns, for example the delivery of 'manualised treatments' by 'graduate therapists' and attempts to restrict interventions to those favoured by a traditional view of evidence, focusing on economically driven outcomes (see Chapter 19 in this volume). The challenges are to influence the shape and delivery of these proposals and to respond to them in a way that maintains an effective and supportive role that attracts new recruits, while providing services that meet the needs and expectations of the population in a rapidly changing society.

TRAINING

The present structure of UK clinical psychology training programmes (see Box 4.2) only came about in the mid-1990s. Previously courses lasted two or three years and were based in universities or the NHS (in-service training). University courses offered a master's degree whereas those based in the NHS were examined by the BPS and offered a Diploma in Applied Psychology, marking a researcher/practitioner split; university courses focused more on academic and research aspects of clinical psychology and in-service training more on practice (see Pilgrim and Treacher, 1992). By the early 1990s, accreditation standards by the BPS Committee on Training in Clinical Psychology, with the requirement that courses provide three years' full-time training for their graduates to be eligible for registration as chartered psychologists, encouraged a homogeneous structure. Some academics (e.g. Carr, 1990) questioned whether a master's degree was the appropriate award for three years of full-time postgraduate study and, by the end of the decade, all courses were of three years' duration and awarded a doctoral degree.

Box 4.2   The structure of clinical psychology training

- Course level: Postgraduate (requires first degree in psychology giving the Graduate Basis for Registration).

- Duration: Three calendar years full time.

- Base: University or affiliated to/validated by university.

- Award: Professional Doctorate (Clin Psy D/DClin Psy).

- Elements: Academic teaching (20%); supervised practice (50%), as registered students become NHS employees of 'host' trust designated by confederation; small-scale service-related and thesis-related research and private study (30%).

The aims of training

At the most general level, programmes aim to provide trainees with systematic opportunities, in teaching and placements, to utilise psychological knowledge in practice so as to be able to gather information, conceptualise, map and implement *interventions* with people presenting a wide range of problems in the various settings in which clinical psychologists work. One major task for programmes is to emphasise enough how the theories taught translate into practice and for supervisors to explicitly articulate the theories driving their practice, since trainees can face problems in matching academic teaching to the real-world problems they are trying to solve (e.g. Jones, 1998). The perceived lack of fit can be partly due to the traditional theory–practice divide, as both are part of the same process or *praxis* (see Freire, 1970). This apparently innocuous divide allows a systematic detachment from the 'real world', hence, narrowness of psychological theory. It gives little prominence to factors that have profound effects on people's lives and well-being such as gender, class, ethnicity, economics and power, while insisting that human behaviour and experience can largely be accounted for through the operation of intra-psychic attributes (e.g. cognitions) and that change can be effected through the manipulation of these attributes. Further, the traditional reliance on psychiatric categories, despite their lack of scientific validity, to conceptualise people's distress and 'abnormal' behaviour (like quantification), overlooks or de-emphasises many aspects of people's lives and relationships relevant to their problems (e.g. Boyle, 1999; Johnstone, 2001; Kutchins and Kirk, 1997). As a result, theories are difficult to match with people's accounts of their relationships or lived experience; and possibly attempts to change people via their intra-psychic attributes founder on those very 'realities' of life about which psychology has said little (Fox et al., 2009; Smail, 2005; Ussher and Nicolson, 1992). Another factor is the narrowness of psychological methods: the long-established limitation of psychological research relying on quantification and statistical inference from group data. Danzinger (1985) called this psychology's 'methodological imperative'; when method is primary in psychology, theory has had to be restricted to that which fits the method – i.e. people have to be conceptualised and outcomes defined in ways that allow measurement. Clearly, there is a mismatch between reliance on quantification, which limits or predetermines what a person can 'say', and clinical practice, which relies on encouraging people to speak freely to give an account of their problems in their own way.

Crucially, programmes also aim to teach trainees how to critically evaluate – reflection is inherent in praxis – their knowledge and practice, including the ethical issues raised by them, and how to communicate their ideas and practice to clients, carers and other professionals, both verbally and in writing. Finally, programmes aim to build on research skills gained on undergraduate courses and, particularly, to facilitate trainees' devising and carrying out research in applied settings.

Selection for training

Due to NHS demand for clinical psychologists over the last few years, a vigorous programme of expansion led to an increasing number of training places, creating five new programmes in England and Wales since 1996. Nevertheless, as seen in Table 4.3, the number of applicants far exceeds the number of places and around 75% of applicants have been rejected in any given year. As has been noted (Papworth, 2004, 2007), many good-quality applicants are not offered a place, raising the suspicion that entry criteria are arbitrary or perversely difficult to achieve, and programme staff are well used to receiving calls from prospective applicants asking: 'If I do [this or that], then will I get a place?'

The answer, however, is complex and has more to do with what is learnt from experience than with simply 'getting' the experience. From their shortlisting and

Table 4.3   Training numbers 2005–2010

Year	Number of places	Number of applicants	Ratio applicants/places
2005	588	2125	1:3.6
2006	554	2442	1:4.4
2007	582	2346	1:4
2008	592	2323	1:3.9
2009	623	2342	1:3.7
2010	617	2969	1:4.8

2011: 29 training programmes in clearing house (30 planned for 2012).

Source: Clearing House for Postgraduate Courses in Clinical Psychology.

selection study, Phillips et al. (2004) concluded that degree class, vocational experience and having a clinical referee predicted selection by 78.3%, although programmes might differ in the relative emphasis placed on particular characteristics (like commitment, knowledge of clinical psychology and the NHS) and personal qualities (such as confidence, reflectiveness, empathy and sensitivity). Programmes involve programme staff and NHS psychologists in a variety of selection procedures conducted over several phases. Most programmes specify their criteria: at least two people will independently rate applications, and individual interviews (often more than one) are relied upon in the final selection; some programmes use group interviews, group tasks, oral presentations or written tasks (e.g. clinical vignettes).

Clinical psychology is numerically dominated by white females – this is much less so at higher levels (e.g. the majority of programme directors are male) – but it is worth noting that undergraduate psychology students are also predominantly white females. Although there is no evidence of direct discrimination in selection, the weight of educational attainment and relevant experience raises a concern about indirect discrimination or, at least, about factors that might discourage applications from more varied demographic groups or make them less likely to be selected. For example, in relation to ethnicity, Boyle et al. (1993) found that applicants to the University of East London (UEL) programme from minority ethnic groups were significantly less likely to have had previous experience as an assistant psychologist. Although it is not a selection requirement, this job is the most likely to provide the kind of experience and knowledge to allow people to present themselves well to selectors. Similarly, the demands of travelling to placements with varied standards of access and facilities might discourage applicants with disabilities, while the tendency of mental health professionals to view their clients as 'other' (Sampson, 1993), and their reluctance to discuss their own experience of psychological problems, can discourage applicants who have experienced mental health problems. Programmes, however, have to take account of the Disability Discrimination Act, and the Special Educational Needs and Disability Act, and there have been wide-ranging discussions of their implications for clinical psychology training.

There are also concerns regarding the validity of short-listing and selection procedures due to a number of factors, which may not be demonstrably related to job performance, even if clearly specified and reliably assessed (e.g. Hatton et al., 2000; Simpson et al., 2010). To address some of these concerns, the Group of Trainers in Clinical Psychology commissioned research to explore the possible benefits of creating a nationwide screening system; recommendations follow a 'competency model' for the development and piloting of such a system (see Baron, 2011). It is not clear how the project will be taken forward now and there is still paucity of research to inform the fine selection that programmes have to make among individuals. There is also a key question regarding whether statements of competencies should rely on judgements from those who do the job, rather than including judgements from those with whom the job is done, i.e. people who use clinical psychology services.

MODELS OF TRAINING

Clearly, it is important that we regularly examine what we are trying to achieve in training clinical psychologists. The popularity of the language of knowledge and skills[1], competencies and training[2] can create the impression that the role of programmes is to teach a discrete set of actions whose implementation will have predictable outcomes, also assuming that these actions are dictated by an established body of knowledge. This is explicit in the core purpose and philosophy of the profession, by which trainees are expected to be committed to decreasing psychological distress and promoting psychological well-being *'through the systematic application of knowledge derived from psychological theory and data'* (BPS/DCP, 2010a: 2, emphasis added). The 'competency model' fits with more general attempts to set occupational standards for 'vocational' education and training (BPS, 1998). Additionally, the large increase in training places (with consequent pressure on placements and supervisors) and organisational changes have disrupted the traditional division of placements into discrete core areas such as adult, child, learning disabilities and older adults. This makes planning training in the traditional way – which emphasised specific experiences to be gained in specific settings rather than learning from those experiences (i.e. competencies) – difficult. Organisational developments have provided the opportunity to plan training much more flexibly, as well as creating the demand that we look more fundamentally and explicitly at what it is that training is trying to achieve, and how these goals might be met through a variety of placement routes.

Similarly, learning outcomes of training programmes include the acquisition of 'knowledge required to underpin clinical research and practice' (BPS/Committee on Training in Clinical Psychology, 2001: 10), involving the adoption of what has become known as the 'scientist-practitioner model' (further discussed in Chapter 3). The implications of the model for training seem straightforward: the task for programmes is to provide trainees with the scientific knowledge base that will, in effect, tell them what to do; provide them with guided opportunities to apply this knowledge; and provide research training to enable trainees to carry out research and interpret the research of others to inform their future practice. Although these aims may seem appropriate, in practice they appear to be unrealised. First, the large majority of clinical psychologists do not carry out research, although there is some disagreement over how 'research' should be defined in this context (Agnew et al., 1995; Milne et al., 1990). Second, and a more serious issue, clinical practice appears not to have been strongly informed by research (Barkham and Mellor-Clark, 2003; Long and Hollin, 1997). For trainees, this situation can present itself as a lack of 'fit' between what is expected of them academically and in practice. Indeed, Schön (1987) strongly criticised the scientist-practitioner

---

[1]Promoted by the Knowledge and Skills Framework (NHS KSF) (Department of Health, 2004).

[2]It is interesting to note that the official NHS language for what courses do is 'education and training' but that the term 'education' almost never appears in course (or wider professional) literature.

model for presenting human problems as technical problems capable of technical solutions, and training as the process of instilling the required technical knowledge. In solving problems, experienced practitioners engage in complex thinking at many levels, they draw on research but also on knowledge from previous, similar work, together with subjective impressions about relationships and context and people's own skills and knowledges. Schön's 'reflective-practitioner' model attempts to guide the articulation and transmission of the qualities of the 'expert' practitioner, and the development in trainees and teachers of the ability to reflect on the processes of learning and practice (see also Chapter 3). This model provides a valuable counter to the idea of practitioners as transmitters of technical knowledge and of training as the process of learning 'what to do'. It does, however, require 'the addition of discipline specific knowledge to be combined with the reflective practitioner's artistry in action' (Clegg, 1998: 9), if the model is not to slide into personalised and unaccountable reflection with no criteria for choosing between one sort of perceived expertise and another.

Based on a major curriculum review, the UEL programme team is recommending to its stakeholders a 'levels-of-intervention model', with year modules arranged according to increasing complexity in roles and opportunities for psychological intervention, health promotion and prevention – (1) individuals and relationships, families and groups; (2) organisations and communities; (3) leadership, social policy and research. Teaching modules would include sessions on the approaches and skills that are typically associated with each of these areas (e.g. group-dynamic and systemic approaches with small groups or organisational development), and skills would be assessed using approach-appropriate methods. Training would address the broad range of health determinants (individual, systems, social) at all levels, as well as orienting trainees to work in service planning, design and delivery, and in health promotion/prevention, by influencing local, national and international policies. The approach does not fit with current trends towards clinical psychology as a 'psychotherapy' profession (dominated by the CBT model), and thus will be unattractive to applicants who wish to become individual psychotherapists, and the services who might recruit them. However, it fits well with much of the existing curriculum and makes more explicit how and where complexity in clinical work – and trainee knowledge and skills – develop over the three years of training. Importantly, by explicitly addressing the 'higher' levels of intervention (service provision, social determinants, health policy) the structure directly connects with, and builds upon, the programme's orienting principles, ethos and critical stance. Further, this approach reintegrates some increasingly marginalised clinical psychology activities, including promotion/prevention, policy development and work in the wide range of (non-psychiatric) health settings and agencies.

Personal and professional development and support systems in training

It is acknowledged that clinical psychology training makes significant personal, practical and material demands on trainees (Cushway, 1992; Scaife, 1995), for example extensive travel to placements, moving placements every six months, time management and meeting multiple assessment deadlines with limited study time. Another source of demand on trainees stems from the nature of clinical psychologists' work. Nichols et al. (1992: 29) note that psychological therapy involves 'continual exposure to the distress, frustration, defeat and heightened emotional functioning of others', together with the need to empathise with the perceptions and feelings of another person *and* reduce his or her distress; thus, carrying out psychological therapy can be seen as a source of continual exposure to low-key stressors. Although there is a limit to how far such demands can be reduced, programmes' organisational and feedback systems can help ensure that these are reviewed often and kept to a realistic level.

Clinical psychology, however, does not have a strong history of recognising the impact of such challenges and providing support to its practitioners. Historically, the reluctance to reveal what might be seen as personal vulnerabilities; the desire to convey to colleagues and employers an image of strength and productivity; and fear of becoming or being seen as a client (linked to our earlier remarks about clinical psychologists constructing their clients as 'other') have hindered the development of adequate peer support systems (Walsh and Cormack, 1994). If these are obstacles for qualified practitioners, they are more so for trainees who may see themselves as risking their qualification by revealing what they fear might be seen as ignorance or weakness. Consequently, 'support' has often implicitly been seen in terms of pathology or crisis management. Walsh and Scaife (1998) argued instead for systems of 'personal and professional development' (PPD) within training programmes, moving away from a focus on trainees' internal psychological needs towards a culture that acknowledges PPD as an ongoing process of learning. These systems would include teaching and PPD group sessions encouraging reflection on the process of training and its emotional implications, covering topics such as stress and time management, dealing with violence in the workplace and using supervision. Personal mentors or advisers (without an assessment role) would be available to trainees, providing additional space for discussion of issues such as the impact of values, expectations and life experiences on practice, and vice versa. Most programmes now have at least some of these elements in place, suggesting a recognition of the need for inbuilt support and of the ways in which the relationship between the personal and the professional can be constructively reflected on and used during training.

A third source of demand on trainees, much less often examined, is psychology's narrow theoretical and methodological base, discussed earlier, which has limited our potential for understanding and alleviating distress. When we add to this the lack of discussion of this issue in mainstream literature, together with the relatively uncritical promotion of 'evidence-based practice' (rather than practice-based evidence) and the scientist-practitioner model, it is almost inevitable that trainees will feel inadequate (and fear their inadequacies will be discovered) if they are not able to do what they are supposed to – e.g. apply psychological knowledge to alleviate a person's problem. As Rudkin (2000: 48) – writing as a trainee – has put it, trainees often have the fantasy that 'graduating from clinical training, we shall be presented with an envelope inside of which The Secret will be written, and for ever more we shall be sure we are doing the right thing'. Personal and professional development programmes are not systematically designed to include discussion of these issues, and their emphasis on the 'personal' (as in psychology itself) could divert attention from the social contexts that shape clinical psychological praxis. We would argue that PPD programmes need to exist alongside curricula with the features we mentioned earlier, including teaching that acknowledges the role of social and environmental factors in psychological distress and psychological well-being, and provides a conceptual framework for critically examining psychology's own theory–practice.

CONCLUSION

The future of clinical psychology training is inevitably affected by the current climate of economic uncertainty, with its implications for future NHS funding of training places (which have already seen a reduction for the 2011 intake), local decisions to open training to paying overseas students, together with cutbacks in higher education institutions, in which training programmes sit, and cutbacks in psychological services, presents new challenges and, indeed, ethical dilemmas, for training programmes (see Winter et al., 2011). Increasingly complex and demanding organisational contexts demand we develop appropriate curricula and teaching methods, critically appraising – and attempting to influence – directives from the government on health care structures and priorities, so that trainees are prepared for their future roles and responsibilities (while meeting the requirements of educational stakeholders responsible for funding, validation and accreditation).

These concerns have a number of implications for training. First, programmes need to provide a broad-based academic curriculum, distancing itself from a reliance on psychiatric diagnosis and taking full account of the social and environmental factors repeatedly shown to be associated with psychological distress. This teaching, however, can also show how traditional theories, which do not explicitly acknowledge factors such as power or social inequality, can still be very relevant – Seligman's (1972) learned helplessness theory of depression is a good example. Second, teaching on research should include both quantitative and qualitative methods within the context of their epistemological assumptions – not uncommonly, qualitative methods are taught in this way, with quantitative methods still presented as a taken-for-granted way of developing psychological theory. Third, programmes should provide a structure for trainees to reflect on their learning and experience as practitioners. Finally, programmes should provide trainees with the conceptual means to analyse psychology and clinical psychology as 'enterprises'; in other words, with the means to turn their analytic gaze on their discipline and profession. Such analyses are now well developed within 'critical psychology' but do not yet form an integral part of most training programmes. Analysing oneself, so to speak, rather than one's clients can, of course, bring doubt and confusion as well as important insights (one UEL trainee described the process as 'like scuba diving – you discover a fascinating world you never knew existed'); it can also act as a counter to the doubt and confusion trainees feel at being unable to find the certainty they are sure must lie somewhere just beyond their reach, as well as encouraging the development of creative and innovative practice (Cheshire, 2000; Harper, 2004).

QUESTIONS FOR REFLECTION AND DISCUSSION

1   Clinical psychology has traditionally neglected issues of difference and oppression in its understandings of people's distress. What may have led to this and is this likely to change in the next twenty years?

2   Clinical psychology training has enjoyed NHS funding and positions of authority in contrast to allied psychologists and other health professionals. Why has this been the case and what might be the foreseeable changes given the current socioeconomic and political context?

3   Clinical psychology is becoming increasingly concerned with the relationship between the personal and the professional. Why might this be and how might this be reflected in theory–practice?

4   It has often been remarked that clinical psychology does not 'market' itself very well. Why might this be the case and what could be done about it?

SUGGESTIONS FOR FURTHER READING

Beinnart, H., Kennedy, P. and Llewelyn, S. (eds) (2009) *Clinical Psychology in Practice*. BPS Blackwell. This book covers what clinical psychologists do across the major settings, as well as wider professional roles, including supervision and leadership.

Bentall, R. (2003) *Madness Explained: Psychosis and Human Nature*. London: Penguin Books. Won the British Psychological Society Book Award 2004. Accessible to non-professionals, this book challenges predominant understandings of mental illness and proposes alternative thinking.

Johnstone, L. (2000) *Users and Abusers of Psychiatry*. London: Routledge. A critical analysis of psychiatric services (mainly those for adults) that also provides a clear account of how a social and psychological analysis of mental health problems differs from a psychiatric account, and what might be the implications for practice.

Martín-Baró, I. (1996) *Writings for a Liberation Psychology*. Cambridge, MA: Harvard University Press. This book presents a collection of the author's writings, which have been central to Latin American psychology and social theory but have been largely neglected in Western psychology.

Paré, A. and Larner, G. (2004) *Collaborative Practice in Psychology and Therapy*. London: Haworth Press. An excellent example of the application of postmodern psychology to research, theory, practice and supervision. The book provides a critical analysis of key issues (such as oppression, ethics and truth claims) to collaborative engagement with the problems people take to therapy.

Patel, N., Bennett, E., Dennis, M., Dosanjh, N., Mahtani, A., Miller, A. and Nadirshaw, Z. (2000) *Clinical Psychology, 'Race' and Culture: A Training Manual*. Leicester: BPS Books. Won first prize in the British Medical Association's 'Book of the Year' mental health category. This is a training manual in that it provides many resources for incorporating material on 'race' and culture into teaching, but it is also an excellent source of information on debates in these areas and their implications for practice.

5

EDUCATIONAL AND CHILD PSYCHOLOGY

Mark Fox

This chapter discusses:

- how educational and child psychologists are positioned by their training and employment to undertake a variety of roles in relationship to vulnerable children;

- an example of a 'day in the life' of an educational psychologist (EP);

- working with children and young people;

- who employs EPs;

- who EPs work for;

- the psychological theory that underpins EPs' work;

- how EPs are trained.

INTRODUCTION

'Educational psychologist' is one of the protected titles of the Health Professions Council (HPC), which means you cannot call yourself an educational psychologist unless you are registered with the HPC. In order to be registered as an EP you have to complete a three-year doctoral programme at one of the HPC-approved university courses that offer this training in the UK. The title that most of these universities give their courses is a Doctorate in Educational and Child Psychology.

So what is an educational and child psychologist? Is the focus on education, or on the child – or is the focus on the education of the child? If the focus is on education, is it on how the child learns or how the teacher teaches? If it is on both, why do EPs only receive referrals about children? Is the basis of the work psychological or educational? These two disciplines come from very different backgrounds and have very different understandings of their positions on the generation of knowledge. There is a dynamic tension between these three areas: education, the child and psychology and the position of EPs.

THE IMPORTANCE OF POSITIONING THEORY

In recent years the concept of 'positioning' has been championed as an alternative to focusing on the role of people (Harre et al., 2009). Instead of talking about the role of the EP as something static it is more helpful to think about how EPs position themselves and are positioned by others to act in particular ways within a continually developing, larger narrative (or story) about society. This larger narrative is among other things about the purpose of education, the funding of schools, the involvement of parents, and the emotional well-being of the nation's children. The narrative about the position of the EP is based upon the attributes that EPs claim to have and also those that others give them. Fundamentally it is the meaning that the EP takes, and is given by, the various activities they do. This chapter will outline the various activities that EPs carry out and the different meanings that are ascribed to these actions. Such activities include for example 'taking on a referral', 'offering a consultation service' and 'undertaking an assessment'. The positioning of EPs to undertake these activities takes place within a particular but larger social world. So changes in public policy on local authorities, the management of schools and the financial climate all impact on the position of the EP.

Educational psychologists' positioning takes place within a moral world – as does the positioning of the other applied psychologists and all professionals. Educational psychologists have clusters of moral and ethical beliefs about their rights and duties on particular contemporary issues. Positioning theory, however, suggests that such moral and ethical positioning is local and transitory in terms of the immediate social world and is interconnected with the positions that others take up. Because of this the moral right of any position can be challenged. It can be challenged by someone taking a different position. For example, EPs were originally often associated with using psychometric intelligence tests. This was positioned as the right thing to do with a cluster of ethical beliefs around promoting social mobility, by ensuring that children who were intelligent but who came from disadvantaged backgrounds would have improved educational opportunities. On the basis of such beliefs, selection (originally through the 11-plus) was enshrined into secondary education. Over time this view was challenged by many who saw intelligence tests in a negative way and the basis of labelling many children as failures at eleven. Intelligence tests were vociferously challenged by many ethnic minority groups who felt the tests were culturally biased, and EPs who used psychometric intelligence tests were positioned as being racist. Latterly this view was challenged by, among others, disability groups, who felt that psychometric assessments are a way of ensuring that the ability of children with severe physical disabilities are not overlooked.

Another illustration of moral positioning is EPs' views on inclusion. For many years EPs have largely championed inclusion in schools. This has been done for a number of reasons, including pragmatic ones such as improving educational attainments and the efficient use of resources. However, the main justification has been on moral grounds – that exclusion is a discriminatory practice and that all children have a right to be educated in their local school. The UK's Coalition Government's position is presently (2012) challenging this with another moral argument – that parents, not professionals, have the right to decide on the most beneficial education placement for their own children with special educational needs. So the moral justification for the position that EPs have taken up on inclusion has now been challenged by a competing moral argument. The positioning and repositioning of EPs in light of conflicting moral positions gradually unfolds over the years. However, it is important to understand that underpinning the position (or role) of the EP will be an explicit or implicit moral position.

Below is a description of a day's work – suitably changed to ensure anonymity. The EP takes up, and is given, a variety of positions during this day.

A DAY IN THE LIFE

The day starts at 8:30 with a drive to the EP Service's office. This is housed in a disused school in the middle of the local authority (LA). Often I will go direct to a school but today I go first to the office as I need to pick up a child file. The files are kept in a locked room. Despite the service now being amalgamated into a number of area teams each original service keeps its own files in its own filing system. So there are separate files for the autism service, the early year service and the educational psychology service. There is very little in the file – a Common Assessment Framework (CAF) referral for Lucy, a thirteen-year-old girl with severe physical difficulties, who has come from Spain. I have only a few minutes to read the files before I am due at the school – a twenty-minute drive away.

The school I am visiting is a large secondary school. Attached to the school is a unit for pupils with physical difficulties. My work this morning consists of undertaking an assessment in order to write the Psychological Advice on a pupil who has moved to the school from Spain. The Psychological Advice will become part of the advice from a range of professionals that will lead to a Statement of this pupil's special educational needs. I have arranged the visit to the school by phone two weeks previously, but when I arrive at the school the Head is surprised as he has not been told. However, the class teacher has been notified of my visit. I spend the first ten minutes observing the classroom assistant working with the child. She is undertaking the physical management programme that has to be done every day to maintain Lucy's physical well-being. Lucy's mum joins us to discuss her daughter's needs. She speaks a little English and I speak no Spanish. However, the classroom assistant speaks Spanish and remains as our interpreter. We discuss Lucy's difficulties. The normative developmental chart that I have brought is of little use as it has been developed for children who can move. Lucy has no control over any part of her body, apart from some control of her eyes and head. She has no speech. I am surprised to find that she has been at the school for approximately eighteen months before this assessment for a Statement started. It transpires that she had been very poorly and the school had felt she needed time to settle. In addition changes in staffing had left the paperwork undone that would have initiated the assessment for a Statement. I feel annoyed that children with her complexity of needs have not had an assessment for a Statement.

As the conversation unfolds it clear that developing a communication system for her is the first step for improving the quality of her life. At the same time it also became apparent that one of the major problems for her and her family is housing. Lucy's parents and the three children are living in a one-bedroom flat. The flat is small and damp with no room for Lucy's basic equipment, including her wheelchair. The living conditions are clearly affecting Lucy's health and well-being. The housing department in the LA have been notified but have done nothing. At about 11:30 Mum leaves. I thank the classroom assistant and sit down with the class teacher to pull our thoughts together and have a cup of tea. We clarify the issues around starting the assessment and the practicalities of implementing a teaching strategy to help Lucy to begin to communicate.

At 1:00 I return to the office, have a sandwich and begin to sort through school reports that I have been sent through on children. Cutbacks in the service mean that there is little administrative support so that now we have to do our own filing. This is a laborious and time-consuming job. I have not yet started writing up the psychological report for Lucy, which will take me another half day to do.

At 3:00 I drive to a school for children with severe and multiple disabilities for a meeting with the special educational needs co-ordinator (SENCO) and psychotherapist. We have been meeting monthly for the past year, working on ways of improving the emotional well-being of the children in the school. As well as their severe learning difficulties, many of the children in the school have emotional and behavioural problems. I have been involved in working with some of these children on an individual basis – as have a range of staff including the SENCO and the psychotherapist. This afternoon, however, the focus of the work is on looking at the school as a system and seeing how each classroom team can create the right emotional relationship with the children. I have worked on a number of issues, for example language, with similar groups in this school. Each group has finished with a report and training for the school staff. We finish at 5:00 and I drive straight home. There is still Lucy's report to write and work from the afternoon group – I have promised to work on developing an observation schedule for children's emotional well-being; but that is for another day. Today has generally been both satisfying and productive.

WORKING WITH CHILDREN AND YOUNG PEOPLE

The above 'day in the life' highlights a number of elements of EP practice that are expanded on below. It would be wrong to describe it as a typical day as the focus of all the work has been on children with severe and complex difficulties. One of the delights of working as an EP is that every day is different. However, it does contain many of the elements that occur on a day-to-day basis. These include: visiting schools, consultations with school staff, meetings with parents, individual assessments, working with groups of teachers and, of course, paperwork.

In 2006 the Department for Education and Skills (DfES) commissioned a report on the function and potential contribution of EPs within the Every Child Matters legislation. The subsequent report (Farrell et al., 2006) set out the role of the EP. The report stressed the importance that teachers attached to the psychology that EPs bring to these different activities. However, a major dilemma that it highlighted was the time EPs were giving to statutory assessment for Statementing – the process that Lucy was going through.

The 1993 Education Act and the subsequent 1994 Code of Practice (revised by the 2001 Code of Practice, Department of Education) introduced the concept of Statementing – the multidisciplinary assessment of a child's learning difficulties or disabilities leading to a Statement of their needs and the provision required to meet those needs. During the 1990s EP had increasingly become enmeshed not only in providing the Psychological Advice for the Statement but also, formally or informally, advising on the drawing-up of the Statement. Local authorities had begun to perceive that the rationale for EPs was simply contributing to Statements. Most EPs spend a considerable portion of each week assessing children in order to provide Psychological Advice for their Statements. Though Lucy clearly has complex and significant needs, the OfSTED report (2010) *A Statement is not Enough*, highlighted major concerns about the number of children who are assessed for Statementing who simply required effective teaching. The dilemma for EPs is that though they feel that too much time goes into this assessment role there is also a belief that if they did not provide assessment and advice the difficulties that many children have in schools would increasingly be left to the vagaries of the system. The recent green paper on special educational needs (Department for Education (DfE), 2011) has signalled the government's intention to move from Statements to a care plan. This change in thinking about the position of Statements will have the intended or unintended consequence of positioning EPs' role in assessment in new ways.

A second major issue about EPs' position in relation to practice is whether the role is to provide assessments and advice or whether it is to provide direct interventions and 'treatment' as well. In the above 'day in the life' none of the time went in working directly with an individual child, providing a psychological intervention such as counselling, cognitive–behavioural or solution-focused therapy. In the 1960s, when EPs moved outside of the child guidance clinics to work in school psychological services in local educational authorities (LEAs) one of the major concerns had been to stop labelling and pathologising the child as having the problem. Instead EPs had re-conceptualised their work as within systems – and in particular had taken on Bronfenbrenner's (1979) ecosytemic perspective. Many EPs believe that the focus of their work needs to be on the system (often the classroom and school) that the child is in. This concern to not pathologise the child has become the moral basis for EPs to question the value of undertaking individual therapeutic work with children.

Dessent (1992) made a strong moral argument for EPs to become more involved in individual work twenty years ago. He highlighted a number of hidden reasons why EPs didn't want to become involved in individual casework. These included: it is undoable, it is difficult work, it is low-status work and it has poor links with psychology as a discipline. To these reasons I would add that EPs are rarely given the space, in terms of time (an adequate number of sessions with a child) or the space (a room to work in) to undertake such work. However, what has changed to strengthen the importance of individual work is the links with psychology as a discipline (Boyle and Lauchlan 2009).

Many EPs use individual behavioural interventions with children. Fundamentally these used to consist of a functional analysis of behaviour and then advising on changing antecedents or reinforcements in the classroom in order to change behaviour (McNamara, 2000). More recently the development of CBT has been taken up by many EPs, combining as it does behaviour analysis with the introduction of a cognitive element (Pugh, 2010). The cognitive element in intervention has always been kept alive through 'personal construct psychology' and the writing of Ravenette (1999) and more recently by Beaver (2003). Since the turn of the century, solution-orientated and solution-focused thinking has been increasingly used by EPs (Stobie et al., 2005). In addition what has also happened is that EPs have conceptually reconciled the position of being able to help individual children while at the same time not pathologising them. There are two strands to this. One has been the development of systemic thinking, working with children, their families and teachers (Fox, 2009). The other development is delivering psychological interventions for vulnerable children through the system – for example by introducing an intervention as part of the curriculum in a school (Liddle and Macmillan, 2010).

There is still considerable debate about how EPs should position themselves around providing individual therapy. Many EPs resist the view, believing that it reinforces the position that the problem is within the child. In contrast many EPs now believe that direct intervention with the individual child is a helpful strategy – especially if the child feels empowered by the intervention. In addition, many EPs would see a key element of their work as helping adults, be they teachers, support staff or parents, to deal emotionally with the demands and difficulties of their role. In this sense an EP acts therapeutically in providing emotional support for these adults. In the 'day in a life' account the piece of work in the afternoon was directly addressing this issue. The work was concerned with the emotional and behavioural difficulties of children with severe learning difficulties. However, the focus of the work was on ensuring the emotional resilience and literacy of all the staff who worked in this school.

In summary, EPs' positioning in relationship to their practice contains two paradoxes. The first of these is the EPs' role in relationship to assessment of children with special educational needs. The paradox is that it takes up too much of EPs' time. However, if it also means EPs are very good at assessing children, and if they don't take up this position the very real difficulties some children have learning in school may be misjudged, overlooked and mismanaged. The second paradox is whether EPs should be doing direct, therapeutic work with vulnerable children. The moral dilemma is that the more successfully the EPs do this, the more they may reinforce the position that unsatisfactory learning environments do not need to change but rather the problem lies within the child.

This positioning of EPs in relationship to practice does not happen in a vacuum but is also affected by their positioning in relationship to employment.

WHO EMPLOYS EPs?

So who do EPs work for? Traditionally the vast majority of EPs were employed by LEAs. The LEAs were part of the LA or county council and had responsibility for providing education – schools for children who lived in the area. The educational psychology service or school psychology service was seen as one of a small number of services that were provided by the LA to support schools. Other services were provided by educational welfare officers, school advisors and behavioural support teachers. These were all employed by the LEA to work with schools to support and advise them. As we have seen, EPs had a central role in the assessment and support of children with special educational needs.

Following the Laming Report (2003) investigating the death of Victoria Climbie the government decided that a fundamental problem with protecting vulnerable children was the splintering of LA services for children into a number of departments. Therefore LAs were reorganised with education and parts of social services becoming amalgamated into 'Children's Services'. There was a shift in the position of the new Children's Services from that of essentially supporting schools to that of safeguarding vulnerable children. Educational psychologists began to use the title 'educational and child psychologists' and, though much of the work remains essentially the same, EPs have increasingly positioned themselves as working with vulnerable children rather than simply pupils with special educational needs. Educational psychology services are now usually incorporated into Children's Services as part of a multidisciplinary team including social workers, advisory teachers and care staff. Working in these multidisciplinary teams has moved EPs into a more community-orientated position though the majority of work still takes place in schools. Within children's services EPs are working with; looked after children in conjunction with social workers; children who have mental health difficulties, through secondment or joint work with children and adolescent mental health services (CAMHS); youth offenders, in conjunction with youth offending teams (YOTS); and a range of other vulnerable children. The Farrell Report (Farrell et al., 2006) highlighted that despite the development of children's services there are still problems with genuine joined-up services for vulnerable children – as we have seen illustrated by the housing needs of Lucy and her family.

The changes in local authorities from education to Children's Services, with work in multidisciplinary teams, have positioned EPs to see themselves increasingly as supporting vulnerable children and young people rather than simply as educational psychologists. The coalition's vision of the 'Big Society' coupled with the reduction of public sector workers in LAs means that opportunities are likely to arise for EPs to position themselves outside LAs. Though EPs will continue to work for LAs, it is likely that some EPs will be employed by voluntary and other non-governmental organisations (NGOs) involved in supporting vulnerable children. In addition parents will continue to buy the services of EPs particularly around the identification of special needs but also to provide advice on common issues of child development, for example sleeping problems.

So what are the implications of these changes in employment? Does it matter who the EP works for? Most EPs take a moral position that their services should be provided free at the point of delivery. That is, a family, or a school, should not have access to a service simply because they can pay, or be denied a service because they cannot pay. However, this moral principle is now being challenged by a social narrative that promotes the rights of individuals (parents) and institutions (schools) to decide how they want to spend their money. In other words if a school (an academy) or a family wishes to choose to spend their money on services from an EP they have a right to access such a service. This is a fundamental change in moral position for many EPs brought up on the principle of equal access to services. Educational psychologists may be moving beyond the concept of a free universal service to one where additional services can be bought.

If the position for whom EPs work changes, does that affect who is their client? Is the client the person or organisation that pays the EP's salary – or is it the child? The position of most EPs is that it remains as the child. Helping the child is seen as the focus of the work of the EP in the same way that the focus of the work of a teacher is on teaching the pupil – not on supporting the school. However, this raises another question. Are EPs positioned as advocates or professionals for the child?

WHO EPs WORK FOR

Professionals' central characteristic has been described as having a lengthy period of training in a body of abstract knowledge and a strong service orientation (Goode, 1960). There is little doubt that this statement is true for EPs. The value of being a professional service is that it is seen to offer a view on a situation based on expert knowledge or skills and that it is not biased by financial considerations. In other words a professional holds a position of truth and should not take up a position that they know not to be true. In that sense much of the credibility of a professional is that their position is not swayed by financial interest. In that sense one would expect the employment status of an EP not to alter their perceptions of, and recommendations about, an issue. It should not matter if the EP is employed by the LA, the Dyslexia Association or a parent: their recommendations about an individual child's needs and the provision required to meet those needs should remain the same.

This can be contrasted with the position of the advocate. The advocate's responsibility is to take up the position of their client and to argue and support their case in the best way they can. The EP's responsibility would then be to identify what their client wants, and to make a case to support them using the law (and local and national policies and procedures) and their expert knowledge. The EP's own personal opinion would not enter into the equation. So the client may want the child to move schools, to get extra support or to have access to therapy. The EPs role as advocate is to make the case for this on behalf of their client (Bateman, 2000).

Advocacy may appear as unprofessional but for some professions, for example social workers, there is a legal expectation that they can take up the position of advocates (The Children Act 1989, HM Government). When employed by LAs, EPs usually position themselves as mediators – trying to ensure that all different views are heard. However, a common criticism by parents is that professionals implicitly position themselves as advocates for the organisation that they are working for (Beresford, 1995). So, for example, EPs can be criticised as only recommending particular provision if the LA provides it rather than if the child would benefit from it.

If EPs continue to see their clients as children they need to decide if they are positioning themselves as professionals or advocates. Advocacy is about speaking up for the child or young person. The EPs' role would then be working in order to secure their rights, to meet their needs and to help them make informed choices. Of course, parents are the first advocates for their children but parents are often put in a powerless position. Parents can feel powerless as they do not have adequate knowledge and information about their child's rights. They may also feel powerless because they do not have the interpersonal skills to express their views and because there are a range of agencies opposing their views. The EP can position themself to support the child through empowerment of not only the child but also their parents.

The changes in employment opportunities mean it is possible that EPs will be increasingly positioned as advocates through employment by voluntary organisations and national charities to support their agendas. There may also be small groups of parents coalescing around a single issue such as setting up a special free school or individual parents concerned about their child's specific reading difficulties. If social policy moves to a more market economy, increasingly EPs are likely to be positioned as advocates by their employers, be they parents, voluntary agencies, schools or LAs. This is likely to be particularly contentious as only a limited amount of the EP work has legislative backing or is evidence based. This means that the issue around the identification of difficulties or needs, and the types of intervention to meet those needs, is often disputed territory. More fundamentally, disputed territory is now seen not as a matter of the limitations of the evidence base for the professional practice of the EP but more fundamentally about whether there can be a single right solution to some of the issues that EPs are asked to deal with.

WHAT IS THE PSYCHOLOGICAL THEORY THAT UNDERPINS EPs' WORK?

There have been significant changes in terms of the positioning of EPs as applied psychologists in relation to theory in the past ten years. Fundamentally there has been a shift in perception about the nature of reality (EPs' ontological position) and the best ways to find out, or investigate, this reality (the epistemological position). Ontology is concerned with the nature of reality whereas epistemology refers to different ways of establishing what is true (cf. Chapter 2).

Traditionally psychologists started from the ontological premise that there is an objective and real world independent of human beliefs, culture and the language that is used to describe it (Hart, 2002). The purpose of psychology is to make sense of this world through the epistemology of scientific research. Science takes a positivist or realist position. Fundamental to this is a belief that there is a reality, and through the scientific method we can come to understand that reality. Hypothetical constructs used by EPs such as motivation, attribution theory and self-concept have been developed as theories to make sense of this world. These theories are developed through scientific research that is characterised by experiments where data is gathered under strictly controlled conditions and analysed to see if it can disprove existing hypotheses. Through these experimental procedures, theories are developed that better explain and make sense of the world.

Though most academic psychologists maintain this positivist scientific tradition, increasingly, applied psychologists have taken up a relativist or constructionist position. Their position is that people construct their own reality in a particular situation. The contrast between a realist and a relativist position can be seen in how EPs make sense of their work with teachers in a classroom. A realist EP would take the position that there is a real classroom, with a teacher who can be objectively described as being an effective or ineffective teacher, and pupils who are learning or not learning. In contrast the relativist EP would claim there is not an objective, real classroom, in so far as the teacher and each of the pupils will have a different understanding of what is going on. There may be a few simple things that can be objectively seen and measured, for example how many pupils and what gender they are. However, a relativist would argue that all the other, more psychologically important aspects of the classroom are not objective realities. The effectiveness of the teaching will differ from one pupil to another. A pupil's learning, motivation and attention will also be constantly shifting and changing. A pupil who cannot read at the age of six in a British school is labelled as having problems with their reading, whereas in another country they would not be conceived of as a poor reader. In other words there is not a reality about a child having a difficulty.

If there is not an objective reality then it can be questioned whether a scientific, deductive, experimental, quantitative way of generating knowledge is the most appropriate. If there are multiple realities then what is important is how different people understand the situation they are in. The starting point for an EP working in a classroom is to see how the people, children and adults, have different understanding or meanings for what is going on. Increasingly, qualitative research is seen as the best way of generating new knowledge (cf. Chapters 2 and 3). In qualitative research, information is usually gathered from observation or interviews and then critically analysed and organised in a systematic way. Qualitative research is usually interested in how people talk about their reality or how they behave in real life. In that sense the theory does not come from controlled experiments but rather from the real experiences of people in a complex situation.

Traditionally, applied psychologists, including EPs, have used psychological theories developed by academics from a positivist position. This has been reinforced in the past decade by governments' insistence on the importance of evidence-based practice (EBP) – especially for health professionals (Sacket et al., 1996). The rationale for EBP is that this professional practice should be based on evidence of what works and that the evidence should come from scientific research. Evidence-based practice takes very much a realist or positivist view of the world, i.e. that there are best ways of educating children, teaching them to read and managing their emotional difficulties. Once these best interventions are known, then they can be applied in the classroom.

From this point of view the EP's position in relation to theory and research is to find the best evidence there is to resolve particular issues and then to apply it. The research drives the professional practice of the EP. However, this only makes sense if you apply a realist positivist perspective. If you take a relativist perspective then this is the wrong direction of travel. From a relativist perspective what makes sense is practice-based evidence. In other words the evidence of what is effective comes from practice – not from research. Out of practice theories about effective interventions can be evidenced (cf. Chapter 3).

This fits in with the position of EPs as working in indeterminate zones of practice (Argyris, 1989; Schön, 1987). In these indeterminate zones, every situation, every classroom is different and there are alternative ways of seeing things. Underpinning these different constructions of reality there are alternative values or moral positions. Educational practitioners need practice-based artistry, not evidence-based rationality, as the basis on which to work. The psychology then behind the practice is the ability of the EP to make meaningful sense of the problems that children, teachers, parents and other involved adults have, and to help them turn these problem-saturated narratives to ones that create opportunities for development.

The question then is how do you train EPs to be practice-based artists?

HOW EPs ARE TRAINED

Changes to EPs' training has also affected the positioning of EPs in relation to psychological theory. With the introduction of doctoral training in 2003, the requirement for having worked as a teacher was removed. Trainees now come from a variety of backgrounds. All have worked with children, some as teachers and most in schools, but some come with experience of working in social care and mental health services. This reinforces the focus of EPs working with vulnerable children rather than solely with pupils with educational difficulties.

Though the requirement for having been a teacher has been removed, the requirement to have an initial degree in psychology has remained. So the profession has become more psychological and less educational. This change of backgrounds of people coming into the profession means that most EPs position themselves now as fundamentally psychologists who work with vulnerable children in schools and the wider community.

There are twelve training courses in England all attached to university departments – once again some education and some psychology departments. Training courses vary but all are accredited by the HPC and the BPS. The government presently pays the training cost of a limited number of places on each course. This means that places for any of the courses are fiercely contested each year.

Educational psychology training at UEL can be seen as consisting of three fundamental components. The first is the development of an understanding of psychological theories to give frameworks for understanding the world (Kelly et al., 2008). This allows the trainee to recognise patterns and themes in their work that can be turned into hypotheses or formulations about the nature of problems and how they can be resolved (Johnstone and Dallos, 2006). The second fundamental component is the ability to apply these theories in practice in the complexity of the real world. This ties back to Argyris and Schön's notion of working in indeterminate areas. Though the trainee can learn the theory about child development or the best way of teaching reading, the reality is that every home and every classroom is different. It is the EP's responsibility to identify the particular factors for this child, in this classroom, in this particular family that will help their reading development. It may be that some of the changes that are needed can be implemented for the whole class but often it is tailoring individual solutions to individual problems. The third component is being able to turn this practice back into theory through research – practice-based evidence.

The first of these components is largely gained through being taught at the university. The majority of the first year is spent at the university developing an understanding of the psychology of teaching and learning, child development, assessment, consultation and intervention. Trainees are introduced to problem-based learning but they also spend time in schools (and the wider community) actually applying this knowledge in practice. In the second and third year additional psychological frameworks are taught specifically on the psychology of groups and organisations. However, in the second and third year the main focus switches to the second fundamental component – the ability to apply these theories in practice in the complexity of the real world. Trainees spend most of these two years working under supervision in educational psychology services. Over these two years they become proficient and reflective practitioners. The third component of turning practice back into research is developed through undertaking a research project in the second and third year. The research that the trainee carries out is based on a real issue for the service. In that sense it is practice led, not theory led. The research may have different purposes. Some students undertake research to evaluate an intervention, some to explore issues, others to promote change (through action research). In this sense the value of the research is to systematically investigate issues and develop knowledge about the most effective ways of applying psychology in practice.

The course at UEL implicitly and explicitly positions trainees as applying psychology to make a positive difference to children and young people. The importance of advocating for children, listening to their views and involving them in decision-making is reinforced by a commitment to improving the quality of life for all vulnerable children.

The programme celebrates the opportunities of being in a diverse part of society in the East End of London. We believe in the importance of recognising different views and therefore different solutions to similar problems.

CONCLUSION

I have tried to use positioning theory in this chapter to stimulate the reader to think about how EPs both position themselves and are positioned by the society we live in. I am acknowledging that the role of the EP will change as successive governments make changes to social structures and policy. However, I am also suggesting that EPs have a responsibility to position ourself and to take up new positions as the world changes. I have highlighted how there is an explicit or implicit moral position that EPs attach to their positions. It is difficult for any of us to change our moral positions as they are usually emotionally, as well as rationally, held. However, over time, the moral position of EPs has shifted and changed as other positions have been taken up in the wider narrative of what is a right and just society. There are many other issues that EPs struggle with on a daily basis, but there has not been space to deal with these in this chapter. However, positioning theory gives a psychological framework to think about these issues and to take up your own moral position as an applied psychologist.

QUESTIONS FOR REFLECTION AND DISCUSSION

1   Is assessing children's difficulties morally defensible?

2   Should EPs be advocates for children and their families?

3   What are the implications of working independently rather than for an LA?

4   Practice-based evidence or evidence-based practice – which is the way forward?

5   What moral position(s) should underpin your practice?

6   What are the key skills and attributes required to be a successful EP?

SUGGESTIONS FOR FURTHER READING

Beaver, R. (2003) *Educational Psychology Casework*. London: Jessica Kingsley. This practical book contains a wealth of ideas for using psychology to work with children. It is one that both trainees and experienced EPs use extensively.

Farrell, P., Woods, K., Lewis, S., Rooney, S., Squires, G. and O'Conner, M. (2006) *Review of Function and Contribution of Educational Psychologists in Light of the 'Every Child Matters: Change for Children' Agenda*. Nottingham: DfES. This is the most recent report on the role and function of EPs. It contains a detailed analysis of how EPs are actually positioned.

Kelly, B., Woolfson, L. and Boyle, J. (2008) *Frameworks for Practice in Educational Psychology: A Textbook for Trainees and Practitioners*. London: Jessica Kingsley. The book describes a range of frameworks that practising EPs use to underpin their practice. Understanding and taking up a position on these frameworks can be seen as a key to effective practice.

Long, M., Wood, C., Littleton, K., Passenger, T. and Sheehy, K. (2011) *The Psychology of Education* (2nd edn). London: Routledge. Provides a contemporary overview of psychological theory and research that relate to education.

6

OCCUPATIONAL PSYCHOLOGY

Carla Gibbes, Mark Holloway and Donald Ridley

This chapter discusses:

- what occupational psychology is;

- how to become a Chartered Occupational Psychologist;

- a case study of the process of becoming a Chartered Occupational Psychologist;

- a day in the life of an occupational psychologist;

- the importance of CPD (continuing professional development);

- who we work for – ethical considerations.

INTRODUCTION

Occupational psychology attempts to understand and explain the behaviour and experience of people at work by applying theory and research from psychology. It is known in different countries by other names, e.g. in the USA it is called industrial/organisational psychology and in Europe it is work and organisational psychology. Moreover, other disciplines also concern themselves with people at work, e.g. human resource management and personnel management, and some practitioners call themselves business psychologists or management psychologists.

Clive Fletcher and Chris Lewis's contributions to Chapter 19 of this book comment on the problems associated with this complexity, and Christine Doyle (2003) used the following comment from an occupational psychologist to illustrate one of them. The psychologist said to her: 'If I tell my clients that I *must* evaluate my interventions in their organisations, they'll just get out *Yellow Pages* and look up the nearest management consultant' (p. 39).

In this chapter, we focus most on the process of becoming an occupational psychologist and on aspects of what we actually do, including examples of ethical dilemmas and judgements about them (cf. Richard Kwiatkowski's contribution to Chapter 19).

HOW TO BECOME A CHARTERED OCCUPATIONAL PSYCHOLOGIST

To become a chartered member of the BPS and a full member of the Division of Occupational Psychology, students must complete the Qualification in Occupational Psychology (Stage 1 and Stage 2). Before this, students must be eligible for the Graduate Basis for Chartership (GBC) and be Graduate Members of the BPS (see Box 6.1 below). Full details can be found at the BPS website (http://www.bps.org.uk/careers-education-training/society-qualifications/occupational-psychology/occupational-psychology).

Box 6.1   Route to becoming a Chartered Occupational Psychologist

1 Graduate Basic for Chartered Membership (GBC) (completion of a society-accredited degree or conversion course).

2 Society-accredited Master's in Occupational Psychology or Stage 1 of the Society's Qualification in Occupational Psychology.

3 Stage 2 of the Society's Qualification in Occupational Psychology (minimum two years' supervised practice). This will lead to full membership of the Division of Occupational Psychology (DOP).

4 Registration with the Health Professions Council (HPC).

Stage 1 is made up of a knowledge and a research dimension. It can be completed in two ways, either through passing a society-accredited MSc in Occupational or Organisational Psychology, or by the DOP Stage 1 examinations. The knowledge dimension covers eight areas:

1 *Human–machine interaction*

   Designing machines (for example, computers) or complex human–machine systems (such as power plants or planes) so that human physical and psychological needs are met in ways that promote maximum efficiency, productivity, safety and well-being. Specialists in this area increasingly deal with human–computer interaction since more and more processes are controlled by computer systems. They are also concerned with preventing accidents and disasters in hazardous industries, e.g. issues connected with risk perception and encouraging a safety culture.

2 *Design of environments and work; health and safety*

   Investigating job design and work spaces to maximise comfort, well-being, safety and efficiency, with particular reference to people's physical and psychological needs. Implicit in this is the notion of stress, or rather how to create jobs and workplaces that do not create too much stress in workers.

3 *Personnel selection and assessment*

Choosing the best person for a job by means that are as reliable, valid and fair as possible, in order (again) to maximise worker well-being and productivity. For instance, someone who has the skills, knowledge and ability to do a complex job is less likely to suffer undue pressure than someone lacking these attributes. Assessment might also be concerned with analysing people's training needs or their potential for promotion.

4 *Performance appraisal and career development*

Measuring people's job performance so that they can be rewarded fairly. Also helping people to develop their skills and improve their performance by, for example, devising personal development and career management plans. Specialists in this area are often engaged in assessing strengths and weaknesses and offering careers guidance to people of all ages.

5 *Counselling and personal development*

Counselling skills are needed in many aspects of occupational psychology from the consulting process itself to developmental forms of appraisal. There has also been a growth in employee assistance programmes that are designed to help workers deal with personal or work-related problems.

The related specialism of coaching is discussed in Chapter 16 of this book.

6 *Training*

Identifying training and development needs, designing and delivering training programmes, and evaluating their effectiveness. Many organisations aspire to be 'learning organisations' where there is a climate of constant learning to promote improved performance and innovation. Such learning may be provided by on-the-job experience and computerised packages as well as by traditional classroom-based training courses. Specialists in this area are skilled in the design of training courses as well as their delivery.

7 *Employee relations and motivation*

Using knowledge of social processes at work to increase worker motivation, well-being and effectiveness. Also industrial relations and conflicts between employers and employees.

8 *Organisational development and change*

Helping organisations and their staff to cope with an increasingly turbulent business environment. Organisations have become more complex and international. Doyle (2003) called them 'effectively "boundary-less"', and also remarked on partnerships, consortia, mergers and acquisitions and a greater felt need to 'celebrate diversity' (p. 42).

The research dimension

Students must demonstrate their knowledge of psychological research within the context of occupational psychology. Students must show their knowledge in the following areas:

- ethical issues in applied research;

- principles of design including different types of data analysis;

- an ability to critically evaluate occupational psychology literature.

The research dimension can be completed in three ways:

1 Successful completion of the exam in Research Methods and Statistics (Stage 1 of the Qualification only).

2 Successful completion of the research proposal (Stage 1of the Qualification only).

3 Successful completion of a Society-accredited MSc in Occupational or Organisational Psychology.

It is possible for students who have completed a non-accredited MSc in Occupational Psychology or equivalent areas to apply for exemption from parts of the Stage 1 qualification (BPS, 2010)

Stage 2: The practice dimension

Students must complete a period of practice as a 'Trainee Occupational Psychologist under the supervision of a Chartered Occupational Psychologist with Full Membership of the Division of Occupational Psychology (DOP) and registered with the Health Professions Council (HPC) as a Practitioner Psychologist' (BPS, 2012). Supervisors must have undergone the qualification's approved supervisor training and also be on the Society's Register of Applied Psychology Practice Supervisors (RAPPS).

The practice dimension is divided into breadth elements and depth elements. Breadth elements require the student to demonstrate their practical competence in five out of the eight areas of the knowledge dimension. Students must also demonstrate their competence in the following process skills:

1 gathering information;

2 testing or analysing the information;

3 evaluating the information;

4 applying the information.

Depth elements require the student to demonstrate their practical competence in the consultancy cycle in one of the four areas below:

1 work and the environment;

2 the individual;

3 the organisation;

4 training.

Evidence of all the stages of the consultancy cycle must be demonstrated within a depth entry:

1 establishing agreements with customers;

2 identifying needs and problems;

3 analysing needs and problems;

4 formulating solutions;

5 implementing and reviewing solutions;

6 evaluating outcomes;

7 reporting and reflecting outcomes.

In addition the following generic skills must be demonstrated at least once in either depth or breadth entries:

1 questionnaire or survey design;

2 interviewing;

3 report writing;

4 presentation skills;

5 statistical skills or qualitative analyses;

6 evaluation techniques.

The minimum duration of the Qualification in Occupational Psychology (Stage 1 and Stage 2) is three years.

A CASE STUDY OF THE PROCESS OF BECOMING A CHARTERED OCCUPATIONAL PSYCHOLOGIST (PRE-2010)

I graduated in 1983 with a BPS-recognised degree in psychology. Being unable to find a suitable job at that time I successfully applied for a Social Science Research Council (SSRC) grant to undertake an MA in Manpower Studies, what we would now recognise as the field of human resource management (HRM). I got my first job in HRM shortly after attaining the MA. I worked in an operational role for a large retail organisation. Two years later I switched roles to work for a top-ten firm of chartered accountants, where I rose up through the ranks quickly, becoming assistant human resources (HR) director in four years.

I was now in my early thirties and my career path appeared set. However, the appointment of a new HR director meant I was quickly out of favour and I was made redundant. I challenged this redundancy decision at an employment tribunal and successfully claimed for wrongful dismissal.

After several thwarted attempts to restart my HR career I accepted a job as a lecturer in a university business school, responsible for the training and education of HR professionals. Three years later I started my MSc Occupational Psychology on a part-time basis, completing it in two years. Half way through the programme I undertook my first 'consultancy' assignment, within a local NHS trust. This led to many other pieces of consultancy work, which were well paid, contributed to the finances of the business school and, critically, helped me develop a significant portfolio of work that not only assisted towards my Chartership but also made me a better lecturer, as I was able to bring real experiences into the classroom.

I now had a BSc Psychology, an MA HRM and an MSc Occupational Psychology, yet I was still working in a business school and not properly using my knowledge of psychology in my job. So when I was contacted in 2000 by my former MSc tutor and encouraged to apply for the vacant post of Programme Director MSc Occupational Psychology I needed little persuading. I got the job, but one of the conditions of the appointment was that I had to attain Chartered Occupational Psychologist status. Up to that point I had no real need to become chartered: my job did not require it and for my growing consultancy client list it was largely an irrelevance. However, my new appointment forced me to address the situation.

It took six months to become chartered. My MSc tutor volunteered to be my supervisor, which was incredibly helpful as she was able to guide me through the process from a position of experience: in other words she knew what the BPS liked to see in the submitted evidence. The chartership process was different then to how it is now. I needed to submit a logbook that demonstrated knowledge and experience at three levels. Level one was knowledge of the eight areas of occupational psychology, achieved by completing the MSc. Level two was supervised practice in a number of these areas, which was achieved by a combination of MSc assignments and experience from my HR career. Level three specified the demonstration of three hundred hours of independent practice in one particular area.

This was the trickiest level because the three hundred hours could not include repeated work. For example, I had designed and run countless assessment centres for clients but could not count them as separate experiences for logbook purposes. So I chose the broadest area, organisational development and change, and managed to piece together a portfolio of consultancy experiences that were sufficiently distinct from each other to be eligible. The hardest part of all of this was finding proof that I had actually undertaken all the assignments I was claiming for. This salutary experience has meant that I now keep a paper trail of all such work.

My first chartership submission was rejected by the BPS, with minor changes required for the logbook. This was disappointing but not unexpected. I made the changes and added more documentary proof, and my application succeeded the second time around.

I have now been a Chartered Occupational Psychologist for ten years. It is obviously important for me to be chartered, as I would not be allowed to do my job without it. As far as clients are concerned, I recall telling my biggest client that I had just become chartered. This news was met with a look of bewilderment, a shrug of the shoulders and a warning that I should not increase my fees. For other client work, however, it has been essential to be chartered. If you are working with fellow occupational psychologists it demonstrates without ambiguity that you can operate at a high level and use psychology ethically and professionally in organisations. The more you rub shoulders with other occupational psychologists the more important chartered status becomes.

A DAY IN THE LIFE OF AN OCCUPATIONAL PSYCHOLOGIST

What is a typical day in the life of an occupational psychologist? That would depend, in part, on the type of occupational psychologist you are. Broadly speaking there are four main career routes available:

- working for a consultancy practice;
- working in the public or private sector;
- working as an academic;
- working for yourself.

Case study

This variety of choices is one of the most appealing aspects of this field of psychology. I have forged a career where I both work as an academic and work for myself. By this I mean that I operate as a Chartered Occupational Psychologist with organisational clients on behalf of the university I work for. This means that, unlike more than half of occupational psychologists who work for themselves, I do not have to rely solely on client work for my income. This also means that I am able to bring my consultancy experiences back into the classroom for the benefit of my students. So what follows is an account, not of a typical day, but of a day where these various identities come together effectively.

I leave home at 7:15 and take the train to London. I am due to meet the Assistant Dean of the School of Psychology at Embankment Station at 8:30. Together we have designed a one-day workshop called 'Occupational Choice and Transitions'.

It is due to be delivered at 9:30 to a small group of Royal Air Force pilots at the Ministry of Defence (MOD). This group have just been informed that they are to be made redundant within the next six months. They are among the earliest casualties of the cuts in the Armed Forces, which will see 20,000 job losses in the next three years.

As we walk to the MOD, my colleague and I go over the last-minute arrangements, checking laptops, memory sticks, workshop handbooks and the like. This is the first time we have run this workshop and we hope to roll it out further in the years to come. We need to make a good impression but we feel confident, as we have invested considerable time in designing the day to suit the needs of the client group. This has involved us talking at length to the client, drafting and redrafting programme designs, conducting extensive desk research and thinking carefully about how to engage the workshop delegates across the day. We feel confident, although there is a nagging concern in my mind that we have been unable to talk in advance to the delegates themselves, so we have only been able to address their development needs through an intermediary, an independent consultant with the remit for handling the transition into civilian life for these and other military personnel under threat of redundancy.

Upon arrival at the MOD, I am reminded of the everyday practical issues involved when working with external organisations. We have a person to meet (our client) who we have never met before, just spoken to over the telephone. We have to prove our identities in order to gain access to the building (luckily we have remembered our passports). We have to hope that the training room has been set out according to our wishes. We have to hope that we have access to the computer systems in the building in order to be able to use our laptops to show the slides, video clips and internet sites we will be using during the day. We have to ensure that we remain professional and composed while negotiating these last-minute glitches, as our delegates are likely to be present in the training room while all this is going on.

In the event, these issues are handled relatively smoothly and the day gets under way. My colleague and I have split the day between us. We have never trained together before and this brings with it other concerns about being observed and judged by colleagues, especially when that colleague happens to be your boss. We support each other effortlessly and seem able to read when the other is in need of our input. This is lucky, as we had not had a chance for a dress rehearsal of any sort.

We have designed the workshop with our relative strengths in mind. I am a Chartered Occupational Psychologist and my colleague is an expert in careers guidance and a Fellow of the BPS. She will be running the following sessions:

- managing career transition effectively;
- leverage in the labour market.

I am responsible for:

- coming to terms with loss and change;
- identifying and working with personal strengths.

I have researched these areas carefully and have drawn upon my knowledge and experience of using principles and techniques from positive psychology to develop the sessions. I have also explored in depth an approach to mindfulness called acceptance and commitment therapy (ACT), which teaches people to notice and accept their thoughts, feelings and memories rather than trying to control them. This is useful in this context as it helps you to clarify your personal values and to work out how to take action on them, thus improving your psychological flexibility and helping you to deal with change more successfully. The reason we have taken this approach is because we believe, correctly as it turns out, that our delegates need time to reflect on, and come to terms with, their new situation (redundancy) rather than simply dust themselves down and get a new job (most of our delegates had aspired to be pilots since their childhood so the sense of loss is real and quite acute).

The ACT example illustrates one of the challenges faced by occupational psychologists, namely to present psychological models and approaches in such a way that they have meaning and usefulness to non-psychologists. I have felt this keenly many times when working with organisations. It does not involve 'dumbing down' the psychology for the lay person, but asks that you try to see the world from the client's point of view and remain mindful of what will help that person towards greater growth and well-being. It also reminds me that, as a profession, we have the comfort of knowing that what we do is backed up by a solid body of good research evidence, and this is something that sets us apart from the average consultant who aspires to tread the same path.

The day itself is extremely well received by our group. Our client is present throughout the day and his contributions are valuable. My colleague and I are experienced enough to 'flex' our approach according to the shifting dynamics of the group and to reflect the different preferences for learning styles present in the room. We know that our delegates will be feeling uncertain upon arrival and that they will want to know that they have considerable input into the way the day pans out. We also know that we have a preferred way of learning that will not be shared by everyone in the room so we need to switch our delivery to engage their attention.

At the end of the day, when the delegates have departed, we have a conversation with our client where we ask him for his perceptions of the day and where, if anywhere, this day may be rolled out further. Our client speaks in very favourable terms about the workshop and tells us how he intends to take things further. This will involve numerous high-level conversations, along with some delicate political negotiating. We have his assurance that he will advocate our workshop on our behalf, as it represents a different approach to the redundancy counselling that they currently use. We offer to be part of any conversations he has and he thanks us for our offer. We leave with a real sense that this humble one-day workshop, which we designed with much thought and care, may well have some future beyond today.

THE IMPORTANCE OF CONTINUING PROFESSIONAL DEVELOPMENT (CPD)

All Chartered Occupational Psychologists have to abide by a code of professional ethics, and part of that code requires them to engage in CPD by keeping abreast of developments in their fields of expertise and by reflecting on their practice. One way of doing this is to embark on a Professional Doctorate in Occupational Psychology.

The Professional Doctorate in Occupational Psychology

Once practitioners are reasonably established, there may come a point when they ask 'where next?' Taking time out to do a PhD is not usually feasible.

The Professional Doctorate at UEL uses a 'work-based challenge framework' and is a research degree that involves the practitioner's ongoing work. All this encourages a focus on real business issues.

During year 1 there is a requirement to undertake taught elements in both research and professional practice. In years 2 and 3 students must undertake two research studies, one quantitative and the other a qualitative study. Using a mixed-methods approach helps to broaden practitioners' research expertise and encourage development as a researcher-practitioner. It may also foster the development of new research strategies and innovative practice. Writing up the research requires an evidence-based approach, while students are encouraged to disseminate their research through attendance at conferences and writing articles for publication in mainstream journals.

The Doctorate can be completed within a minimum of three years and takes place within a mutually supportive climate. The model is one of a collaboration of equals in this endeavour and this, and monthly support seminars, help to counteract the 'loneliness of the long-distance scholar'.

The main aim of the programme is to advance practice and the profession as a whole. Perhaps one way it can do this is by a Doctorate raising the status of practitioners and making them distinctive from rival professionals. This collaboration between the researcher and practitioner arms of the profession may also help to heal rifts.

WHO WE WORK FOR: ETHICAL CONSIDERATIONS

The ethics of a practising occupational psychologist can be complex. Here are some examples.

First an example from the field of ergonomics. While assessing the safety of a hazardous fuel-handling system as part of a large engineering project, some engineers from the project team come along with a problem. The deadline for a key part of the work is now five days away and they need a probability of the likelihood of human failure in the system. In fact the answer they need, they tell you, was one error in every one hundred executions of a particularly complex task. This would give them an acceptable overall system reliability. They want you to fudge it. You reply, 'Sorry, I cannot do that in five days; we need to do a proper analysis that will take several weeks.' They insist, and your boss and engineer put pressure on you. You say that it's not correct and point out that to give an answer without doing the work properly would put you in breach of BPS regulations. Ultimately your boss, who is not qualified, makes an estimate and signs it off. The documentation is hidden in project files and the matter is not discussed. The project manager thinks you have been unhelpful and is noticeably gruff. As you are up for promotion soon and he is chairing the interview panel you reflect that doing the right thing has costs attached to it.

Now let's look at an example where you are working for a large firm of consultants. You are retained to do an analysis of stress in a large privatised organisation. You are asked to do the analysis by the management because they think the reason the staff are stressed is because the equipment they have to use is very old. They are seeking a government capital grant to replace the equipment with a more modern version that will need fewer staff. It is a nationwide study. You have been asked to explain to the trade union that represents the operators what you are doing and include them in the loop. You measure cortisol levels as well as using self-report measures of stress. You are conducting interviews and using broader questionnaires as well.

It becomes quite clear as you proceed that the stress experienced by the system operators has little to do with their aged equipment but quite a lot to do with working practices and management style. Your line manager is busy and does not meet your request to have a meeting to discuss the draft results. You present these results at the pre-arranged time. Your manager is surprised. The managers of the organisation are horrified. One of them verbally attacks you and questions your competence. You are very taken aback but slowly recover your composure and refer them to the agreed remit.

They say that there has obviously been a misunderstanding. These results are interesting but not relevant and you have been asking the wrong question. It's not your fault as you are young and enthusiastic. They have a meeting with your manager, where they say they are not going to pay for these results. Your manager goes over your findings and produces a much thinner report that appears to say that the operators are not very stressed, and that what little stress is experienced is caused by the equipment. You have been thinking about this over the weekend as well. When the manager shows you the new thinner report, you say that is fine, but unfortunately you sent a draft copy of the original results to the trade union representatives, as previously agreed. Your manager groans. You actually post the copy to the union that evening.

These two examples illustrate a number of points regarding ethical issues. First is that you may have two masters: your professional standards and the person who is paying for the work. Does the person who is paying the bill have a right to influence the outcome or be selective about the results that they wish to take notice of? Do you have a duty or a right to disseminate findings that your client may wish to suppress?

In these two examples, the issue is relatively clear cut. In the first case you obviously should not tell lies for professional convenience. In the second case you certainly have a right to present the results. You do not deserve to be treated rudely. You manager is clearly behaving questionably and without any moral fibre. His argument is that if we damage the relationship we have with this client, contracts and then jobs will be lost. Did you have a right to post that copy of the results to the union? It might have been OK had you done it before the meeting, but is it OK afterwards? You know that if the clients found out they would be very angry. Now these two examples sound extreme, but in their essential details they are both true. These situations actually occurred though enough details have been changed to anonymise the organisations and participants. In both examples you find that the need to be impartial is often compromised by the view of the person paying the bill. It is not at all unusual for findings to be tweaked and manipulated to suit public relations and internal political issues.

Do not feel glum though. Part of your professional development as an occupational psychologist is about learning how to position yourself at the beginning of a contract where you make it clear that you will be operating under certain professional parameters and that although you have your client's interests very much at heart, you know that your clients will agree that openness and honesty are best for the organisation. In the second case there was a lesson there for the management that they did not want to hear. In the first case, ten years later, someone could have died. Luckily the system that was being planned was never fully commissioned, so that issue did not arise.

CONCLUSION

Occupational psychologists can specialise in one or more of eight areas, which overlap significantly with other branches of applied psychology as currently defined. They also come from very diverse backgrounds and have very varied working lives, as illustrated in the case study and the 'day in the life' respectively. The work often involves complex ethical dilemmas and judgements as vividly shown in the two detailed case studies.

QUESTIONS FOR REFLECTION AND DISCUSSION

1   Are there other people with related skill sets who I might be working with?

2   How might I best work with other professionals in a team?

3   How should I define my working relationship with a client and with other stakeholders?

4   Who is my client? Is it the person who is paying the bill or is it the entire organisation?

5   What do I do if a piece of work changes and I am not confident of my competence?

6   What should I say to a line manager who is not a psychologist?

7   How might I develop myself professionally while I am working?

8   If I do not think I am 'adding value', should I be doing the work in the first place?

SUGGESTIONS FOR FURTHER READING

There are many excellent general introductions to occupational psychology. A small selection follows.

Arnold, J., Randall, R., Patterson, F., Silvester, J., Robertson, I.T., Cooper, C., Burnes, B., Harries, D., Axtell, C. and Den Hartog, D. (2010) *Work Psychology: Understanding Human Behaviour in the Workplace* (5th edn). Harlow: Financial Times/Prentice Hall. A well-established textbook, currently in its fifth edition, which tackles contemporary issues in an engaging and readable way.

Chmiel, N. (ed.) (2008) *Introduction to Work and Organizational Psychology: A European Perspective* (2nd edn). Oxford: Blackwell. A collection of thought-provoking chapters by experts in their fields, this book gives ergonomics the coverage it deserves and which is often lacking.

Doyle, C.E. (2002) *Work and Organizational Psychology: An Introduction with Attitude.* Hove: Psychology Press. Groundbreaking at the time of publication, this book still manages to rattle a few cages with its brash and opinionated tone.

7

HEALTH PSYCHOLOGY

Paula Nicolson

This chapter discusses:

- the background and history of the development of health psychology in the UK in particular;

- the development of processes and procedures that have led to the registration of health psychologists (HPs) with the Health Professions Council (HPC);

- what is considered health psychology research and how some researchers have accomplished their work;

- what it means to be a critical HP.

INTRODUCTION

Health psychology emphasises the role of psychological factors in the cause, progression and consequences of health and illness.

(Ogden, 2001: 6)

Placing psychology at the heart of contemporary understandings of health and illness may seem self-evident now during the second decade of the twenty-first century. However, the presumption that mind and body are interconnected in relation to health and illness confirms the impact that psychologists and psychological knowledge have made upon medicine and public discourses of health and well-being despite health psychology itself being one of the youngest branches of the discipline.

The assumption that health psychology is positioned *in some relation* to the biomedical model of health (and illness) is at the core of ongoing debates around health psychology. Is it the case that disease and illness originates from outside the body or from an involuntary physical change within the body? Is the body a biological entity whereby health and illness are outside a person's control? Are the human body and mind integrated in ways that an interaction between them has an impact upon health and well-being? Does health have a contextual meaning?

'Internal' critics, such as Kerry Chamberlain, suggest that health psychology (academically and professionally) could have achieved more than simply challenging the mind–body split. He believes that health psychology has been too willing to take up medical agendas preferring to focus upon how psychological issues can be understood in relation to treatments of, and coping with, illness rather than challenging the hegemony of the medical model (Workman, 2011). Chamberlain, and other *critical* health psychologists (HPs) (Nicolson, 2003a), argue that a critical HP has the potential, and possibly the responsibility, to question the underlying ideologies of health, illness and medical practice, working towards a community health psychology with a radical agenda to improve the experience of public well-being including access to health information and care (Campbell and Murray, 2004; Hutton, 2011)

In this chapter therefore I outline what health psychology is (or at least how it might be understood), and provide a brief account of its genesis and the recent changes in regulation and training in the UK. I then consider the role of critical and community health psychology in the present-day theory, research and practitioner 'mix', accompanied by a case example based around my own work.

WHAT IS HEALTH PSYCHOLOGY?

It was the psychiatrist George Engel (Engel, 1977) who first introduced the argument for a biopsychosocial model of health and illness, incorporating biological, social, cultural and behavioural factors, thereby challenging the dominant biomedical model. However, the contemporary origins of health psychology as a distinct enterprise are mostly traced back to a paper by Matarazzo (1980) following a review by a task force of the American Psychological Association (APA). Matarazzo saw a future for health psychology as a discipline involved in research and professional practice with the potential to explain, maintain, treat and promote health specifically acknowledging the role of the mind in the cause and reduction of physical ill health. This differed from clinical psychology, where the focus was mostly on psychological aspects of mental illness. Some of the first practitioner HPs were clinical psychologists who identified themselves as clinical HPs working with patients suffering from emotional trauma, depression or distress following injury or illness.

In the UK, as health psychology moved from 'infancy' to 'adolescence', David Marks was one of the first to shine the light on the subdiscipline's development, suggesting the time had come for its own theories to move health psychology away from (mostly) cognitive psychology and reliance on its inter-relation to the medical model (Marks, 1996).

Becoming an HP

As an applied, professional branch of psychology the route to becoming qualified is regulated academically by the BPS and professionally by the HPC.

The BPS, who regulated British health psychology practice until 2009, set out the original disciplinary aims and now focus more on the means of becoming a health psychologist.[1] The aim of health psychology, they suggest, is broadly to study scientifically the psychological processes of health, illness and health care, and apply psychology to the promotion and maintenance of health, the analysis and improvement of the health care system and health policy formation, and the enhancement of well-being in those affected by illness or disability. It is secondly to develop professional skills in research, consultancy and teaching/training. The Health Professions Council (HPC), the regulatory body, sets out the aims and responsibilities in detail.

The APA (Division 38/HP) similarly stated:

> The Division of Health Psychology of the American Psychological Association (APA) facilitates collaboration among psychologists interested in the psychological and behavioral aspects of physical and mental health. We are committed to providing information about current practice and research, and connecting our members and creating opportunities for professional growth. Through our professional meetings and publications, we bring further focus on quality research to inform clinical practice.[2]

In other words, in both the USA and the UK, health psychology is at heart an applied subdiscipline of academic psychology and psychological practice drawing upon a recognised evidence base, reinforcing the point that HPs need research and evaluation as well as therapeutic/consultancy skills.

Before explaining the contemporary process of regulation and registration of HPs I present a case study of my own career in health psychology by way of the BPS 'grandparent' route.

CASE STUDY

Reflections of a critical HP

I became a full member of the BPS Division of Health Psychology, based upon the topic and methods of my PhD – a study of postnatal depression. When the opportunities arose I registered as a Chartered Health Psychologist (then CPsychol Health) and am now a Chartered Psychologist (CPsychol) but registered as a Practitioner Health Psychologist with the HPC.

This process initially took place through what was lovingly called the 'grandparent' route, a time-limited transitional period during which full members of the BPS could submit their qualifications for scrutiny. At the time most of us who took that path were academics doing research and teaching in the area, but who sometimes undertook consultancy in health care settings. I doubt many were employed as HPs by the NHS then unless they were from a background of accredited clinical psychology training, specialising in working with physical rather than mental health issues.

---

[1]http://www.bps.org.uk/careers-education-training/how-become-psychologist/types-psychologists/becoming-health-psychologis-0

[2]http://www.health-psych.org/AboutWhatWeDo.cfm

I recall in particular, from the earlier days of the specialism, hearing feedback from Louise Wallace, commissioned by the BPS (Wallace, 2000) to look at the careers of those who had taken master's degrees in health psychology, which she presented then as having a gloomy outlook. There was rarely a role labelled HP in the NHS or pharmaceutical companies, who might be thought of as the obvious employers. The master's graduates could be found working in research and development or in health service management and occasionally as internal consultants in the NHS. The majority of those in the Division were academics working on health-related topics. Walsh and McDermott provide a brief overview of the subsequent directions in which non-academics and some academics moved – public health psychology, health policy, outcomes research or further training in clinical or counselling psychology were among the favoured options (Walsh and McDermott, 2003).

For me (as with others, I suspect) health psychology was serendipitous. My PhD on postnatal depression was meant as a challenge to the traditional psychological and psychiatric model of women's reproductive health. I certainly did not see a potential for health psychology (in its infancy at the time) although gradually I found that as a non-clinician it became difficult to position myself in any influential way, nor was it easy to secure research funding, until I became involved in health-services research (HSR) around 1994. Although I found the pragmatism and multidisciplinary focus of HSR off-putting at first, I had found myself a niche from where I could develop ideas.

Psychologists involved in HSR were mostly drawn from those who broadly accepted the medical model, and adopted a quantitative approach to their work. In the early days of my involvement I experienced the ire of one such psychologist who believed my proposed in-depth interviews and focus groups were a waste of money; she literally screamed this at me in front of a room full of medical researchers, statisticians and health economists – some of whom were a lot more sympathetic to my work than she was.

Through persisting in my involvement in HSR I gained opportunities to do other things – collect in-depth interview and focus group data from patients and health care staff. It then became possible to find a place for qualitative data to accompany information about clinical and economic effectiveness. This was at the time described as 'unintended consequences' of cost or clinically efficient systems or as supporting data to measures of health status and quality of life. But there was far more to the work I did than that.

Pharmaceutical companies began to realise the potential of the human stories behind chronic illness, and I conducted studies of chronic bronchitis (Nicolson and Anderson, 2003), overactive bladder (Nicolson et al., 2008) and multiple sclerosis (Nicolson and Anderson, 2001) that also became the focus of health campaigns. I still recall that some participants in the study of chronic bronchitis who had volunteered to participate in a public relations campaign were discovered by the back door of the British Medical Association building, smoking. What they told me later was that smoking was one of their few remaining pleasures.

As part of my work I interviewed many senior medical and nursing professionals who had become managers. They frequently told stories of work stresses and anxieties that were not necessarily part of the story I was seeking. One man for example told me how he had been looking forward to the visit from the 'psychologist', as there were things worrying him about the pressure of work, the strain on his marriage and his fear that if he failed to seek further promotion he would be letting his parents down (Nicolson, 2003b). Another told me of how, following his return to work after a serious operation, he felt diminished and that he was unable to admit this even to his family but that it was affecting his performance. Another told of how she could not sleep for fear of being removed from her post if a junior colleague were to make a mistake – something that had happened to some of her contemporaries.

I was struck by all of this 'peripheral' information in two ways. Why were these highly competent and senior people keeping so much anxiety to themselves? What did it say about the health of the health carers and the systems they worked in? What was it about me in my role as a researcher and psychologist that made them tell *me* these important 'secrets'?

As a consequence of this I trained as an organisational consultant at the Tavistock Centre at the Tavistock and Portman NHS Foundation Trust. It is probably unnecessary to say that this qualified me to take a psychoanalytic and systemic approach to role consultancy, coaching and working with groups and organisations, and as a registered practitioner HP I run reflective groups for managers and other staff as well as seeing people individually to help them consider their own relationships and positions in their organisations.

REGULATION OF HEALTH PSYCHOLOGY

The regulatory process has changed dramatically in recent years. Health psychology was granted Divisional status by the BPS in 1997 (Walsh and McDermott, 2003). This provided recognition that this area of knowledge underpinned a clearly defined application of psychology with acknowledged professional and academic standards.

Until 2009 the BPS had been the only regulating body for Chartered Health Psychologists in both public and private practices. Now regulation of practice is by the HPC, who also regulate other 'allied' health professions. Thus, since 2009 the title Chartered Health Psychologist was replaced by that of Registered Practitioner Psychologist (Health Psychology), although 'Chartered Psychologist' may also be used if the HP is a BPS member recognised to have chartered status.

Although this move to regulation by the HPC has in many ways been unpopular within the discipline, and reduced the role and influence of the BPS in certain ways, it has also strengthened the professional identity and career opportunities for HPs working in health care settings. The HPC is more specific in its rules than the BPS had been although the objectives are similar. Under the HPC rules HPs need to be able to plan, design and deliver teaching and training, support the learning of others and plan and implement assessment and training programmes. To do this they are expected to be able to use standardised psychometric tests, conduct interviews and develop appropriate psychological assessments based on an appraisal of the influence of the social context. Health psychologists are expected to have the skills to develop psychological formulations drawing on theory, research and explanatory models. Finally HPs need to be able to critically evaluate models of behaviour change and develop effective interventions to promote well-being and engage in consultancy and service delivery (HPC, 2009).

The BPS still regulates and accredits HP *academic* training programmes in the UK in partnership with the HPC. It has also taken on a role to promote the profession.[3] In March 2011 the BPS produced leaflets and PowerPoint presentations generally available to members of the Division of Health Psychology (DHP) members to enable them to inform employers, employees, potential students and members of the public about health psychology.

To qualify requires training to at least master's level followed by staged and supervised practice. An accredited MSc in Health Psychology equates with Stage 1 training, having ensured the student admitted to the programme has the basic requirements for graduate recognition. The BPS requires that core modules cover topics such as psychological research methods, psychology and health, biopsychosocial aspects of health and illness, disabilities and health inequalities. Programmes also have optional modules, which include a range of related areas such as introduction to psychological therapies, communication skills, chronic illness, stress and anxiety, health care organisations, critical approaches, gender and health, and advanced research and evaluation methods (there are others depending on relevant staff specialisations) (Walsh and McDermott, 2003).

These courses are taught and examined through a mixture of course work, written unseen examinations and a dissertation demonstrating research capability. Programmes vary in some of the detail but not substantively in the content. The dissertation carries a high proportion of the final marks.

Professional doctorates in health psychology include both Stages 1 and 2, the latter focusing on supervised practice in an 'appropriate' supervised health setting that is assessed by a portfolio of practice. Students are called 'trainees', similar to those training in clinical psychology. City University assessment requirements for example include:

- a supervision log;
- a supplementary report summarising the practice and supervision log (3,000 words);
- a research thesis (40,000 words);
- a systematic review (6,000 words);
- and four case studies (approximately 3,000 words each) with relevant appendices.

The academic work for the professional doctorate is clearly intellectually demanding and the trainee has to demonstrate the ability not only to practise effectively to a high

[3]http://bps.org.uk/dhp/php/php_home.cfm

standard but also to record and reflect on their practice. Further the thesis demands a high level of research capability and commitment. Ultimately, the qualified HP has also demonstrated sustained professional development, practiced implementing interventions, and has a clear grasp of research skills including systematic reviews, development and use of questionnaires, surveys and interviews, and consultancy skills.

RESEARCH AND HEALTH PSYCHOLOGY

Mainstream health psychology research concerns itself with the relationship between psychological well-being and biological health. This work is now well-established in the UK, Europe and North America as an applied professional branch of psychological practice with a recognised place in undergraduate and postgraduate education. There are also regular conferences supported by bodies such as the BPS Division of Health Psychology, the European Health Psychology Society and Division 38 of the APA. There are also biennial meetings of the International Society of Critical Health Psychology (ISCHP).

Health psychology is also an increasingly important area of applied research, brought closer to the spotlight through formal funding initiatives, such as those in the UK proposed by the Economic and Social Research Council (ESRC). Until recently health and well-being were specifically identified as priority areas for funding. However, health psychology remains part of the ESRC's overall strategic plan within their initiative on influencing behaviour and informing interventions.[4] The National Institute for Health Research (NIHR), however, has been strengthened to provide a broad brief covering health technologies (i.e. interventions in health care ranging from psychotherapy to interventions with drugs or equipment such as magnetic resonance imaging (MRI) scanners) and service delivery and organisation.[5] The aim of these funding streams is to identify and evaluate means of ensuring public health, well-being and effective and beneficial health care delivery.

It is only relatively recently that health psychology (research and practice) as such has been accepted as a core approach to the study of well-being. This follows the recognition of the growing body of empirical evidence of the role that psychological factors play in understanding patients suffering from chronic pain (Hoffman et al., 2007) or chronic ill health such as multiple sclerosis (P. Nicolson and Anderson, 2003), chronic bronchitis (P. Nicolson and Anderson, 2000) or diabetes (Macrodimitris and Endler, 2001), or measuring quality of life and health status (Bradley, 2001). Furthermore, psychologists have involved themselves in multidisciplinary research projects working with medical academics, epidemiologists, medical statisticians and health economists in particular, and although this was initially 'broad brush' psychology applied to HSR, rather than health psychology *per se*, increasingly there is

---

[4]http://www.esrc.ac.uk/about-esrc/what-we-do/mission-strategy-priorities/refining-priorities/influencing-behaviour.aspx

[5]http://www.ccf.nihr.ac.uk/PGfAR/Pages/Home.aspx

acknowledgement of a distinct health psychology similar to the previous recognition of *health* economics and *medical* statistics.

Examples of health psychology research

The well-defined flavour of health psychology over and above HSR research includes the following areas.

- The exploration of causation and the development and evaluation of interventions to change unhealthy behaviours such as obesity, anorexia/bulimia, drug and alcohol abuse, smoking and unprotected sex in the face of HIV/AIDS (e.g. Adams and Neville, 2009; Jeffery et al., 2000; Mulveen and Hepworth, 2006; Vanable et al., 2000; West et al., 2000).

- Understanding the impact of anxiety and stress at work, particularly pertinent for thinking about the psychological strains on health care providers (Lokman et al., 2011).

- Work–life balance (Cooper, 2003).

- The organisation of health care institutions and how that has an impact on staff well-being and the delivery of patient care (Michie and West, 2004; Nicolson et al., 2011).

CASE EXAMPLE

Chronic bronchitis

This study conducted by myself and Pippa Anderson (a health economist) was funded by a pharmaceutical company and published in the *British Journal of Health Psychology* – as well as in medically oriented journals (Nicolson and Anderson, 2000, 2003). The task set by the funder was to discover how sufferers of chronic bronchitis coped with exacerbations of the illness. All sufferers of chronic obstructive pulmonary diseases (COPD), of which chronic bronchitis is one, experience shortness of breath most of the time, which severely limits their capacity for physical exertion of any sort. This includes walking any distance, climbing stairs, carrying shopping, gentle gardening and many everyday activities that most of us take for granted. In some cases even carrying babies or picking up toddlers is very difficult. During an exacerbation the person would find it almost impossible to move because their lungs were so restricted by congestion. Most would be prescribed strong antibiotics, and the pharmaceutical companies were always bringing new versions on the market.

However, although psychologists had collected quantitative information on quality of life and COPD, there was very little information on what it was actually like to live with this type of disease. Thus we were commissioned to collect in-depth data from those who suffered. As you will see from the paper, we set up focus groups and, in co-operation with local GPs, ran them in Glasgow (known for high levels of COPD – often associated with poverty, smoking and social exclusion) and Sheffield (parts of which comprised a similar population).

We found distressing evidence from elderly and surprisingly young people – young parents – of the way their lives and potential were constrained, and with the heartbreak of not being able to be active parents and grandparents in particular. We also identified a contradictory relationship to smoking. Stopping smoking does reduce the level and frequency of exacerbations and improves general well-being in this population. However, the sufferers who were unable to stop said they felt a cigarette cleared and 'disinfected' their lungs. This is not the case, of course, but some respondents thought this was important information. Also it was clear that long-term smokers did stop when a doctor told them it was 'Stop smoking or die a painful death'.

As part of the study a film was made for doctors using interviews with some of the respondents, and a study day was set up at the headquarters of the British Medical Association that some of the respondents addressed.

CRITICAL HEALTH PSYCHOLOGY

Whereas some commentators had identified health psychology as a potentially radical project extending the scope of investigation of health and illness beyond that of bio-medicine, others continue to charge it with being deeply conservative and merely adding 'psychology' to a model of health and illness. Michael Murray expresses this well:

> The advent of health psychology, less than 30 years ago, offered much promise. It was heralded as an opportunity for psychology to expand our understanding of the experience of health and illness and to contribute to the great task of improving the health of society. In the eager rush to establish its credentials this new sub-discipline largely adopted the theories, methods and disciplining techniques of its parent discipline. (Murray, 2004: 1)

Over the past thirty years the position of mainstream, traditional, positivist academic psychology as the sole scientific evidence base to the discipline has been challenged, and this challenge applies to health psychology as much as any other academic or applied branch of the discipline. The emergence of methods using a variety of qualitative, textual or word-based data sets such as narrative psychology (Murray, 2000), grounded theory (Chamberlain et al., 2003), thematic analysis (Braun and Clarke, 2006) and phenomenology and discourse analysis (Kugelmann, 2003; Willig, 2000) have demonstrated in different ways that there is more to knowledge and evidence than objective, observable 'facts' and there is more to the practice of health care than complementing the biomedical model. The importance of context, such as the psychosocial and historical–political, potentially opens up thinking about what constitutes well-being, whose account is prioritised, or what health 'means' for practitioners who want to promote the well-being of individuals and populations.

The development of 'community' psychology has gone some way towards putting a critical perspective into practice to work with communities to combat inequalities and promote health through collective action (Campbell and Murray, 2004). Jennifer Hutton proposed that the nature of the health care organisation makes a difference to the health psychology service offered. She describes how her move from the NHS to Lanarkshire Council meant that she was in a position to advance the health of the community by promoting 'mental flourishing' for the population from infancy to older age (Hutton, 2011).

Feminist psychology also played an important role in challenging 'whose knowledge counts?' about the psychology of women's health particularly in the areas of reproductive (see Brown Travis and Compton, 2001; Ussher, 2003; Ussher and Perz, 2008) and family health, including domestic violence and abuse (Nicolson, 2010). In many cases there is an overlap between critical health psychology and sociology (Fox et al., 2005) that returns us full circle to Marks' plea for health psychology to consider the nature of its interdisciplinarity (Marks, 1996).

CASE EXAMPLE

Leadership: a critical psychodynamic–systemic health psychology

This was a major study funded by the NHS National Institute for Health Research as part of the Service Delivery and Organisation funding stream (Nicolson et al., 2011). Although there were (among the very many) qualitative and mixed-method studies of leadership (Alvesson, 1992; Balkundi and Kilduff, 2005), critical ones were less frequent (Bryman, 2004; Ford, 2010). Our study did involve using an organisational climate questionnaire, but we also used ethnographic observation, ethnographic 'shadowing', in-depth interviews and focus groups (see Figures 7.1 and 7.2). The data were analysed using a psychodynamic–systemic framework – with reference to social constructionist ideas as well – not common in this type of work. Subsequent presentations to various NHS senior clinicians and managers received mixed receptions. At that level the NHS staff tend to be interested in results that tell them how to do something rather than make them think about what is going on. Boiling down three-and-a-half years of work to a sentence, we found that leaders exercising emotional intelligence were most effective in keeping up staff morale and implementing change, but those with no emotional intelligence had major difficulties managing staff.

I became 'enchanted' by the use of ethnographic methods for exploring social interactions in depth and particularly noted how these methods exposed the behaviours underneath the interview data (good and bad). Also, using psychoanalysis as a means of data analysis replicated how anxiety saturates the everyday lives of clinicians – even, and probably especially, those trained to distance themselves from emotional involvement with patients (Lokman et al., 2011). The details of the methods we used and the analysis can be found online.[6]

---

[6]http://www.netscc.ac.uk/hsdr/projdetails.php?ref=08-1601-137

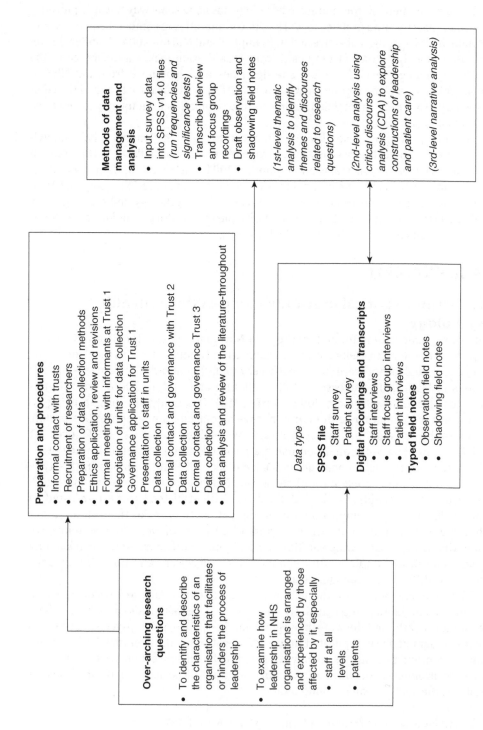

Preparation and procedures
- Informal contact with trusts
- Recruitment of researchers
- Preparation of data collection methods
- Ethics application, review and revisions
- Formal meetings with informants at Trust 1
- Negotiation of units for data collection
- Governance application for Trust 1
- Presentation to staff in units
- Data collection
- Formal contact and governance with Trust 2
- Data collection
- Formal contact and governance Trust 3
- Data collection
- Data analysis and review of the literature–throughout

Over-arching research questions
- To identify and describe the characteristics of an organisation that facilitates or hinders the process of leadership
- To examine how leadership in NHS organisations is arranged and experienced by those affected by it, especially
  - staff at all levels
  - patients

Data type

SPSS file
- Staff survey
- Patient survey

Digital recordings and transcripts
- Staff interviews
- Staff focus group interviews
- Patient interviews

Typed field notes
- Observation field notes
- Shadowing field notes

Methods of data management and analysis
- Input survey data into SPSS v14.0 files *(run frequencies and significance tests)*
- Transcribe interview and focus group recordings
- Draft observation and shadowing field notes

(1st-level thematic analysis to identify themes and discourses related to research questions)

(2nd-level analysis using critical discourse analysis (CDA) to explore constructions of leadership and patient care)

(3rd-level narrative analysis)

Figure 7.1 Outline of study procedures and methods

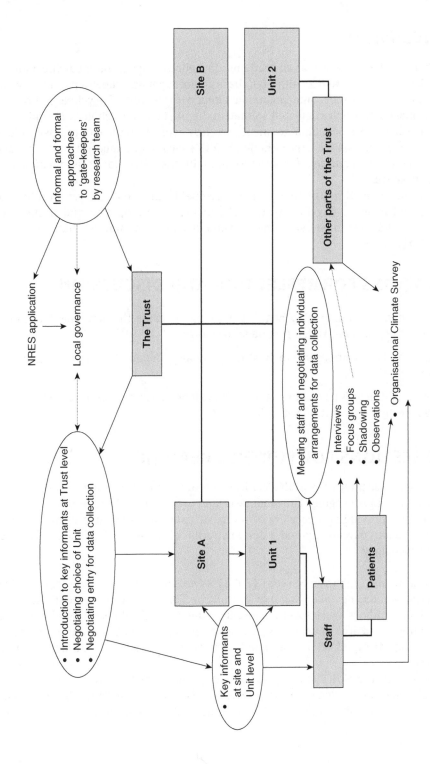

Figure 7.2 'Access pathways', sampling procedure and data-collection process

CONCLUSION

Health psychology emerged as an academic discipline alongside biomedicine with the potential for radical practice. Although the academic agenda of health psychology has broadened, it has also become 'polarised' along with the rest of psychology. Practice has become increasingly regulated so that, in the UK, health psychology is equivalent to a health profession allied to medicine. However, as with clinical psychology this shift in regulation has strengthened health psychology's identity and expanded employment opportunities for practitioners in the NHS, local authorities and private practice.

Training in health psychology has become formalised – corresponding to clinical and forensic psychology training in the duration, type and number of assessment hurdles to be overcome – although salaries do not yet match those of clinical psychology.

QUESTIONS FOR REFLECTION AND DISCUSSION

1   How far has contemporary health psychology become the 'handmaiden' to the medical profession? And does it need to change?

2   Might a critical approach to health psychology benefit the well-being of the population?

3   How might health psychology and HSR evidence become integrated into health practice and organisational development?

SUGGESTIONS FOR FURTHER READING

As my particular interest is at the 'critical' end of health psychology I would recommend some of the engaging critical material and in particular three sets of edited collections that provide an overview of the basic concepts, a critique of mainstream academic health psychology and a demonstration of the breadth of focus of critical health psychology.

Horrocks, C. and Johnson, S. (eds) (2012) *Advances in Health Psychology: Critical Approaches*. Basingstoke: Palgrave Macmillian. This book brings practitioners and academic authors' work together, emphasising that critical health psychology is a growing, broad area of health psychology focusing on the contemporary concerns in the age of rapidly changing health care delivery structures and demographic changes.

Marks, D.F., Murray, M.P., Evans, B., Willig, C., Woodall, C. and Sykes, C.M. (2005) *Health Psychology: Theory, Research and Practice* (2nd edn). London: Sage. This edited collection is a companion to Marks' edited reader (2002b) and contains chapters from all contemporary health psychology perspectives and from most of the major authors in the field.

Murray, M. and Chamberlain, K. (1999) *Qualitative Health Psychology: Theories and Methods*. London: Sage. This volume demonstrates how the concepts, theories and epistemologies are inseparable so that critical health psychology is by definition best understood through a qualitative lens. Each chapter examines different ways of conceptualising, collecting and analysing data. There are examples of feminist health psychology, Foucauldian discourse analysis, material-discursive understandings, grounded theory, and story-telling and narrative accounts of health, illness and well-being.

8

MARKETING PSYCHOLOGY

Chris Hackley

This chapter discusses:

- how psychological theory has been applied in marketing practice and research;

- to what extent psychological approaches to understanding marketing are viable;

- whether the contribution of psychology to marketing is fully acknowledged;

- how psychology graduates might apply their knowledge in careers in marketing, advertising and management.

INTRODUCTION

There are relatively few designated psychology roles or structured career development programmes for psychology graduates in marketing. Yet virtually all professional marketing roles would benefit from psychological knowledge and skills. In this chapter I will discuss the role of psychology in marketing from a broad perspective, in order to outline the kinds of career in marketing a psychology graduate might aspire to, whether or not psychological knowledge is explicitly seen as an element of the job role. There are many varieties of professional career in marketing, and the chapter will outline some of these in order to point to the very wide relevance of psychology in the field. I will also mention some of the reasons why psychology, as a knowledge base informing marketing techniques and strategies, has a controversial history in marketing. It is important that psychology graduates who are considering a career in marketing understand the sensitivity that can surround the use of psychological science in marketing, as well as its potential for informing management decisions and improving marketing effectiveness. Finally, the chapter will discuss the nature of day-to-day work in two marketing roles in which psychology graduates are most often found – market research and advertising.

THE RELEVANCE OF PSYCHOLOGY IN MARKETING

Marketing is an extremely broad and varied field with many professional designations. It involves communication and persuasion, among many other things, and therefore often operates at a psychological level. For example, advertising design and planning, package design, pricing, marketing strategy development, marketing metrics analysis, merchandising and in-store displays, contract negotiation, product design, sales promotion, brand strategy, personal selling and service operations, not to mention activities in allied fields such as public relations, media planning and industrial marketing, all have their psychological elements. Marketing operates psychologically at the level of the individual, and also of the group. Marketing initiatives seek to gain consumers' attention, to exploit biases in perception, to embed brands and brand 'values' into short- and long-term memory, to link brands with reference groups, and, through mass communication, to change attitudes and behaviour in particular contexts (Box 8.1). The psychologies of group influence, social learning, cognition, reasoning and decision-making, communication, identity and self-perception all seem particularly relevant to marketing. It is not an overstatement to say that, in a broad sense, marketing could be conceived as a branch of applied psychology. Today, the extent of psychological research in marketing practice is seen in the pursuit of 'neuro marketing', by using neuropsychological techniques to try to reveal the physio-psychological bases of choice, attitude and preference.

Box 8.1   A selection of marketing tasks with implicit psychological elements

- Advertising (creative/copywriting and planning)
- Brand planning
- Package design
- Pricing
- Market and consumer research
- Merchandising, store design
- Strategic marketing planning
- Product design
- Sales promotion
- Public relations

(Continued)

(Continued)

- Personal selling

- Product placement and promotion

- 'Neuromarketing' neuropsychology

Since there are so few designated, specialist psychological roles in marketing, psychology graduates interested in marketing often gravitate towards careers that use their research skills, most obviously in the marketing and consumer research functions that underpin and inter-penetrate all organisational marketing activities. Aspects of these roles will be discussed in greater detail later in the chapter. Psychological knowledge could, then, be useful in any area of marketing, while marketing itself is a field that enjoys a huge scope of activity.

THE SCOPE OF MARKETING

Marketing textbooks are fond of asserting that marketing is not only the job of marketing professionals but also of many other staff in an organisation, sometimes called 'part-time' marketers (Gummesson, 1991), all of whom have a role in applying marketing as an organisational philosophy that places the customer at the heart of the organisation's activities and its purpose (Drucker, 1954). These roles can include any 'front line' service personnel who interact with customers, people with internal marketing responsibility who deliver services within the organisation, or indeed any employee whose decisions and actions have an impact on the external presentation of the organisation. As a consequence, defining just exactly who the marketing professional is, is by no means clear cut. Besides the specialist subfields of marketing, many marketing management careers in organisations entail general management skills such as analysing, communicating, presenting, writing reports, commissioning research, building and working in teams, enlisting support and advocating – all skills that psychology graduates should have. Psychology graduates with a postgraduate management qualification, in particular, have a potent combination of knowledge and skills they can potentially apply in virtually any area of marketing and general management.

MARKETING ROLES IN NON-PROFIT SECTORS

As if this was not complicated enough, a further issue in designating marketing careers is that, since the concept of marketing was broadened to include non-profit, charitable and public sector organisations (Kotler and Levy, 1969), a marketing professional's scope of responsibility may encompass not only commercial transactions and relationships, but public service and charity work. The vocabulary of marketing has reached well beyond the commercial world, to the extent that it is hard to think of a job role in either the public or private sectors in which employees are not enjoined to apply a market rationality to the service of customers. As one mass-selling marketing textbook proclaims, 'We are all customers now' (Hackley, 2003a). But, if one can get past marketing's over-use of hyperbolic clichés, the idea of using one's psychological knowledge in a marketing career is not necessarily a matter of opting for superficiality over substance, nor of putting profit before people. Many marketing academics would sincerely argue that better marketing brings increases in general social welfare through more efficient organisations and (therefore) more effective use of resources, more competitive markets (and more competitive prices), and greater consumer choice and convenience, so effective marketing adds to the general quality of life. For the ethically engaged, most major charitable bodies now have marketing directors (often recruited from the commercial sector) running established marketing departments. Along with museums, LA (local authority) services, universities and other public sector organisations that have to compete both for public funds and private revenue, most charities have developed dedicated marketing departments over the past twenty years. Having a heart, or indeed a brain, does not necessarily disqualify one from a marketing career.

LACK OF RECOGNITION FOR PSYCHOLOGY IN MARKETING

The legitimate scope of the marketing discipline might well be exaggerated by its proponents (e.g. Hackley, 2009) but it is hard to deny, first, that there is enormous variety in the number of marketing and marketing-related careers now available, and second, that psychological knowledge and skills are highly relevant for these careers. Now we can turn to the question of exactly why, when so much of marketing seems inherently psychological, so few marketing roles are designated as psychological roles. This question seems even more perplexing when one considers that some academic marketing disciplines, which supposedly reflect marketing practice, have been directly influenced by psychology paradigms (Foxall, 1997). For example, according to many university marketing management courses, consumers 'behave' in response to environmental stimuli, internal traits and dispositions in the 'black box' of cognition (e.g. Bagozzi et al, 2002; Engel et al., 2000). What is more, many marketing academics apply psychological paradigms to their research, and publish in psychology journals. Yet the number of careers within professional marketing that are designated as consumer psychology remain relatively few.

There may be two main reasons for the lack of explicit recognition of the value of psychology in marketing. One is that, in spite of its status as a major subject of university teaching and research, marketing practice is not based on an agreed set of research-based principles, knowledge of which is enforced through professional certification. There is no requirement for marketing professionals to be professionally qualified or certified, and many would assert that common sense and experience are all one needs to work in marketing. Marketing does have professional bodies, lots of them. The (UK) Chartered Institute of Marketing (CIM), and the American Marketing Association are probably the two biggest general marketing associations, with membership in many scores of thousands. They provide professional development courses and, in the case of the CIM, structured educational programmes for enhancing professional knowledge and skills, so that members can attain Chartered Marketer status. Each marketing subfield has its own trade and professional associations, such as the Institute for Practitioners in Advertising (widely known as the IPA), the Market Research Society (MRS) and the Institute of Direct Marketing (IDM). Each has a system of professional registration and qualifications, and membership for marketing professionals is common, but by no means compulsory. But in spite of the professional associations in the field, the role of professional knowledge in marketing, and in particular its status as a discipline informed by social science, is contested in practice. Professionals in marketing have many different educational backgrounds; there are trained engineers, chemists and maths graduates, as well as literature, geography, psychology graduates and many more. Many non-graduates work in marketing as well. So there is a striking lack of common grounding in education or practical principles.

MARKETING – THE DARK ART?

A second reason for the relative lack of recognition for psychology in marketing professions, probably connected to the first, is that marketing's role as an art and science of persuasion has sometimes raised public disquiet and suspicion for its apparently low standards of ethics. The idea, in particular, that psychological science is being deployed to persuade consumers to buy things we do not need is particularly sensitive. I will discuss this further below. Finally, a third reason may be to do with the institutional politics of universities. Marketing has had to fight for space as an independent university discipline and, perhaps, tends to play down its own reliance on theories from other branches of social science. Academic research in marketing is said to have developed from roots in microeconomics and economic history (Hackley, 2009), but contemporary research in the area makes use of theories, concepts and methods from sociology, statistics, econometrics and anthropology, in as well as from psychology (Box 8.2).

Box 8.2   Marketing's informing social sciences

- Microeconomics (e.g. utility, rationality, demand elasticity).

- Psychology (e.g. consumer needs and wants, motivation, attitudes, attention, affect, decisions, behaviour).

- Sociology (e.g. socio-economic groups, class, segmentation).

- Anthropology (e.g. brand symbolism, status, consumer ritual).

Given the contested place of social science in general, and of psychology in particular, in marketing research and practice, it might be helpful to look briefly at the role psychology has played in the development of marketing, before looking more closely at a selection of marketing careers that may particularly fit the skills and knowledge of psychology graduates.

PSYCHOLOGY IN MARKETING – SOME HIGHLIGHTS AND LOWLIGHTS

The centrality of psychology to marketing may seem self-evident, yet, as I have noted, marketing as a profession has been slow to explicitly acknowledge its value. The role of psychological skills and knowledge in marketing is political, sensitive and sometimes controversial. This section will outline something of the problematic history of psychology in marketing in order to contextualise the ways in which psychological roles are played out in the marketing field.

Perhaps of all the management disciplines, marketing has made most use of psychology – if sometimes it has been misguided or self-serving, or both. For example, Abraham Maslow's hierarchy-of-needs theory is shamelessly misapplied in practically every introductory marketing textbook (Hackley, 2007). Maslow would, no doubt, have been grimly amused at the irony of having his humanistic theory of self-realisation presented as a rationale for a consumption-dominated lifestyle. No doubt many marketing authors found his ideas useful for lending a sheen of intellectual credibility to their prescriptive aphorisms. Advertising agencies have been particularly enthusiastic in using Maslow's hierarchy to categorise consumers. In another example of marketing pseudo-psychology, advertisers even invented their own version of psychometrics, called psychographics, to 'segment' consumers into stereotyped groups according to their attitudes and lifestyle, the more easily to target and sell to them. The technique is sensible enough – it involves collating demographic, economic and attitudinal information on consumers for the purpose of categorising them. The categories are then spiced up with acronyms: DINKIES (dual income no kids) or YUPPIES (young upwardly mobile professionals) are among the more well-known categories. But the psychology of psychographics is less than robust. It must be admitted that not all uses of psychology in marketing have been quite so self-serving. For example, a small number of studies have looked at the psychological downsides of marketing, for example with respect to addictive consumption (Elliott, 1994). But psychology has typically been used to try to help managers sell us more stuff.

BEHAVIOURISM AND THE MAD MEN

John B. Watson (1924) is possibly the most well-known psychologist to turn his scientific knowledge to the dark art of persuasion, though he certainly was not the last. Watson enjoyed a successful career as an advertising man with JWT after his academic career as a psychology professor ended, applying his theory of behaviourism to the promotion of Pond's cold cream and other famous brands (Bogart, 1966). Watson's career was touched by controversy, not least over his notorious encounter with baby 'Little Albert', a story that should be familiar to psychology students. Watson came up with a telling experiment to illustrate operant conditioning. The eponymous baby seemed quite fond of Watson's white rat, that is, until Watson conditioned poor Albert to regard the rat with terror by making a loud frightening noise every time the rat appeared. It has been said that, at the time, there was more public outcry about the treatment of the rat than of the baby. But Watson's attempts to eliminate cognition from psychology attracted more criticism as the years passed. Nonetheless, his work on behavioural conditioning still resonates when we see advertising that is repetitive, brash, direct and annoying, but impossible to ignore. Perhaps, there is indeed an element of conditioning in the mundane, everyday purchases that we make because our critical faculties have disintegrated under the welter of banal but repetitive advertising. When was the last time you ate at McDonald's? Did you even notice what it tasted like? The influence of behaviourism remains strong in marketing not only as an implicit but under-acknowledged presence in much consumer behaviour theory, but also as an explicit research agenda (e.g. Foxall, 2000).

In the early part of the century there were attempts to draw on psychology to create theories of personal selling. Books like Edward Strong's (1929) *The Psychology of Selling* and Harry D. Kitson's (1921) *The Mind of the Buyer* set out a linear sequence of persuasion in successful personal selling as a process of getting the consumer's attention, eliciting interest, provoking desire for the product or service and, finally, generating action in the form of a purchase (see Figure 8.1). These theories were eagerly adopted by the advertising industry and remain highly popular today. American copywriter John E. Kennedy (1924), working at the famous Lord and Thomas agency, decided that advertising ought to be 'salesmanship in print' and adapted the linear model of persuasion for mass media (known today in basic marketing textbooks by its acronym of AIDA). Kennedy's assumption that the psychology of mass communication is the same as that of personal communication remains influential in mass communication theory and in 'hierarchy-of-effects' advertising theory (Hackley, 2010a). Kennedy was most famous for his 'reason why' approach to advertising strategy, which advocated a straightforward, rational approach to persuasion, focusing on the benefits of purchase (Fox, 1984). Kennedy's 'reason why' idea was reinvented as the 'unique selling proposition' (USP) several decades later by Rosser Reeves (McDonald and Scott, 2007). Reason why and USP, though, played up the consumer's economic rationality. They assumed that we carefully evaluate product features and price and make a reasoned decision when we buy. New marketing theories were to emerge that emphasised the emotional and symbolic elements of the motivation to consume. Of course, these, too, drew heavily on experiential, psychoanalytic and humanistic traditions of psychology.

Exposure to the advertisement ⟶ Attention ⟶ Interest ⟶ Desire ⟶ Action (purchase)

Figure 8.1   Strong's AIDA model of advertising persuasion

MOTIVATION RESEARCH AND PACKARD'S HIDDEN PERSUADERS

Ernest Dichter (1949) pioneered the use of qualitative psychology to focus not on the surface rationality of consumers but on our deeper motivations. Dichter's (1949) genre of 'motivation research' has gone out of fashion but many of its principles can be seen in modern marketing practice in the use of group discussions, observation, depth interviews and projective techniques designed to generate qualitative insights into consumers' subjective experience of brands and consumption. Dichter (1949) seems to have been whitewashed from modern marketing theory (see Tadajewski, 2006), perhaps because the idea that consumers are not necessarily rational, and furthermore that marketers exploit this irrationality, is problematic for the idea of a scientific, and ethical, marketing discipline. The point that consumer motivations can be mood-induced, sexual, symbolic, fantasy-driven and hedonistic is made frequently (see, for example, Levy, 1959; and, later, Hirschman and Holbrook, 1982; Hirschman, 1986; Holbrook and Hirschman, 1982) but academic research in marketing, like research in psychology, remains divided along ontological and epistemological lines. Each enterprise, the 'hard' scientific with its experiments and rigorous statistical analyses, and the humanistic with its qualitative data-sets and ideographic approaches, thrives independently, but inter-penetration of theories and methods is still relatively rare.

The use of science in marketing has been known to raise public suspicion. In 1957 Vance Packard did Dichter's (1949) legacy no favours when he won notoriety by whipping up public hysteria in response to what he saw as the underhand and sinister role of psychological research in marketing, and especially in advertising. In his book *The Hidden Persuaders*, Packard (1957/1984) described the uses of depth interviews, observation, focus groups and experiments to reveal consumers' deep motivations, for exploitation by the rapacious marketing machine. Even children were (and indeed are) subject to this psychic invasion, much to Packard's ire. The idea of subliminal suggestion, through images or sounds broadcast in moving images beneath the threshold of conscious awareness, passed into popular consciousness. Partly as a result of Packard's work, the role of psychology in marketing was inflected with a sense of the unseen and illegitimate use of scientific power (Hackley, 2007). This public suspicion of marketing, especially when it is allied with psychology, remains today.

IMPLICIT ADVERTISING AND PRODUCT PLACEMENT

For example, many people feel that product placement, the inclusion of brands in the plot, scene or script of television (TV) shows, is an inherently deceitful promotional method, and said so when the UK media regulator, Ofcom, proposed to allow it for the first time on UK television. There was a lobby against allowing the practice on UK TV on the grounds that, as an implicit promotion technique, it was regarded as deceitful or manipulative. Notwithstanding worries about the ethics of product placement, since February 2011 UK television companies are now permitted to earn revenue from agreements with companies who pay to have their brands featured in shows. Although 'subliminal' images are not allowed on television, there is ample opportunity for brands to prime television viewing with the ostensibly incidental and contextualised appearance of brands in scenes and scripts. This can indeed be seen to be a subtle and powerful way of normalizing brands as accessories to everyday living and identity production (Hackley, 2010a). Whether the persuasive effect is in fact psychological or sociocultural is open to debate.

CONTEMPORARY PSYCHOLOGICAL RESEARCH IN MARKETING

Today, as noted earlier, the marketing industry has grasped at the idea of neuro-marketing in its pursuit of a science of consumer control. Some major global consumer-goods conglomerates fund their own research programmes using MRI scanners. Drawing on cognitive neuroscience, neuro-marketing investigates how people evaluate factors to make decisions on purchases. Neuroimaging evidence has suggested that distinct neural circuits are involved in the estimation of anticipated gain or loss as a result of purchase or non-purchase and therefore offer a route to predicting purchase decisions more accurately than self-reports (Knutson et al., 2007). In spite of its promise, there is little clear evidence to date of neuro-marketing research findings having a tangible influence on marketing strategies.

The research agenda of many business-school marketing academics also follows an experimental and cognitive psychological paradigm, although equally there are many management and business academics who pursue a consumer research agenda theoretically grounded in the liberal arts and qualitative sociology (Hackley, 2010b; see also Foxall, 1997). In contrast to the pursuit of marketing science, on whatever model of science, many professionals working in the field would keenly assert that practical experience and common sense are far more important than academic psychological knowledge. In advertising, for example, an area where one might think that social scientific knowledge is universally respected, many creative professionals are frank about their disdain for research of any kind (Hackley, 2000; Hackley and Kover, 2007). The intellectual legitimacy of psychology as a source of insight and understanding into marketing phenomena is by no means universally accepted. That is not to say that such knowledge is not sought. Many account planners in advertising agencies have first and sometimes second degrees in psychology. Their job is to be experts in commissioning and interpreting consumer research, both quantitative and qualitative, in order to integrate research-based insights into the creative development of advertising. Yet their insights into consumer culture and behaviour may be rejected outright by the creative professionals (the 'creatives') who often feel that their own creative intuition and informal observation of human behaviour gives them all the understanding they need.

This, in outline, is a snapshot of the peculiar status of psychology in marketing. Intuitively, marketing can be seen as applied psychology in a thoroughgoing and far-reaching way. This commonality between the disciplines is fully acknowledged in academic marketing teaching and research, which draws heavily on psychological methods and theories. Indeed, if one takes a historical and critical perspective on the development of marketing theory, it can be seen that marketing is a magpie of a discipline, taking concepts, theories and methods wholesale from psychology, sociology and anthropology, and often failing to fully contextualise that adaptation. For example, much marketing research into consumer emotion takes metrics and constructs from psychology emotion research and applies it to consumption situations, without necessarily asking whether emotions are culturally constructed and therefore rather different in quality between, say, one's experience of true love, and one's first car. Male readers may not want to reflect for too long on that comparison.

PSYCHOLOGY AND CAREERS IN ADVERTISING AND MARKETING RESEARCH

It is to be hoped that psychology students have not been put off marketing careers by the foregoing. It must be admitted that most people with a psychology training who work in marketing would not recognise Packard's dystopian vision of a culturally dominant psychology discipline slavishly serving big business by cynically manipulating consumers. Marketing is generally much more difficult than that. In any case, although the influence of psychology on marketing theory and practice is great, the corporate goal of scientific control over consumer decision-making seems, to most commentators, as far away as it was in Packard's day. Both science and art can contribute powerful insights to marketing management but neither can eliminate the role of human judgement or sheer luck in the success or failure of marketing interventions.

THE ETHICS OF MARKETING CAREERS

If you still have reservations about the ethics of a career in marketing, consider what the world would look like if all marketing were incompetent, dishonest or destructive. When we buy something, the chances are that it solves a problem for us or brings pleasure. Marketing law in the UK is pretty robust and most things we see advertised do pretty much what they claim. Advanced economies have a sophisticated infrastructure for marketing in common, generating wealth, creating jobs and improving the quality of life. Industries that have highly developed marketing functions are more competitive and more successful, and they can bring many benefits to the local region and to the national economy. In spite of the bad press that marketing often gets, there is a robust integrity to a great deal of practice in the field. Marketing employees are generally sincere and often highly qualified professionals who are fascinated by human behaviour and who feel that their role is worthwhile and important.

For some who gravitate towards the marketing field, its reputation for shadiness, venality and self-indulgence are by no means a deterrent. In fact, some perceive there to be a touch of glamour about marketing careers, conferring a *frisson* of excitement to the idea of being a psychologist of persuasion, a svengali of spin, a 'hidden persuader'. Psychology students seeking marketing careers might be ribbed for turning to the dark side, but for many this might make marketing sound all the more fun. Advertising, in particular, is a source of fascination for its apparent psychological influence. The media portrayals of advertising types as charming, suave, ruthless, devious, brilliant and wealthy mavericks (Hackley and Kover, 2007) is hardly off-putting to the impecunious graduate. There is always room in marketing for a more robust approach to psychology.

CAREERS FOR PSYCHOLOGY GRADUATES IN ADVERTISING

So, having set out the problematic context for psychology in marketing, we can turn to a consideration of the day-to-day work in a selection of marketing roles. I will focus on two areas: advertising and marketing research. It will be useful to outline something of the working practices of advertising before discussing the psychology elements of advertising careers (see also Hackley 2010a for a fuller account of advertising agency roles and processes). It should not be forgotten, though, that advertising is a small sector and there are many other opportunities in similar roles working for media agencies, digital agencies, direct marketing, public relations and sales promotion agencies, to name a few.

If you watch the TV show *Mad Men*, you might already have an idea about agency life. But things are not really like that any more. Ad agencies today tend to be relaxed but businesslike places, fun but also driven and goal-oriented. Suits and ties are optional in most UK agencies – the culture of an agency can be very different, and far more formal, in other countries. Advertising is designed by a team working in close co-operation. The days when a star creative ran the whole show and made key strategic decisions on impulse are, I understand, gone. Agencies now have formal processes and paper trails for accountability. A career in advertising, although not quite the glamorous life it once was, remains highly sought after by a great many graduates (Box 8.3).

Box 8.3   The UK's top advertising agencies (by billings) 2011

Abbott Mead Vickers, BBDO, Euro RSCG London, Gratterpalm, McCann Erickson, DDB London, Fallon London, RKCR/Y&R, Publicis, Adam & Eve, Leo Burnett, JWT, Beattie McGuinness Bungay, M&C Saatchi, The Red Brick Road, Dare, WCRS, Bartle Bogle Hegarty, Mother, Karmarama, DLKW Lowe, CHI & Partners, VCCP, Wieden & Kennedy, Ogilvy & Mather, Grey London, Saatchi & Saatchi, SapientNitro, Brothers and Sisters, TBWA London, AV Browne.

Source: Nielsen / Campaign Top 100, 2012, adbrands.net,
http://www.adbrands.net/uk/top_uk_advertising_agencies.html

When a client appoints an agency to handle a campaign, the client is assigned to an account team. If the account is a major one then several account teams might be working for the same client, or even on the same campaign. An account team typically consists of three main roles: account management, account planning and creative. Traditionally, there are two people on the creative team. There are also ancillary roles such as media planning and buying, TV and art production, digital planning and project management or 'traffic'. It should be noted, though, that digital planning is working its way into a more central role in the top agencies. The traffic person monitors and project-manages the progress of all accounts and ensures that work is project-managed effectively.

In some ad agencies, there is also a separate function for market and consumer research. In the 1960s, a role called account planning was created to try to bring the research function fully within the advertising development process (Hackley, 2003b). The account planner is the agency 'boffin' who is supposed to be comfortable with the design and interpretation of social research, both qualitative or quantitative. They are usually responsible not only for research that informs the creative strategy and design but also for designing pre- and post-campaign testing. Creative research tends to be qualitative, consisting of discussion or focus groups, interviews, observation or ethnographies that generate insights that can be incorporated into the creative advertising development process. Pre- or post-campaign research (called copy-testing) is often experimental in design. Copy-testing can be undertaken prior to campaign launch to reassure the client that there is nothing catastrophically wrong with the finished ad. During and after the campaign, combinations of experimental, survey and statistical methods are used to evaluate the effectiveness of campaigns against their objectives. A psychology training is extremely useful in the account planning role.

The account manager is responsible for client liaison and in overall charge of the account, although in some agencies the account planner holds equal status with the account manager. Account managers (often called 'suits', whether or not they wear one to work) are essentially managing the business side of things. They are, in effect, the voice of the client in the agency, whereas the account planner is said to be the voice of the consumer in the agency. Advertising creative staff (called 'creatives') come from many different educational backgrounds (McLeod et al., 2009) although many do graduate through specialist colleges. Stereotypically, account managers might have business qualifications, account planners or researchers might have advanced social science qualifications, and creatives might have no qualifications at all. But as is the way with stereotypes, many advertising professionals do not fit into these categories.

HOW TO MAKE ADVERTISING

To offer a simplification of the process of making an ad, in the first instance a client awards the agency the business, often after a competitive 'pitch'. In many cases, by the time this happens, the agency has already done a couple of weeks of primary and secondary research into the brand, the market and the target consumers. The client tells the agency what the campaign needs to achieve. Many people, if asked to say what advertising does, would say something like 'it raises awareness' or 'it sells stuff'. In fact, what advertising does is far from agreed upon. Some in the business are convinced that it can persuade us to change our attitudes and/or behaviour. Others feel that it more often reassures us that the brands we like are the right choice. Still others point to advertising's role in creating an image for a brand, so that consumers can link it to their sense of self- and social identity. In the industry, the objectives for advertising campaigns tend to be expressed in down-to-earth and practical ways. Advertising in all its forms can be used to support many different kinds of marketing objective (Box 8.4). For example, an advertising campaign can increase market share, ward off competition from a rival, launch a new brand, change attitudes or behaviour, attract a new market segment to the brand, link the brand with particular values or imagery (called 'positioning' in marketing jargon), or revive falling sales.

Box 8.4   Marketing objectives that can be supported by advertising

Increase market share; position or re-position the brand; communicate price offers; launch a new brand; attract a new market segment for an existing brand; defend against competition; generate short-term sales increases; change attitudes; communicate with stakeholders such as shareholders or employees; defend against negative public relations; help support the direct sales force; link a brand with relevant themes, values or events.

The marketing objectives are then transformed by the agency into a set of communication objectives. The client and agency agree a communication strategy, which is what they want the campaign to say in order to support the desired marketing objective. For example, one agency working for a major car brand found in their qualitative research that consumers thought the cars were more expensive than they actually were. The brand wanted to increase its presence and market share in its sector within Europe. The fact that you can buy such a car for less than you might think became the key theme in a very long-running campaign. The agency creatives found all manner of amusing ways to show consumers being surprised at how reasonably the cars are priced. This simple, low-key communication strategy (for Volkswagen, by DDB Needham) helped achieve increases in market share for the brand, and the campaign has won many awards for the agency over the years. Other advertising successes have been more spectacular. For example, Bartle Bogle Hegarty's iconic 'Launderette' ad for Levi 501s in the mid-1980s was thought to have increased the denim jeans market as a whole by some 800% over the next decade.

Once the communication strategy has been devised, the account planner will write a creative brief. This is the document the creatives have to work from, and it should capture the strategy, the main audience characteristics, the media channels to be used and the campaign objectives in a stimulating and succinct way. Then the creatives have ten ideas, all of which are trashed either by the agency creative director or by the client. After a suitable hiatus for tantrums they have ten more. One of these gets made, it wins multiple awards, everyone becomes famous and the client is thrilled. Remarkably, this sometimes actually happens. More typically, the creatives labour over the detail and the implementation of the key creative ideas. In today's digitally integrated advertising world, having a digital platform (social media, website, mobile, etc.) that is integrated with the principal campaign theme is becoming a necessary element of most campaigns, so creatives have to spend much time thinking about how creative executions that work well on one media channel might be extended to work as well on another. Translating creative ideas from print or TV to digital media can be more complex and difficult than you might think.

PSYCHOLOGISTS IN AD AGENCIES

So, what of the psychology content of these roles? In my experience of talking to agency people I have found psychology graduates in all three main roles – account planning, account management and creative. Most agencies really do not care too much about what one's first degree is in. British advertising is full of maths, classics and English graduates as well as graduates in management, economics and social science. I would guess that the highest concentration of psychology graduates would be in the account planning area. This role seems to combine intellectual curiosity and analytical ability, people and communication skills. It is a difficult and complex role, but, as I note above, psychology graduates have a good range of skills they can bring to it. Most agencies offer a structured training programme to graduate trainees with professional examinations; some of these examinations are offered by the Communication, Advertising and Marketing Education Foundation (CAM).

HOW TO GET INTO ADVERTISING

The next question is: how do you get into advertising? It is not easy. Many agencies have quirky and perplexing application processes for their general graduate traineeships. One college that offers an advertising course for aspiring creative professionals[1] asks applicants to complete a creative test for entry to its copywriting/art direction course. The questions are typical of many one finds on general graduate trainee application forms for advertising, for example:

Why do birds suddenly appear?

How would you increase the sales of lard?

Why should you never underestimate a handsome bear?

How would you make the world a better place?

---

[1]Some good advice on becoming a creative professional in advertising is http://www.tonycullingham .com/howtogetawatfordplace.htm (accessed 29 March 2011).

My students sometimes show me questions like these and ask my advice. I tell them the agency does not want my answer, even if I knew what the answer was. Agencies do not have a fixed idea of what they want in a graduate trainee, but they do feel that if they ask people to demonstrate that they can have ideas and articulate them creatively, that they love advertising, and that they are engaged with culture on many levels (e.g. popular, commercial, classical) then the right people will appear.

Advertising is a small industry with few employment opportunities in the small number of top agencies, but many graduates who are fascinated by it get into roles in connected areas of marketing communication, media and public relations. For example, some of my own former students have gone into careers in top advertising agencies, but others have gone into direct mail or sales promotion agencies and found them just as exciting as mainstream advertising agencies. In recent years the distinction between the industry disciplines has begun to blur and formerly specialist agencies encroach on each other's domain. So digital, media and direct mail agencies have been making broadcast ads, mainstream agencies have been getting into digital, and so on. The various disciplines are merging within a convergent media industry, and skills and knowledge, along with career structures, are having to become more mobile as a result.

PSYCHOLOGY CAREERS IN MARKETING RESEARCH

Finally, a word about careers in market research. There is far more to market research than door-to-door or high street surveys, or annoying phone calls asking whether you were satisfied, very satisfied or in paroxysms of joy after your recent encounter with Kwik Fit. Although psychological knowledge and skill is mainly implicit in advertising, there is more recognition of it in market and consumer research. It is probably fair to say that of the many subfields in marketing, research careers are a bit more structured and professionalised than most. This is partly due, in the UK, to the long-established and respected influence of the Market Research Society (MRS). The MRS, incidentally, has helpful information on graduate careers on its website.[2]

Research is more important in marketing than ever. Advertising, marketing and branding agencies today rarely make decisions in an *ad hoc* or impressionistic way. Clients usually demand evidence for strategic decisions, and research gathers that evidence. The most important qualities for an aspiring career market researcher are curiosity about people and the world, a drive to find and solve problems, skill in communicating and presenting ideas and an ability to think creatively. Specialist psychology knowledge and skills can go a long way here. A market research career could begin as a graduate entrant at one of the many market research agencies, or it could begin in another organisation's in-house market research unit. Talented market researchers can progress through the ranks very quickly if they are independent thinkers with good project management skills.

There are many different kinds of research in marketing, although many of these share common methods and theoretical principles. I have already touched on some

---

[2]http://www.mrs.org.uk/careers/career.htm

examples from advertising, namely creative research (exploring the meanings of a brand and its consumption for a given target audience) and copy-testing (showing a finished advertisement to a sample of the target audience to gauge their response before campaign launch). Agency account planners would also often be engaged in general market research studies on behalf of clients, for example in the early stages of a campaign when they want to understand the competitive issues in a market as well as consumers' underlying motivations.

Market researchers' roles would depend on their seniority. A junior researcher would normally be responsible for executing a research design, or parts of it. They might, for example, be asked to assist in designing a survey questionnaire, or to help in interpreting the results. They might be required to facilitate group discussions, assist in an experiment or conduct depth interviews. As a senior researcher, they might be asked to design the research study itself, oversee the execution of all its components, and present the findings to the client. In short, think of virtually any research design you have studied or taken part in within your psychological studies, and that could be adapted for a specific purpose in market or consumer research.

CONCLUSION

Much of this chapter has explored reasons why the practical value of applied psychology is not acknowledged in marketing as much as it ought to be. This may be disappointing news for psychology graduates, but it is also an opportunity. There is tremendous scope for psychology graduates to apply their skills and knowledge, implicitly or explicitly, to a huge range of marketing roles. Much marketing theory is based implicitly on psychological principles, yet psychology is seldom taught as an explicit component of marketing management courses. All this means that marketing holds many potential opportunities for psychology graduates. One final piece of advice is worth mentioning. Only apply for a career in marketing if you are highly committed, energetic and robust. Marketing professionals are, usually, very busy indeed. In return for the unforgiving deadlines and demanding clients, marketing careers can be fascinating and fulfilling for psychology graduates.

QUESTIONS FOR REFLECTION AND DISCUSSION

1   List the areas of psychology that might be relevant to advertising and marketing, and give an example for each (e.g. attention research, because advertising has to get a consumer's attention in order to communicate its message).

2   How *would* you increase the sales of lard?

3   Evaluate different marketing roles for the potential value of psychological knowledge in executing them effectively.

4   Discuss reasons why psychology is not explicitly valued more for its potential in marketing. Is it all Vance Packard's fault?

5   What contributions could psychological knowledge make to increasing the effectiveness and professionalism of marketing roles such as advertising account planner, industrial sales manager, retail store merchandiser or brand communications director?

6   Reflect on how you would 'sell' your psychology knowledge and skills to a marketing employer. Draw up a list of arguments that would convince them to hire you in a marketing role.

SUGGESTIONS FOR FURTHER READING

There are many useful books and journals that offer a flavour of some of the uses of psychology in marketing. For example, Gordon Foxall's work applies a radical behaviourist approach, the precursor of which still has a strong tradition in mainstream consumer behaviour textbooks. The academic periodical *Journal of Consumer Research* (*JCR*) contains many examples of experimental cognitive psychology research studies, along with some economic and qualitative/cultural psychology. *JCR* is also well known for opening up consumer research to humanistic and also cultural psychology perspectives. Mainstream marketing texts include selected concepts from psychology, but usually without discussing the psychological context from which they were derived. Psychology graduates who can bring their social scientific insight to bear on marketing applications may have a head start in the marketing game.

Foxall, G. (1997) *Marketing Psychology: The Paradigm in the Wings*. London: Macmillan.

Useful websites
Institute of Direct Marketing: http://www.theidm.com/
Chartered Institute of Marketing: http://www.cim.co.uk/home.aspx
American Marketing Association: http://www.marketingpower.com/Pages/default.aspx
Market Research Society: http://www.mrs.org.uk/
Institute for Practitioners in Advertising: http://www.ipa.co.uk/
Advertising Association: http://www.adassoc.org.uk/Home
Communication Advertising and Marketing Foundation: http://www.camfoundation.com/

Academic journals
Psychology and Marketing
Journal of Consumer Research
Journal of Marketing Management
Journal of Advertising Research
Journal of Economic Psychology

9

FORENSIC PSYCHOLOGY

Brian R. Clifford

This chapter discusses:

- the evolution of forensic psychology;

- the numerous and varied aspects of current forensic psychology;

- how one becomes a forensic psychologist;

- law and psychology's similarities and differences in philosophy and practice;

- the increasing professionalism of forensic psychology.

INTRODUCTION

This chapter documents in broad terms the evolution of forensic psychology and its current growth and future trends. It then indicates how forensic psychologists work in all phases of the criminal justice system: investigation, trial, post-trial and release phases, as well as the aetiology of criminal behaviour. It then discusses the education and training of forensic psychologists, pointing out that the BPS is progressively tightening its rules for Chartership. Pay, prospects and conditions are next presented. Professional issues, stresses and strains, and ongoing areas of disputation or professional unease are presented at some length. Forensic psychology is then argued to be a broad church with ample scope for subspecialisms. The chapter ends by stating clearly what professional expertise is expected if the obligations and responsibilities of forensic psychology are to be fully discharged.

DEFINITIONAL ISSUES

Arguments rage about the *precise* meaning of the term 'forensic psychology'. *The Oxford English Dictionary* defines 'forensic' as 'pertaining to, connected with, or used in courts of law'. Others are accused of using the terms 'criminological psychology' and 'forensic psychology' interchangeably (Brown, 1998; Coolican et al., 1996). The definition employed here is that offered by the BPS. In their view forensic psychology is the application of psychological theories, research and techniques to the criminological and law areas. This definition obviously serves to increase the scope of the forensic psychologist well beyond the confines of the court and the matter of judicial evidence.

EVOLUTION OF FORENSIC PSYCHOLOGY

Psychologists have been aware of the possible importance of their knowledge, skills and expertise, and their application, since the turn of the twentieth century. In 1908 Hugo Munsterberg (see Clifford, 1997) called upon the legal profession to appreciate the relevance, and apply the findings, of psychology to their profession in his book *On the Witness Stand*. In the 1920s Burt (1925) produced his book *The Young Delinquent*, and in the 1940s and 1950s Bowlby's (1944, 1951) work on attachment argued that a lack of attachment to a maternal figure 'caused', or at least was a critical factor in, criminal behaviour. These early works served to keep the relation between psychology and law in the forefront of the interested layperson's mind. In 1964 Eysenck produced his well-publicised theory of criminality whereby neurotic extraverts were argued to be more likely to become criminals as they were less conditionable and therefore less likely to learn and adopt the social norms and rules of society. A more specific reference point is that of Haward's (1981) book, *Forensic Psychology*, which sought to detail how a psychologist should behave in their role as a forensic psychologist.

Of more recent origin, Brown (1998) suggests that critical incidents in society served to 'throw' psychologists and criminal justice system personnel together, especially in the case of the police, and thus contributed to the 'unplanned' evolution of the discipline.

CURRENT CONTEXT AND FUTURE TRENDS

Clearly then psychology has always felt that it had something to offer the legal and criminal justice system. Of late, however, this perception has become an imperative. Crime rates have soared and recidivism is endemic in all industrialised society. Something has to be done. Pure punishment – incarceration and 'throwing away the key' – is seen as neither a practical, logical nor a moral option. Rather, a stress on prevention and rehabilitation has to be wedded to the immediately satisfying, but ultimately demoralising, socially acceptable incarceration response. It is now realised that simple protection of the populace by incarceration is not a long-term solution that is sustainable. From this proposition, the current growth in forensic psychology can be traced.

Forensic psychology is one of the most popular areas of applied psychology. There is both a supply and a demand side to this situation. In terms of the supply of recruits, there can be little doubt that the explosion of interest in forensic psychology demonstrated by undergraduates has been fuelled by the increasingly ubiquitous presence of crime both on the small and big screens. In addition to books, films and dramas, such as *Red Dragon*, *Silence of the Lambs*, *Cracker*, *Silent Witness*, *Wire in the Blood*, and *CSI* (crime scene investigation), and many other dramatic portrayals of 'forensic success' over 'evil', numerous fact-based television programmes have focused upon offender profilers as they either interact with the police to produce profiles of current perpetrators, or engage in retrospective profiling ('psychological autopsy') of deceased persons, or discuss sensational real-life murders – whether they be serial, mass or sexual-sadistic killers. These media portrayals serve to increase the demand for undergraduate units, modules, options or even full degrees variously named forensic psychology, criminological psychology or investigative psychology.

The demand side is the past and present government's espoused aim of being 'tough on crime and on the causes of crime'. The implications of this assertion are that the prison population will continue to increase (as it is doing); that sentences other than custodial will continue to proliferate (as they are doing); and that prevention will be seen as the most economically and humanely viable strategy. Thus, there will be an increasing demand for forensic psychologists to research the precursors of crime and criminal behaviour and to produce policy-orientated and best-practice guidance in the prevention of crime and the prevention of recidivistic behaviour.

There will be a concomitant demand for forensic psychologists to organise, monitor and manage non-custodial sentenced offenders, and an ever-increasing demand to service the increasing prison population by innovations and evaluations of existing and potential rehabilitation treatments that ensure earlier release dates and decreased levels of recidivism. At the court phase, increasingly pressure will be brought to bear upon forensic psychologists to offer advice and guidance on how best to handle defendants that come before the courts, and to prioritise categories of criminals in terms of the various and myriad options confronting judges, or more likely magistrates, who have to pass sentence, against the backdrop of sentencing policies and frameworks, government diktats and ever-changing societal patterns.

As an example of this increased expansion of the forensic psychologist's role, the 54 autonomous probation services in England and Wales amalgamated into the new National Probation Service in April 2001, at the same time as amalgamating with the Prisons Psychology Service. A key driver in this joint venture was the delivery of an offender behaviour programme in both prisons and the probation service, and the development of the 'offender assessment system' as a joint risk-assessment tool. It is clear that forensic psychologists will become central players in the multidisciplinary delivery and management of these programmes. This development promises to enlarge the working roles of forensic psychologists and introduce different routes for career progression. In addition, forensic psychologists are increasingly being employed in the health service (including rehabilitation units and secure hospitals) and the social services (including the police service and young offender units).

SPHERES OF INFLUENCE AND GROWTH POINTS

Increasingly then, psychologists have become involved in all stages of the criminal justice system: the investigatory phases of the criminal justice system, where police are the main beneficiaries of psychology; at the trial phase; at the post-trial (penal) phase; and eventually at the release phase. A major area of activity of forensic psychologists is at a still earlier phase – the investigation of the causes, contexts and risk factors associated with crime and criminal behaviour. That is, a significant number of forensic psychologists, located within universities, facilitate, at least potentially, the criminal justice system by trying to document and understand criminological behaviour and evolve policy recommendations that will progressively decrease the need for pre-trial, trial and post-trial phases. These multiple areas of operation mean that the concept of a forensic psychologist is multifarious and their sphere of influence is varied and diverse.

Academic forensic psychologists are found in academe where a major focus is empirical research into precursors of crime (genetic, biological, psychological, sociological). They are also found working with police in terms of selection procedures, organisational change, stress management and improvements in operational efficiency. They also engage with training and education.

In the field they can be found offering guidance and research critiques on interviewing suspects, victims and witnesses, and critiquing line-up (identification parade) procedures that maximise the likelihood of achieving a valid identification while minimising the possibility of obtaining a wrongful identification. As an example of this area of operation, the author is currently engaged with exploring the benefits and drawbacks of the recently introduced video identification parade electronic recording (VIPER) method of identification, funded by the Scottish Institute of Policing Research. Perhaps the best known, but in reality, infrequently utilised, role of forensic psychologists is offering an 'offender profile' that aids police in reducing their search-space, increasing their awareness of what (and who) to look for, and providing additional insights into the case and how to question the perpetrator once apprehended.

Another area of possible increasing involvement, pre-dating the trial process but crucially involved with evidence, is the interviewing of children and other vulnerable witnesses under the *Achieving Best Evidence* (Home Office, 2002, 2007) guidelines. Research has indicated that this crucial evidential-interview, and its precursor, the *Memorandum of Good Practice* (Home Office, 1992), is poorly understood, managed, staged and executed. At the moment it is conducted primarily by the investigating police officer, supported by a social worker. A forensic psychologist, with a deep knowledge of child development, linguistic and cognitive development, and an appreciation of how the law requires questions to be put, would seem ideally suited to unburden the police with this task and ensure the best quality of evidence is produced in court.

A role that forensic psychologists may come to play increasingly in the future is as court- or evidence-facilitator. Children who come before the courts as witnesses, victims or defendants have been shown to benefit greatly from receiving prior information about, and visits to, the court. Guidelines have been produced by the National Society for the Prevention of Cruelty to Children (NSPCC) but what research clearly indicates is that such pre-trial preparation is piecemeal and in need of professionalisation. This would be a natural role for a forensic psychologist to fulfil, given their background in psychology.

At the trial phase, forensic psychologists are normally involved in providing reports on a variety of questions that are central to either the trial being conducted or the sentence to be handed down. Thus, forensic reports will be readily accepted on educational, clinical or occupational issues that are currently before the court. Much less frequently they can appear as expert witnesses. Now this is a highly contentious issue (see Clifford, 2008, 2010, 2012). In descending order of acceptability, courts have little problem with experts who testify on physical as opposed to human matters (e.g. a ballistics expert), because bullet markings and properties are beyond the knowledge of the jury. Second, courts have little problem with physical trauma or illnesses as opposed to mental abnormality as a topic for expert opinion (e.g. the potential or actual damage caused by a blow to the head). Third, courts have little problem with expert testimony on mental abnormality as opposed to mental normalcy (e.g. paranoid schizophrenia as a condition causing atypical behavioural dispositions). What the courts have a real problem with are experts who testify (offer opinions) on what are regarded by the court as normal mental processes such as memory and perception. These normal mental processes are assumed to be within the knowledge and experience of the jury, and thus the introduction of an expert offering an opinion on their operation is held to be more prejudicial than probative. That is, such testimony acts against the offering of evidential proof that helps the jury to reach a reasoned and reasonable decision. As such, this type of evidence is much more likely to be rejected or disallowed than accepted.

Thus, the courts have, generally, baulked at admitting evidence from experimental forensic psychologists giving opinions as experts on matters of, for example, disputed identification evidence (Box 9.1). However, the two-hundred-plus cases of wrongful conviction uncovered by the Innocence Project (2011) by means of post-conviction deoxyribonucleic acid (DNA) evidence, some 75% of which were based on faulty eyewitness testimony, suggests that this rejection by the courts of normal-mental-state expert witnessing is a fight that forensic psychologists should not abandon.

Box 9.1   A cautionary tale: an episode in the life of an expert witness

The email arrived out of the blue. 'As a recognised expert witness who had been pivotal in a successful high-profile Appeal Case in Scotland, the Queen's Counsel involved in that case would like to engage you in another High Court case involving perjury and the possible issue of mistaken voice identification'. The solicitor in the case wished to instruct me to prepare a report and appear as an expert witness in the up-coming trial. After careful consideration of the possible probative input from experimental psychology I accepted the instruction. There then followed a blizzard of papers constituting the evidence in the case, several DVDs of full and edited interviews and transcripts of police interviews with the defendant that served as the standard sample of speech output, and a DVD of an alleged conversation involving the defendant (the comparison sample of speech) admitting to an act that had been previously denied under oath – thus constituting perjury. My stated tasks

(Continued)

(Continued)

were to (1) provide a critical review of the known literature on voice recognition by humans, with special reference to recognition of a familiar voice; (2) compare and contrast the approaches to voice recognition and identification of experimental psychologists, phonological experts and machine-based voice recognition experts, indicating the strengths and weaknesses of all three approaches. Last, I was requested to listen to the standard and comparison speech samples to form an opinion as to the probability that the alleged critical voice was that of the defendant. In addition to all this, I was asked to review and comment upon several reports by prosecution expert witnesses.

After many days work fulfilling the wishes of the instruction, and having submitted my report and met the QC and instructing solicitor to discuss the report, the day of the trial was fast approaching. I had booked and paid for a hotel in Glasgow, had Googled the route to the High Court from the hotel, packed my bags and was 'good to go'. As the last thing 'to do' I checked my emails on Sunday at six o'clock, and there it was! The defendant had informed the instructing solicitor that he did not wish my voice identification evidence to be entered at trial, thus my attendance (and the many hours of work I had put into the case) was not required.

The moral of this episode is you win some and you lose some, but as a forensic psychologist you must always interact with the law in good faith, albeit in the full knowledge that, in this partnership, law is the master and not psychology.

In the post-trial phase, once a defendant has been 'sent down', forensic psychologists will be found in the prison system, special secure hospitals, remand homes or youth offender institutions, assessing offenders' needs, their likelihood of reoffending (risk assessment) and devising, executing and evaluating various treatment regimes and programmes. It is a fact that the majority of forensic psychologists are found in the prison service. Here their chief role is as treatment officers: piloting and implementing treatment programmes. The range of therapeutic offerings is wide, stretching from one-to-one psychoanalytical therapy to group discussions, and involving behavioural, cognitive–behavioural and/or cognitive techniques. Cognitive restructuring, anger management and social skills are key objectives of all treatment and rehabilitation regimes. Whereas it used to be believed that 'nothing works' (Martinson, 1974) it is now firmly believed that some treatments work for some inmates, some of the time (e.g. Hatcher, 2008). Forensic psychologists are prime movers in organising, monitoring, delivering and evaluating this treatment philosophy. In addition to their focus on prisoners, forensic psychologists may be responsible for the development and delivery to prison staff of programmes on stress management, understanding bullying and techniques of hostage negotiation.

EDUCATION AND TRAINING

So how does one become a forensic psychologist? If you have not yet started your training or you started your training after 1 May 2001, to become a Chartered Forensic Psychologist you must follow the forensic psychology training route. This entails the following qualifications.

1 Graduate Basis for Chartered Membership (GBC–previously known as GBR). This is achieved by completing a Society-accredited degree or a conversion course, at undergraduate level.

2 Society-accredited Master's in Forensic Psychology, or Stage 1 of the Society's Diploma in Forensic Psychology, designed to assess the trainee's academic knowledge base and research competence.

3 Stage 2 of the Society's Diploma in Forensic Psychology, which involves two years' supervised practice, designed to develop key role experience.

4 In order to use the title Forensic Psychologist you will need to be registered with the Health Professions Council (HPC). This will involve completing Stage 2 of the Society's Diploma in Forensic Psychology or equivalent qualification that has been approved by the HPC.

Although there are numerous undergraduate courses that either offer joint, or major and minor honours (of psychology and law or other cognate disciplines), or at least modules or units in forensic psychology, to date there are only a few masters' courses that provide BPS- accredited courses. At the time of writing, Masters courses are offered at Birkbeck, Birmingham (2 courses), Central Lancashire, Coventry (2 courses), Glasgow Caledonian, Gloucestershire, Institute of Psychiatry, Kent, Leicester (3 courses), Liverpool (2 courses), London Metropolitan, Manchester Metropolitan, Middlesex, Portsmouth, Surrey, Teesside and York. Several of these run part-time as well as distance learning courses in addition to their full-time one-year courses. Birmingham University runs a Doctorate in Forensic Psychology Practice, which covers both Stage 1 and 2 of the Society's Diploma in Forensic Psychology.

As with educational psychology and clinical psychology before it, forensic psychology currently suffers from this 'bottleneck' problem. Many hundreds of undergraduates leave with the intention of pursuing a Master's in Forensic Psychology but find places extremely restricted. How can you best maximise your chances of getting on a Master's Course in Forensic Psychology – a *sine qua non* of becoming a Chartered Forensic Psychologist?

As has been said, the bottleneck appears between undergraduate and postgraduate masters'. A sifting device that has been used in both educational and clinical psychology is to ask for a specific number of years of relevant experience, as with forensic masters'. This is the infamous 'Catch 22' problem – you cannot get work because you do not have the qualifications: you can't get the qualifications because you haven't got relevant experience. This will not cease to apply, but current study patterns in higher education make it possible – and acceptable – to mix full-time undergraduate study with part-time (or even flexible time) employment. If you are set on forensic psychology as a career then you must choose work that relates to forensic concerns. In this way you can accumulate work experience that can go some way to overcoming the sieve that is applied by masters' courses to keep numbers of applicants within manageable bounds.

In terms of study, you must select courses from among options/units that relate clearly to forensic concerns (research methods, cognitive psychology, social psychology, child development, personality and individual differences, etc.). Obviously you must select any and all options that contain forensic material. Your undergraduate project (individually determined research) should be forensically related as you are likely to present this at interview for a forensic master's place. In the event of obtaining a 2:2 undergraduate degree, this will have to be rehabilitated by undertaking a research-based master's, ideally in a forensic-related field, before an admissions tutor for a forensic master's will entertain your application.

An important consideration is the possibility that an employer may pay for your master's degree as part of continuing professional development (CPD). This is the case with many government agencies or statutory bodies. To go to an interview able to say that you will be funded by your employer puts you well ahead of any equally good, but unfunded, rivals for that scarce place.

The requirement that you be mentored/guided/supervised by a Chartered Forensic Psychologist, on balance, is a desirable innovation. As long as the mentoring aspect is played up, and the line-management control aspect is played down, the availability of an experienced person who 'has seen it all before' can be a great help as you struggle to find your feet in what could be an alien environment.

PAY, PROSPECTS AND CONDITIONS

Forensic psychologists who work in the prison service have the same conditions of employment as other civil servants. Those working in special hospitals and regional secure units are employed under NHS conditions. Both these bodies pay higher rates than university lecturer scales. Pay scales can range from £20,000+ to £60,000+. All systems have ladders of promotion with clear guidelines as to principles and procedures for advancement up the promotional scales.

Increasingly, forensic psychologists are becoming self-employed consultants. Consultants charge fees and these are commensurate with training, expertise and reputation. Consultancies will employ novice (trainee) or newly qualified Chartered Forensic Psychologists and salaries will be paid in line with negotiated schemes. Clearly, consultancy is a 'middle' or 'late' career consideration, but it is an option that should be countenanced at the earliest opportunity. Consequently, any and all generic and/or transferable skills-curricula offerings should be grasped whenever and wherever possible. Continuing professional development is now an integral, and often mandatory, part of any profession and professional advancement.

PROFESSIONAL ISSUES IN FORENSIC PSYCHOLOGY AS A PROFESSION

There is no doubt that forensic psychology, like all other professions, contains hidden stresses and strains. Some are overt – such as case load, oppressive environments, the nature of the clients who have to be dealt with, and frustration with the lack of perceived best-practice, evidence-based, or at least evidence-guided, policy implementation.

There are, however, latent, more value-laden, philosophical issues that need to be considered before entering the forensic psychology arena. As I (Clifford, 1995, 2002) and others (Carson, 1995), have argued elsewhere, while psychology's premises, methods and values are not necessarily antithetical to those of law, nonetheless they are different from them. At particular times, and in particular situations, within the psychology–law interface that is forensic psychology, these differences can surface and be a source of contention, dispute and contestation. So what are these differences (Table 9.1)?

Table 9.1   Contrasting premises, methods and values of law and psychology[1]

Contrasts	Law	Psychology
Control	Immediate	Long term
Persons	Individuates	Generalises
Behaviour	Reasons	Causes
Emphasise	Common sense	Facts
Requirements	Dichotomies	Dimensions
Areas of operation	Litigation	Legislation

[1]See text for explanations of these contrasts.

Although both law and psychology have human behaviour and its control as a central focus, the law's control tends to be immediate, direct and explicit. Psychology's control, on the other hand, is indirect, long term and implicit. Thus, the courts control a defendant's behaviour, once found guilty, by directly imposing an immediate sentence that is explicitly extracted or enacted (fines, community sentence or imprisonment). Psychology attempts to control either unwelcome or undesirable behaviour by indirectly changing that behaviour over an extended period of time by changing thought processes or perceptions, or by empowerment via social skills training and anger management. In this way, it is hoped that implicit cognitive restructuring, training or treatment will eventuate in explicit behavioural change. The inherent conflict between law and psychology here tends to be handled temporally – once the courts have passed sentence the forensic psychologists can begin to ply their trade, although this conflicting view on how to control behaviour can surface pre-sentencing, where forensic reports can recommend strategies other than incarceration.

Law individuates; psychology generalises. This is a fundamental difference between the two disciplines. While the law has to make decisions about a particular individual, psychology's knowledge, which could serve to inform that decision, emanates from experimental or empirical findings. However, these findings almost always refer to *group* means, not *individual* scores. This immediately raises issues in courts of law where specific decisions have to be arrived at about the specific defendant in the case. It also becomes an issue when risk or dangerousness has to be decided upon, or allocation of a specific treatment or rehabilitation programme has to be made to a specific prisoner. This conflict can manifest itself when expert testimony is offered in court, where the expert has not had contact with the particular person from whom the disputed fact or facts have issued. However, if contact has been mandated by the court then the conflict is attenuated because individual scores on a relevant test or psychometric instrument can be referred to.

Another running battle forensic psychologists frequently have with legal personnel is the issue of reasons versus causes of behaviour. The law operates on the principle of free-will, and thus talks of humans having reasons for behaviour. Psychology on the other hand talks of causes of behaviour in the sense of multiple causes eventuating in the behaviour at issue. Free-will and determinism are uncomfortable bedfellows, underpinned as they are by intentional versus causal explanations of behaviour. Yet this issue frequently has to be resolved in courts of law where defences involving pre-menstrual tension, postnatal depression, post-traumatic stress disorder (PTSD) and battered-wife-syndrome are advanced as explanations and thus mitigating circumstances in cases of infanticide, manslaughter and even murder.

Related to, but distinct from, free-will versus determinism, is law's emphasis on common sense and psychology's emphasis on empirical fact. The 'person on the Clapham Omnibus' is often the touchstone of law's reasoning, i.e. common sense. Psychology's emphasis on inter-subjective verifiability of object fact frequently does not agree with common sense (Furnham, 1992). When it does agree with common sense, law tends to scoff at the redundancy of psychology: when it does not, psychology is usually ignored. One of the frequently espoused reasons given by Appeal Court judges for refusing the entry of psychological findings into the proceedings is that psychology is a pseudo-science. This was the explicit statement made in a case I was involved in with the Scottish Criminal Cases Review Commission. Now, although it may be that judges are simply confusing the subject matter of science (if it is physics, then it is science; if it is human behaviour, then it is pseudo-science) with the *approach* and *method* of science (where both animate and inanimate entities can be investigated by the same methods of science), nonetheless, the fact that people in high positions of authority can still make these pronouncements, and presumably believe them, should worry any would-be forensic psychologist.

Another area of potential disputation is where the law requires dichotomies – guilty or not, culpable or not, suggestible or not, treatable or not – but psychologists suggest dimensions (of for example, intelligence, suggestibility, capacity, competence). Many issues that forensic psychologists become involved in are underpinned by this conflicting conceptualisation. A good example is in the assessment of risk and dangerousness. There are simply no universal predictors of future behaviour, and the factors associated with predicting different types of behaviour are different. Hodgins (1997) also draws out the important distinction between predictors and causes. Predictors of dangerousness are often simple – e.g. age and previous criminal history; the causes of dangerous behaviour are complex and multicausal. At present there are two fundamental approaches to risk and dangerousness assessment: clinical judgement, and statistical or actuarial assessment. Neither of these assessment methods eventuates in categorical dichotomies of certainty; at best they are probabilistic 'guesses'.

The last area to be discussed where law and psychology can conflict is in policy-making and policy implementation. The law argues that litigation is a matter purely for the law: psychology has no place. Where psychology does have a place is in legislation, that is, the formulation of law that is then litigated. If the primary motivation for entering forensic psychology is to make a difference (in what, and to whom, being left unspecified) then this acceptance by law of psychology's role is gratifying. And certainly there are areas of law and legislation where psychologists have made a difference.

To take just one example, let us look at how academic forensic psychologists have been instrumental in bringing about massive changes in one particular aspect of law and litigation. Until a few decades ago child witnesses were not welcomed by the courts. If they did appear they had to pass competency tests and their evidence had to be corroborated by other witnesses. For a variety of reasons, chief among which was the increased number of cases of sexual abuse coming before the courts, the law was faced with a problem. They distrusted the reliability and validity of children's testimony, yet cases involving such evidence were increasingly being presented for adjudication.

Co-terminous with this social movement, experimental psychologists were producing empirical data that showed that children could give reliable testimony, especially if supported by the court, its setting and its procedures. By making representation to Royal Commissions, by 'giving psychology away' (Miller, 1969: 9), by writing in popular journals, newspapers and appearing on radio and TV, and by engaging with the legal profession at conferences, symposia and meetings, successive acts of legislation have both increasingly allowed children to be heard and progressively eased their passage and facilitated their delivery (e.g. live-link, pre-exposure to the court and its procedures, removal of wigs and gowns, videoed evidence-in-chief, special measures, etc.). At the time of writing, allowing children to give their evidence-in-chief *and* to be cross-examined outside the court setting is a battle still to be universally won, but which is nonetheless being fought tenaciously by psychologists.

This case study, and many others like it (for example, interviewing of both witnesses and suspects, false confessions, best-practice identification procedures) across the law–psychology interface, bodes well for the future of forensic psychology and its practitioners.

A BROAD CHURCH

Forensic psychology is a very interesting profession to be in, and promises to be even more so in the future. Some of the most exciting topics in undergraduate psychology are actually real-life, everyday topics or issues that arise in legal disputation and therefore forensic psychology. Almost any recognised area of psychological expertise can be 'transported' to forensic psychology.

Thus, an educational psychologist could expect to research and inform the legal profession on such matters as, *inter alia*, educational subnormality, language, and fitness to stand trial, or recovered memories. A clinical psychologist could be interested in such matters as the psychopathology of crime, mental disorders and states of mind, dangerousness, violence and sexual disorders. Occupational or organisational psychologists can be involved in training and civil suits involving damages, liability and compensation.

Academic psychologists with a background in developmental psychology would have expertise in juvenile delinquency, attention-deficit disorders, moral development, hyperactivity and knowledge of right and wrong. Experimental cognitive psychologists, as we have seen, are already heavily involved in investigation of suggestibility, false memory syndrome, identification evidence, witness/victim questioning, false confessions and lie detection techniques.

From the above it can be seen that many of the issues that engage psychologists are issues that the law struggles with daily. The melding of law and psychology in the production of forensic psychology is a development that promises to be a win–win–win situation. Psychology wins by being confronted by real-life situations and issues that can be resolved by the knowledge that psychology already has accumulated, or can be investigated by robust research methods. Law wins by gaining insights and new perspectives on what appear as intractable issues. And the defendants and appellants win by making legal procedures more of a process predicated upon reason, fact and justice rather than blind precedent, rhetoric and persuasion, and appeals to common sense.

INCREASING RIGOUR IN PROFESSIONALISM

However, as a profession the gatekeepers have to be vigilant. Until a few years ago anyone could set themselves up as a forensic psychologist and sell their wares. The BPS has closed the door on this danger. As we saw above, to become a Chartered Forensic Psychologist requires an extensive education and training. They (the BPS: *Qualifications in Forensic Psychology (Stage 2). Candidate Handbook*, 2011) believe that chartered status, with all that that entails, should only be conferred on members who are able to demonstrate the following.

1   A sound conceptual basis and understanding of the context within which they practise, involving both criminal behaviour and the legal framework of the law and the civil and criminal justice systems.

2   A sound understanding of the contribution of applied psychology to the criminal justice system as it involves investigative, trial, custodial, treatment and resettlement processes.

3   A detailed understanding of key individuals in the criminal justice system, including offenders, victims, witnesses and investigators, to whom interventions may be applied.

4   A sound understanding of forensic psychology in practice including the nature and style of communication required in assessment, processes of investigation, treatment and rehabilitation, professional criteria for report production and giving of testimony, and extensive practical experience in engaging in at least one area of forensic psychology.

Broadly one to three above is covered by your first and second degree. The last is covered by the two-year supervised practice. In its entirety the training package is designed to give experience in at least four key roles of a forensic psychologist: (1) conducting psychological applications and interventions; (2) conducting research; (3) communicating psychological knowledge and advice to other professionals; and, eventually, (4) training other professionals in psychological skills and knowledge. Although it may seem a somewhat protracted process this duration is necessitated by the nature of the job and the sensitivity of issues that a forensic psychologist would be expected to meet. The nature and duration of training is also mandated by the critical consideration that only the highest level of professional expertise should be brought to bear on issues of life-changing importance to the clients you will be dealing with.

CONCLUSION

Forensic psychology is a relatively young profession undergoing unprecedented growth. This is predicated upon both supply- and demand-side economics. It has been shown to be a broad church involving many potentially contributing subdisciplines. While currently experiencing bottlenecks between undergraduate and postgraduate educational provision, the entry qualification to chartered status is becoming ever more stringent. Yet, if these hurdles can be overcome, successful candidates can look forward to an exciting, varied and ultimately rewarding career, punctuated by wrestling with, and hopefully resolution of, several deep-seated philosophical and discipline-specific dilemmas.

QUESTIONS FOR REFLECTION AND DISCUSSION

1   How realistic do you feel the various dramatic representations are of psychology's interaction with the police and crime solution? Give reasons for your answer.

2   Which of the various work locations of forensic psychologists would you find *most* and *least* convivial? Give your reasons for both choices.

3   How sensible is it to always explain human behaviour as *either* the result of free will *or* as the result of biological, psychological or social causes?

4   The prediction of risk of reoffending is easy: the prediction of actually reoffending is complex. What do you understand by this assertion?

5   Why do people commit murder?

6   'Once a criminal always a criminal.' What do you think?

SUGGESTIONS FOR FURTHER READING

Adler, J.R. (ed.) (2004) *Forensic Psychology: Concepts, Debates and Practice.* Cullompton: Willan Publishing. 'As it says on the tin', an excellent collection of chapters that covers issues and topics of current interest in the field of forensic psychology.

Howitt, D. (2011) *Introduction to Forensic and Criminal Psychology* (4th edn). London: Pearson. A volume on forensic psychology that serves to illustrate the range and scope of the discipline. It covers all phases of the criminal justice system and spheres of influence of the forensic psychologist, in good depth.

Davies, G.H., Hollin, C. and Bull, R. (eds) (2008) *Forensic Psychology*. Chichester: John Wiley & Sons.

Towel, G.T. and Crighton, D.A. (eds) (2010) *Forensic Psychology*. London: BPS and Blackwell Publishing.

These two books cover in much greater detail several of the issues raised in this chapter.

10

CLINICAL NEUROPSYCHOLOGY

Ashok Jansari

This chapter discusses:

- a list of the main requirements of being a clinical neuropsychologist;

- the history of clinical neuropsychology;

- why an understanding of cognitive psychology is at the heart of the job;

- neuroscientific techniques that can aid the work of a clinician;

- the different stages involved in conducting a cognitive assessment;

- the emerging field of neuropsychological rehabilitation;

- how to become a clinical neuropsychologist.

INTRODUCTION

Clinical neuropsychology is a speciality within clinical psychology that involves assessing and helping to treat people who have had injuries or illnesses that have affected the brain and general behaviour. Due to the variations across the systems in place in different countries, depending on where a person receives their training, they may or may not have to train first as a clinical psychologist before further specialist training. In general, a clinical neuropsychologist would need to be able to do the following.

1 *Consider the individual patient as a whole as well as part of a bigger system.*

Although a patient may have a brain abnormality, it is important to understand that there are social, environmental and psychosocial impacts on their behaviour and therefore considering them just at the level of the brain would be missing out important aspects of the job. Similarly, each person is part of a bigger system in terms of their relationships, family and work situations so therefore it is important to take these into consideration when attempting to evaluate or help the patient.

2 *Understand the difference between the behavioural and psychopathological aspects to behaviour.*

Although brain damage can have a severe impact on behaviour, behaviour can also be affected by psychopathology. So for example due to major emotional trauma, in some cases, an individual's memory may be totally impaired, resulting in what is known as a 'fugue' state. However, although on the surface this may look like amnesia caused by brain damage (see below), the cause is very different. Recognising the difference between these two forms of memory problem will result in referring the fugue patient to a psychiatrist rather than following a clinical neuropsychological course of assessment and treatment.

3 *Have an understanding of cognition and how this can evolve over time as well as the impact of factors such as disease and brain damage.*

Cognitive psychology is the bedrock of clinical neuropsychology since an important aspect of the work involves assessing the patient's mental abilities following some form of trauma. An analogy would be that a medical doctor has to have, as the basis of any work they do, an understanding of biochemistry since without an appreciation of how the chemistry of living cells functions, it would be impossible to work in almost any field within medicine. Therefore, a good clinical neuropsychologist would need to have a firm grounding in cognitive psychology.

4 *Understand some aspects of the neurosciences to the extent that they can be used in evaluating an individual's performance.*

Since the 1980s, understanding brain functions has been greatly influenced by an explosion in a range of different neuroscientific techniques. If these are available as part of a clinical service, they can add significantly to the information that a neuropsychologist can use in their assessment. Therefore, having an understanding of some aspects of the neurosciences can be extremely beneficial.

5 *Conduct specialised assessments of cognitive functions.*

Related to the understanding of cognitive functions, a neuropsychologist needs to be able to conduct assessments. These are all related to different cognitive functions such as short-term memory, long-term memory, visual recognition and problem-solving.

6 *Plan rehabilitation where appropriate and possible.*

Depending on the extent of a patient's problem, it is sometimes possible to use the abilities that have not been negatively affected, to develop interventions to improve the quality of life of the individual.

This 'tool kit' is an idealised set of tasks that would be desired for a clinical neuropsychologist. However, whether or not an individual neuropsychologist will be able to work at each of these levels will depend on a number of factors such as their initial training, the availability of resources, the type of environment they are working within and time constraints. Even where it is not possible to engage with each of these levels, through engagement with ongoing developments (by attending conferences and training workshops or keeping updated with the latest published literature) it is possible to have an appreciation of all the different types of work. Tasks one and two above are common to all clinical psychologists so please refer to Chapter 4. Tasks three to six above are specific to clinical neuropsychology and will be addressed in more depth here.

The remainder of this chapter will begin with a brief history of clinical neuropsychology since the evolution of this has shaped both the professional position of practitioners and also determined the major tasks outlined above. Following this history, tasks three to six will be addressed individually and then the chapter will conclude with a brief description of how to become a clinical neuropsychologist.

THE HISTORY OF CLINICAL NEUROPSYCHOLOGY

One of the most pivotal moments in the history of clinical neuropsychology came in 1861 when a French neurologist called Paul Broca worked with a patient who had suffered a stroke. Following the stroke, the patient was only able to utter the sound 'tan' and therefore became known as patient Tan. Despite this profound problem in making speech, Tan was still able to understand what was said to him, his memory worked normally and other functions such as vision also seemed quite unimpaired. As a result of this very specific problem, Broca hypothesised that mental functions such as making language, understanding language, memory and vision were all located in different parts of the brain; further he proposed that Tan's stroke had damaged the speech centres while leaving all the other areas intact. When Tan eventually died, an autopsy of his brain showed that, indeed, the whole of his brain was intact with the exception of an area in the left frontal lobe. Following similar cases of patients who also had problems with creating speech and who were also found to have damage to a similar part of the brain, this area of the brain became known as Broca's area (see Figure 10.1).

The work of Broca and other neurologists in the late 1800s such as Carl Wernicke and Ludwig Lichteim set the foundation for what is now a widely held belief that mental functions are localised in specific parts of the brain and therefore that damage or abnormality will result in problems with these functions.

The next important phase was the work of Alexandra Luria in Russia, Oliver Zangwill in the UK and Norman Geschwind in the USA. These men were either neurologists or worked with behavioural neurologists, and for the purpose of standard assessment, they pioneered the development of tests that could be reproduced from one hospital, clinic or research centre to the other and thereby laid the foundations for modern neuropsychology.

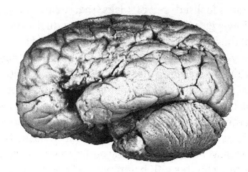

Nature Reviews | Neuroscience

Figure 10.1   Diagram of the brain showing Broca's area

Source: Chris Rorden & Hans-Otto Karnath 'Using human brain lesions to infer function: a relic from a past era in the fMRI age?' *Nature Reviews Neuroscience* 5, 812–819 (October 2004)

A rather strange and unfortunate contribution to the field was made by the Second World War. Previous to this, the majority of patients seen by neurologists were older and had suffered strokes within a particular set of arteries. The damage caused by these strokes resulted in a set of symptoms that were relatively common. Therefore, similar to the work carried out by Broca and others, neurologists tended to see patients with many disorders of language and motor control. However, the brutalities of the Second World War saw young men being shot with bullets that tended to be small. If they were hit in the head, because of the speed of the bullets, they managed to penetrate the skull and cause damage that was limited to relatively small areas. Also, rather than being in specific areas, the point of entry of the bullet could be almost anywhere and so neurologists now began dealing with areas of brain damage that were relatively new to them. As a result, for example, patients with specific visual problems caused by damage to the posterior parts of the brain now began to emerge; this then had an impact on developing understanding of a relatively uncharted area. As well as this, another very important issue was that since the soldiers were relatively young, they could still have a number of decades of healthy life ahead of them. This meant that the need to develop methods to help them cope with their new life became paramount. Consequently, exploring methods of rehabilitation became important.

Meanwhile, in mainstream psychology, the birth of cognitive psychology in the 1960s had a major impact within the field and also upon neuropsychology. This new method used an information-processing system analogy in which, like a computer, there is an input system, physical hardware, software (the programs that run on the computer) and an output. In human behaviour, the five senses take in information from the world, the brain is the hardware and the output is a thought process that usually results in speech or physical action. Using this analogy, cognitive psychology set out to understand the 'missing' bit; that is, the software or programs that, for example, allow the brain to take in sound waves to derive an understanding of what your friend tells you and to take visual information in front of you to interpret a text message on your mobile phone.

The birth of cognitive psychology greatly influenced neuropsychology because the two fields developed having a strong reciprocal relationship. For example, an influential model of memory, the modal (or multistore) model of memory proposed by Atkinson and Shiffrin (1968), had suggested a difference between memory that lasts for a few minutes (short-term memory: STM) and that which lasts for anything from a few minutes to a lifetime (long-term memory: LTM). A seminal study published in 1957 of the most famous brain-damaged patient in history, HM, showed that it was possible to severely damage the ability to create new LTMs while leaving STM intact (Scoville and Milner, 1957). Such corroborative evidence greatly strengthened the modal model. Similarly with cognitive psychologists developing ever more refined models of mental functions such as memory and language, this offered clinicians a better method of understanding the problems presented by their patients. So now, rather than simple assessment, they were able to look at the theoretical basis of their work. This bridge between the two disciplines created a new hybrid of cognitive neuropsychology that is the interpretation of disorders of cognition using formal information-processing models of the intact system. A landmark in this field was the creation in 1984 of the journal *Cognitive Neuropsychology*.

The final important step that has had an impact on the work of at least some clinical neuropsychologists is the development of better methods of looking 'inside' the brain. When Broca worked with Tan, he had to wait until Tan eventually passed away before he could attempt to look at what the stroke had done to his patient's brain. Since the 1980s, then especially in the 1990s and the twenty-first century, ever more elaborate ways of looking at the brain have emerged from the field of medical physics. Below I will cover in more detail how this has affected the field.

As an example of how much the field has moved since Broca first *described* Tan's problems, a century-and-a-half later, in 2004, the first ever international neuropsychological rehabilitation symposium was held at Uluru in Australia. This conference brought together mainly clinical neuropsychologists but also cognitive neuropsychologists all with the same purpose. Rather than merely describing and quantifying patients' problems, the focus for this conference was very much on the application of research to improve the lives of patients. As will be shown later, this new field is an exciting development for the future of the field.

The importance of understanding cognition and how brain damage can have an impact on it

Cognitive psychology as described above is the study of mental processes involving the creation of functional models of processes common to us all such as how we remember, how we read, how we visually recognise objects or other people, etc. Some of these models have had a great impact on the way that the impairments experienced by patients are understood. So for example, as described above, the severe deficit in creating new LTMs while leaving the ability to hold onto information in STM could be explained within the modal model of memory that had been derived largely from research conducted on brain-intact individuals. Conversely, the opposite pattern of a patient with an impaired STM but seemingly intact LTM, as found in the patient KF who had suffered a closed head injury (Shallice and Warrington, 1970), could not be accommodated within the modal model. This 'double dissociation' greatly weakened the model as originally proposed (see Jansari (2005) for a fuller explanation of double dissociations that serve as a bedrock of certain aspects of neuropsychological research). Further, it was found that it was not all of KF's STM that was impaired but instead only that which involved recall of auditory–verbal information such as a string of digits. His ability to hold onto information that was visually or spatially based, however, was completely unaffected. This dissociation within STM, coupled with other findings emerging from cognitive psychology led to the development of the highly influential working memory model (Baddeley and Hitch, 1974) that separates out visual from verbal STM.

Cognitive research has further shown that the way in which memory is tested is important. Therefore, although some individuals may have problems in free recall where no cues are provided, they may perform relatively well on a recognition test. This implies that the impairment lies in attempting to retrieve information that is stored; however, once it is presented, some form of memory can express itself. Findings like this have a dual role because they both drive forward cognitive models of the functions involved and also result in the development of appropriate assessments that clinicians can use in their practice. Therefore, a good battery of STM tests should include both verbal and visual subtests as well as the facility to address both free recall and recognition memory.

The reciprocal relationships between experimental research, functional models of cognition, findings from patients with specific impairments and clinical assessments are found across cognitive psychology. These have driven an ever more refined understanding of memory, spoken language, written language, visual recognition and face recognition. Therefore, having a firm grounding in cognitive psychology is of central importance to the budding clinical neuropsychologist.

NEUROSCIENCES

As a result of the huge expansion of methods of looking at both the structure and neural processing within the brain, a neuropsychologist will come across an array of neuroscientific information about a patient. Having a broad understanding of the neurosciences therefore can have a significant impact in the management of a patient. To look at physical structures, a number of techniques are available. The two most common ones are computerised axial tomography (CAT) and MRI scans. Depending on how these are taken, areas of physical damage (resulting from tissue cell death) can be clearly visible. More recently, other forms of neuroimaging have been developed such as diffusion tensor imaging (DTI), which goes beyond looking at physical structures and shows how different brain regions are connected to one another. This method is largely used in experimental research but, with time, is likely to become part of the toolkit of clinical neuroscience.

Even if a structure of the brain looks physically intact on an MRI scan, this does not necessarily mean that the functioning is normal. A classic example would be if an individual has a small area of damaged cells that have begun to malfunction, resulting in epileptic seizures. How this occurs is not well understood but the main point is that an MRI scan is not necessarily going to reveal this abnormality. However, an electro-encephalogram (EEG) is a method whereby a number of electrodes are placed on specific parts of a person's scalp that can then measure very small changes in electrical activity. Enough is understood about this activity to know what the patterns of discharge should be for a normally functioning brain. Therefore, a significant deviation from this would suggest abnormal activity somewhere beneath that specific electrode. This method is often used if it is suspected that someone has epilepsy. Depending on the results, the patient may need to be prescribed anti-epileptic medication or, in severe cases, surgery to remove the damaged area. Other techniques that can look at how the brain is functioning include fMRI (functional MRI), PET (positron emission tomography) and MEG (magneto encephalography).

It is important to note that although an understanding of the neurosciences can be useful, apart from cases involving surgery for epilepsy, it is not vital. Further, it should be noted that scanning is not a substitute for a detailed cognitive assessment; it should be seen as a tool that supplements the main assessment. One major reason for this is that whereas cognitive testing assesses functions, neuroimaging addresses issues such as blood flow, size of physical structures, patterns of electrical activity, etc. There is not a one-to-one mapping from one of these to the other and since in clinical work it is the patient's everyday functioning in the world that the clinician should be concerned with, cognitive testing should take precedence.

ASSESSMENTS

Depending on the particular setting that a clinician works in, a significant aspect of their work will involve conducting specialised assessments of patients referred to them from other health professionals. For example, a patient seen in an accident-and-emergency ward who has been in a car crash might be referred by an emergency physician to see the impact of the closed head injury that they suffered. Or a neurologist who is treating someone who may have suffered a small stroke may want to find out whether it had any permanent impact on the patient's functioning. A neurosurgeon who is going to perform surgery to remove damaged brain tissue in the right hemisphere that is causing epileptic seizures may want to know what the patient's functioning is like before the surgery so that, post-surgery, it is possible to make sure that there has been minimal functional damage. In some quite advanced centres, the neuropsychologist conducts an assessment in the operating theatre while the patient is awake during the surgery: due to the way that sensation is processed, it is actually possible for a patient not to feel pain while their brain is being operated on. This is because it is possible for the surgeon to temporarily anaesthetise very small areas of the brain that they wants to remove because of their possible involvement in the epilepsy. Since language is such a vital skill in human communication, it is crucial that the surgeon's knife does not leave the patient as impaired as Tan above. In such cases, the neuropsychologist would perform assessments during the operation to allow the neurosurgeon to determine the extent of what they feel comfortable in removing. These examples are just a small fraction of the range of scenarios where the neuropsychologist's expert training will be called upon.

There are four broad questions that a clinician needs to address when conducting an assessment.

1   Why am I conducting this assessment?

2   How do I conduct the assessment?

3   What sorts of assessments can I conduct?

4   How do I interpret the findings from the assessment?

Each of these will be addressed in turn.

Why am I conducting this assessment?

A patient can be referred to a clinician for a number of different reasons, and what these are can determine what is done, how it is done and even how the results are interpreted. The most straightforward reason would be to give another medical professional (e.g. a GP or a neurologist) an overall report of the patient's functioning to allow them to consider the best course of treatment. On the other hand, a neurosurgeon may want to determine the impact of removing damaged tissue (e.g. a tumour or areas of damage involved in epileptic seizures). In these latter cases, the range of assessments may be focused on those that are known to require the areas removed by the surgeon to be fully intact. In legal cases, the neuropsychologist may be involved in making a decision on a patient's competency for making informed choices. Each of these scenarios may result in a different choice of tests that are conducted and even how they may be interpreted.

How do I conduct the assessment?

The most important aspect of an assessment is to gather as much information as possible. While the performance on the cognitive assessments (see below) forms the basis for the work with the patient, before that, it is important to develop a comprehensive picture of the patient's background and condition. To begin with, all demographics such as age, gender, schooling and current occupation should be recorded. Age and gender can have a great impact on performance, while someone's educational or employment background can be important for interpreting test results.

The patient's medical history, including use of drugs, needs to be taken. If the patient has had any other neuropsychological investigations including neuroimaging, this should be recorded. Sometimes, such information should be available but if a patient has moved home, it may not. This information is important because the findings from previous investigations can have an impact on the choice of tests conducted now (see below). Details should be taken of any accidents involving head injury or loss of consciousness since such incidents can precipitate slowly progressing brain damage that only becomes obvious much later on. Once a comprehensive background has been taken, the formal assessments can begin.

What sorts of assessments can I conduct?

As stated at the beginning of the chapter, a clinical neuropsychologist should also have general training as a clinical psychologist and therefore many of the general assessments relevant in that field would be among the armoury of tests that could be applied. However, specific to the area of brain–behaviour relationships, there are two main types of assessments that can be performed, cognitive and brain-imaging (see above). The latter is not something that a neuropsychologist would be directly involved in – since it is conducted by radiologists and medical physicists – but, depending on the type of setting a neuropsychologist works in, these may or may not be available – for example, in a large hospital, brain scanning or EEG monitoring may be possible but not in a small community setting. However, even if these are not available, a report of a patient's previous assessments may include such information or it may be possible to recommend that the patient could benefit from such procedures.

The majority of the neuropsychologist's work will be based on assessing a patient's cognitive ability. During their training, based on a firm grounding in cognitive psychology, they should learn how to administer and interpret the results of a large array of different tests. The list of these is exhaustive but examples would be the Wechsler Adult Intelligence Scale (WAIS) for general intelligence, the Wechsler Memory Test – Revised for memory, the Birmingham Object Recognition Battery for visual processing and the Wisconsin Card Sorting Test for frontal functioning. Some tests are administered simply with paper and pencil whereas others may involve computer presentation or more sophisticated means. But all tests should have been created such that the instructions for administration are strictly standardised with precise guidelines on what to say to the participant, what (if any) feedback is to be given, how to score performance and finally how to interpret the results.

The first decision that needs to be made is the choice of tests to be used. The answer to this somewhat depends on the answer to the first question above, i.e. why the assessment is being conducted. Also depending on external factors such as resources (some tests are very expensive and so not every centre will have every single available test) and time constraints (there can be a large range in the amount of time allowed with a patient, depending on the system one is working within), the clinician may have more or less flexibility in the choices they can make. In some cases, the patient may have been referred for a very specific problem, for example a visual recognition problem and so, from the outset, it is possible to narrow down the range of tests that need to be considered.

Another factor that can help in deciding choice of tests is the patient's history. If they have undergone neuropsychological assessment before, then it may be useful to look at the areas of weakness that had been identified previously to see if there has been a change over time. In some areas, for example visual attention, it is possible to use the same test a number of times – the line bisection task can be used many times and it can be possible to see whether the patient's visual attention problems have improved from the acute phase of brain damage into the chronic longer term. However, some other tests, particularly those that involve some sort of memory component, should not be used on multiple occasions because having been exposed to items may make the patient perform better the second time even if there has been no actual improvement in their ability. For this reason, some tests have parallel or alternative forms to allow two valid assessments at different time points.

An important contribution to the decision-making process of which assessments to use is keeping updated with the development of new tools. As part of the standard CPD that all clinicians should engage in, the main way of keeping updated is by belonging to professional societies, participating in training workshops and attending conferences where new knowledge is disseminated.

How do I interpret the findings from the assessment?

After conducting an assessment, the clinician now needs to put together the various forms of background information (patient history, notes about previous assessments, their demographic characteristics) to interpret their performance on the cognitive tests. Part of this interpretation will be based on the first question above, of why the assessment was being conducted since the report they write may be very specific about a particular issue (for example for a speech pathologist working with a patient who has suffered a stroke) or it may be a generic one. The report should contain results from all tests performed because even if the clinician does not feel that some findings are particularly interesting, someone else may notice a pattern that they may miss.

A very crucial point is not to over-interpret the findings since test results are not absolute. In a nutshell, a test is only as good as the thinking that went behind its construction. Since science is a dynamic process and theories are constantly being modified or even replaced by new theories, it may well be that a particular test may not find a deficit that a patient is experiencing. For example, the majority of tests of memory are based on the idea that information moves from a very temporary STM to a LTM where it may remain for a very long time (see above). Further, it was assumed that this was a one-stage process so that once the information moved from STM to LTM, it could last there relatively permanently. Based on this assumption, most tests involve presentation of information followed by immediate recall (to test that the information has actually entered STM) and then delayed recall perhaps half an hour later (to test whether or not it has transferred to LTM). Patients such as HM (see above) with significant memory impairments tend to do well on immediate recall but very poorly at delayed recall.

However, there is a group of patients that complain of marked memory problems who pass both these tests and also on standard MRI scans show no obvious brain damage; based on this, *some* clinicians diagnose them as having normal memory. Unfortunately, it has been found that these patients *do* have profound memory problems but these only become apparent a number of days later, a condition known as 'accelerated long-term forgetting' (ALF) which can be associated with some forms of temporal lobe epilepsy (e.g. Jansari et al., 2010). Currently there is no clinical test that can detect ALF, and researchers are attempting to create one as well as investigate the implications for theories of LTM formation. This is a classic example of what Teuber (1969: 19) warned against, namely, 'confusing absence of evidence with evidence of absence' – just because a deficit cannot be seen from test results, this does not mean that it does not exist.

In summary, conducting specialised cognitive assessments is at the heart of the work that a clinical neuropsychologist performs. By careful application of set procedures and using established principles about how to interpret a patient's past history, in combination with their performance on standard tests, a comprehensive picture can be built up of areas of impairment as well as islands of preserved abilities.

REHABILITATION

Unless a patient has extremely widespread brain damage, a very obvious finding from a comprehensive assessment will be that there are many cognitive functions that are fully intact. As understanding of brain–behaviour relationships and the impact of damage to the brain improve, the management of patients is becoming increasingly more sophisticated. In terms of having an impact on the patient, a major contribution would be an attempt to improve their quality of life. Such 'rehabilitation' could be in one of three broad areas – restoration of function, amelioration of difficulties and compensation. Unfortunately, there is very little research that has shown that restoration of function to pre-morbid levels is possible for the main cognitive domains. This is because although some regrowth of brain tissues can occur, there is very little evidence of it growing in areas that are involved in the main cognitive functions. So for example, brain damage in the medial temporal lobes that are vital for memory functions seems to be permanent and therefore, certainly at the moment, hoping for restoration of these abilities is premature. However, by having an understanding of what a patient can and cannot do, it is possible for allied health professionals to use this to ameliorate their day-to-day lives. For example, occupational therapists who work to aid the patient in this everyday living could use the knowledge that the patient's memory is severely affected to change the layout of their kitchen to make it easier for them to find utensils and crockery.

One great avenue for helping patients post-trauma is in the area of developing compensatory strategies. This work relies upon capitalising on what is left intact after brain damage to allow the individual to perform to at least some degree of normality. An analogy would be that if someone who was right-handed lost that arm, it would be possible to gradually teach them to write with their left hand; although the end result would not be the same as writing with the right hand it would allow a certain degree of everyday functioning. An example in the cognitive sphere comes from memory. Extensive work that began with the case of HM (described above) and developed through the past fifty years with numerous other patients has shown that memory can be subdivided into a number of different forms. The main subdivisions are between STM and LTM (as described above) and then, within the latter, between procedural memory which is skill-based learning, and declarative memory which is memory for facts. Finally, within declarative memory there is a subdivision between episodic memory for events and semantic memory for facts; however, this latter division is not important for the discussion here (see Figure 10.2).

In terms of rehabilitation, the most important issue is that in addition to STM, procedural memory tends to be unaffected in amnesia. For example, HM was able to incrementally learn new motor skills without ever being able to remember from one session to another the event (episodic memory) of having had the earlier learning

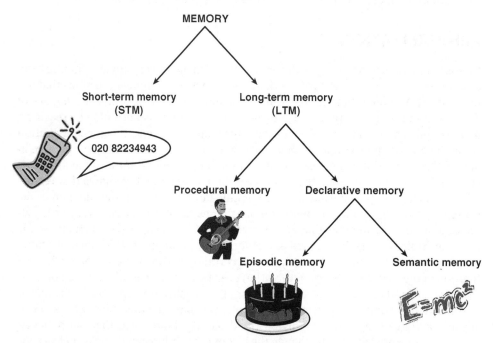

Figure 10.2 Memory tree showing dissociations within human memory. Short-term memory (STM) is temporary memory for up to two minutes; long-term memory (LTM) is memory for anything beyond two minutes; procedural memory is memory for skills such as playing an instrument; declarative memory is memory for facts; episodic memory is for remembering events such as one's birthday party; semantic memory is memory for facts such as mathematical equations

session. Capitalising on this, and using a technique known as 'errorless learning', Professor Barbara Wilson and her team have developed a system called 'NeuroPage' by which patients with memory problems are taught how to use a simple paging device on which they receive pre-programmed reminders of things that they need to do – much like a reminder function on a standard mobile phone. In one study Wilson and colleagues (1997) measured how often patients were able to remember to per-form everyday activities (e.g. remembering to take their medication) before any train-ing (baseline), then used errorless learning to teach the patients to use NeuroPage and found that success improved dramatically (treatment phase). Most importantly, to show that this effect was not simply due to the impact of the intense training regime, they tested the patients long after the training had been stopped and found that success now at this post-treatment stage was double that of the original baseline levels (see Figure 10.3).

This is a classic example of the 'scientist-practitioner' model that clinicians work under. As practitioners, they are ideally placed to know the behavioural and cogni-tive problems experienced by their patients as well as knowing which aspects of eve-ryday life they would like to improve. As scientists who are trained in understanding current literature, through research, they can gradually develop methods to improve the quality of life of their client; this may be improving certain functional abilities or it may simply be enhancing their quality of life as well as that of significant others living with them.

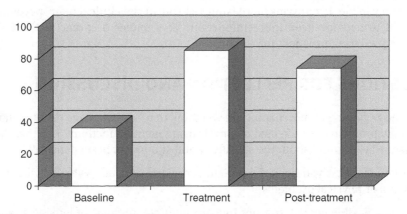

Figure 10.3   Percent success rate of performing activities of daily living by patients with memory problems before (baseline), during (treatment) and after (post-treatment) NeuroPage training

Source: Adapted from Wilson, B.A., Evans, J.J., Emslie H. and Malinek, V. (1997) 'Evaluation of Neu-roPage: a new memory aid', *Journal of Neurology, Neurosurgery and Psychiatry,* 63: 113–5.

HOW DO I BECOME A CLINICAL NEUROPSYCHOLOGIST?

The system for becoming a clinical neuropsychologist varies between different coun-tries, with some countries requiring training to doctoral level, others to master's level and others simply to degree level. In the UK, it is necessary to complete a Professional Doctorate in Clinical Psychology. These doctorates are largely funded by the NHS and places are highly competitive. To greatly improve the chances of achieving one of these places, voluntary work in fields working with individuals that seek clinical ser-vices is extremely beneficial; even better is a job as an assistant psychologist within the NHS. Following qualification from the clinical psychology doctorate, it is neces-sary to specialise in working in neuropsychological settings. The BPS has a special subsection called the Division of Neuropsychology. Membership of this division is in flux at the moment so a trainee psychologist interested in working as a clinical neu-ropsychologist should look at the website http://don.bps.org.uk/.

CONCLUSION

This chapter has reviewed the work of a clinical neuropsychologist, showing that there are a number of different aspects involved. By taking a historical perspec-tive, it was shown that the different elements to the job have evolved as the role of the neuropsychologist has changed from pure assessment to being involved in guiding patient management and possible rehabilitation. This role will continue developing as the techniques and tools available for use on a day-to-day basis improve. Further, as research in cognitive neuropsychology reveals a better understanding of disorders such as age-related dementias, coupled with life expectancy in most countries increasing, the role of the clinical neuropsychologist is bound to become even more important. This makes a career in the field an extremely exciting prospect for the future.

QUESTIONS FOR REFLECTION AND DISCUSSION

1   At the beginning of this chapter did you think that brain damage resulted in wide-spread problems that affected *all* physical and mental functions? Has this chapter changed your mind about the specificity and subtlety of brain damage?

2   Do you feel that you have the patience to work clinically with individuals with mental or physical problems?

3   Are you flexible enough to want to learn multiple methods of looking at an indi-vidual's behaviour ranging from the emotional consequences of brain damage to how the site of lesions may predict the particular problems that an individual exhibits?

4   Are you inquisitive enough to want to examine the pattern of intact and impaired abilities exhibited by a patient to attempt to develop methods of rehabilitation?

SUGGESTIONS FOR FURTHER READING

Goldstein, L.H. and McNeil, J.E. (2008) *Clinical Neuropsychology: A Practical Guide to Assessment and Management for Clinicians*. Chichester: John Wiley & Sons. This is a very thorough book covering an extensive range of topics and is used widely by those who specialise in the field.

Gurd, J.M., Kischka, U. and Marshall, J.C. (2010) *The Handbook of Clinical Neuropsychology* (2nd edn). Oxford: Oxford University Press. This book is similar to the Goldstein and McNeil book above but with different authors. There are slight differences in approach so it is useful to read both.

Jansari, A. (2005) 'Cognitive neuropsychology', in N. Braisby (ed.), *Cognitive Psychology: A Methods Companion*. Oxford: Oxford University Press. This is a book chapter that gives a more in-depth description of the use of cognitive neuropsychology as a research methodology (and its most important principles) than is possible in the current chapter.

Ramachandran, V.S. and Blakeslee, S. (1998) *Phantoms in the Brain: Human Nature and the Architecture of the Mind*. London: Fourth Estate. The first author is a neurologist and neuroscientist who gives fantastic descriptions of patients with quite intriguing brain disorders that reveal the complexity of the human mind. Although Ramachandran is not a neuropsychologist and the patients are sometimes extreme examples, the book is a wonderful insight into brain damage.

11

SPORT PSYCHOLOGY

James Beale and Marcia Wilson

This chapter discusses:

- what is sport psychology?

- how sport psychology is governed within the UK;

- the process of recognition for those working within sport psychology in the UK;

- three key ways of working within sport psychology;

- a case study of the application of sport psychology;

- training for people who are interested in sport psychology but who do not have a psychology degree.

INTRODUCTION

Sport psychology has received considerable attention in recent years, from a range of different areas including the media, the applied field and the academic sphere. This interest is demonstrated through an increase in the number of media reports referring to sport psychology and directly requesting sport psychology comment; the number of athletes utilising sport psychology services and skills (still considerably lower than most expect); and the number of sport science and psychology courses either directly naming sport psychology within the title or including a sport psychology component. Despite this there is no widely accepted definition of sport psychology. For this reason we describe sport psychology here as the study of psychological factors within sport, with the aim of developing an ever-increasing understanding of how psychological factors have an impact on behaviour, across both different sports and different cultures. It is important to mention that there is another very vibrant area of 'exercise psychology' which is often used interchangeably or combined with sport psychology (sport and exercise psychology). It is beyond the scope of this chapter to address exercise psychology specifically and we will focus on sport only. Should you wish to consider the area of exercise psychology there are a number of excellent reviews that are easily available (see Biddle and Mutrie, 2008; Buckworth and Dishman, 2002).

The term 'sport psychologist' is used to mean different things by different people. The term is often used in the media with different connotations and there is as yet no standard way to practise. In effect 'sport psychologist' is an umbrella term for a variety of different ways of doing things. These differences often come down to the core professional philosophy that the practitioner adopts.

'Professional philosophy' is a term used interchangeably with 'professional framework', 'theoretical persuasion' and 'mode of practice' to refer to the preferred manner of conducting sessions by the practitioner. There is very limited evidence on the relative effectiveness of each approach and what is demonstrated consistently within the literature is that the relationship with the client (the therapeutic alliance) is the key issue for the effectiveness of the sessions, above and beyond which professional framework is adopted (McLeod, 2003).

The professional philosophy is still highly relevant in terms of what a sport psychologist actually does. Two different sport psychologists may approach a client in very different ways, but could be equally effective. The *psychological skills-based* sport psychologist would tend to see their role in terms of what happens in the sport setting only, and on many (but not all) occasions would consider this to be limited to training and competition. They would be consultants who in effect have a toolbox of techniques that are performance focused. Techniques such as goal-setting, imagery and confidence-building would often form the basis of an intervention by a sport psychology consultant working with this professional philosophy.

In contrast to this, the *humanistic* practitioner would not normally rely on a series of techniques as the basis of the sessions but would consider their ability to enable the client to reflect on their sport through conversation to be a key area of practice. An ability to listen and strike up a therapeutic alliance will enable the client to discuss things openly and honestly with the practitioner. This then enables the client to develop their awareness and be amenable to challenging in relation to their thinking, attitudes, feelings and concepts. The idea underpinning the humanistic approach is that the practitioner creates an environment that is supportive but challenging through demonstrating the three therapeutic core conditions described by Carl Rogers: empathy, genuineness and unconditional positive regard. This area is very much aligned to the traditional counselling approach (see chapter 15) and was popularised within sport psychology through Timothy Gallwey's series of inner-game books, for example *The Inner Game of Tennis* (Gallwey, 1974). Practitioners from this perspective would be interested in more than the competition and training, and would allow the client to lead on exploring the factors that are relevant to them at the time.

SPORT PSYCHOLOGY TRAINING AND QUALIFICATIONS IN THE UK

As a result of combining the domains of sport and psychology there was always some debate as to the ownership and governance of sport psychology within the UK. This has undergone radical change over the past five years, and appears to have settled now with both sides of the debate seeming to have a clear position.

The sport science governing body, the British Association of Sport and Exercise Sciences (BASES) has for many years had a system of 'accreditation' within all of the key areas of sport and exercise science, of which sport and exercise psychology was one area. The BASES accreditation system recognises both applied practitioners and researchers and there are systems for each of those domains. The BASES system was initially a three-year part-time training programme that normally took place after completion of a relevant postgraduate programme, for example a master's degree in sport psychology. In October 2009 the system for accreditation was revamped and reduced to a two-year part-time post-postgraduate training programme to come more in line with other similar health professions. A key difference between the new and the old system is the generic accreditation as a 'sport and exercise scientist' (not as a sport psychologist) where the key areas of sport science, physiology, biomechanics and psychology are required to a higher minimum level than before, across all of the different specialisms within the programme. Students under the BASES accreditation system go through a process known as 'supervised experience'. While students undertake this process they are advised by BASES to refer to themselves as 'probationary sport and exercise scientists'. The system of supervised experience works through students presenting a portfolio to cover several different areas that are supposed to gradually develop over the two-year period. The key area of applied practice is central to the system and to the supervision process. Over the two years students are expected to undertake five hundred hours of one-to-one consultations with clients. Out of these consultations, four hundred hours are expected to be within the specialist area that the person is working within, and a minimum of twenty hours are expected to be directly supervised.

Students who have a sport science undergraduate degree, recognised under the BASES Undergraduate Endorsement Scheme (BUES) are advantaged in this system. A number of the key components are automatically assumed; for example, the underlying biomechanics and physiology knowledge are automatically accepted for students with a BUES-recognised undergraduate degree.

On completion of supervised experience then accreditation is awarded for a period of five years, after which re-accreditation is required. This process continues every five years. Re-accreditation requires that practitioners spend a minimum of one hundred and fifty hours per year or four hours per week working with individual clients in sport psychology. The process also requires CPD to a minimum of one hundred and twenty hours per year over the time period with a minimum of twenty hours having to come through the BASES system, i.e. BASES workshop attendance/facilitation or BASES conference presentations/attendance.

In both accreditation and re-accreditation, a portfolio of work is submitted and independently reviewed by two reviewers, before being processed through a reviewer panel meeting. There is a clear way of becoming a reviewer within the BASES system, and for re-accreditation it is essentially a process of peer review.

The psychology governing body, the BPS, have developed in recent years to include the recognition of sport and exercise psychologists operating a process leading to chartered status. The BPS have a clear route for chartering psychologists that is consistent within all areas of psychology that have a 'division' within the society. This includes clinical psychologists, counselling psychologists, occupational psychologists, health psychologists and forensic psychologists. There are intricacies within each system. Before starting the process, individuals are expected to have a BPS-recognised undergraduate degree, what was previously known as a degree with GBR and now known as a GBC. The BPS then have a two-stage process that leads on to chartered status as a sport and exercise psychologist and enables the successful student to use the abbreviation CPsychol after their name. The initial stage can be completed in two ways. First, students can go through a BPS-accredited master's degree programme. These programmes can be found on the BPS website. The second way for students with a relevant degree in psychology is to carry out the Stage 1 process, under supervision from a previously chartered psychologist with an up-to-date trainer certificate (a full list is available on the BPS website). Stage 2 is a minimum of a two-year process that involves developing a portfolio around four key roles: ethical practice, applied practice, research and finally dissemination of sport psychology principles. The applied practice section involves a minimum of one hundred and sixty days' work. Within this, a Stage 2 student can include preparation, data-gathering, reflection and design of evidence-based interventions, as well as one-to-one consultancy hours with individual clients.

The Health Professions Council (HPC) now own the terms 'practitioner psychologist' and 'sport and exercise psychologist' and regulate their use and any derivative of them within the UK. The process of BPS chartership does enable successful candidates to apply for inclusion on the HPC register. Within the HPC there is a clear method for application to the register for applicants with international qualifications, so that if a practitioner were to move to the UK from, for example, Australia and wished to practise here, they could apply to the register through the international route. Potential applicants should contact the HPC directly.

KEY AREAS

There are essentially three core areas that sport psychologists find themselves working in. These are:

- researcher
- applied practitioner
- lecturer.

These will be discussed here independently; however, the likelihood is that should readers follow a career in sport psychology, they would find themselves working in a combined role. There are a number of reasons for this, mostly concerned with the ways the roles can complement each other. It is really useful if you are a lecturer to have experience of applying the theory and skills that you present to students. Likewise, to have an up-to-date knowledge of current literature is essential if you are to be an effective practitioner. That same interdependence is evident whichever angle you choose to examine. If you work predominantly as an applied practitioner it is useful to do research and teach, and if you work predominantly as a researcher it is useful to teach and to practise, at least occasionally. This chapter will now examine each of these roles independently.

Researchers in sport psychology range from PhD students, lecturers and post-doctoral researchers to readers and professors. Researchers are most likely to have a dual research–teaching role with a large amount of time spent carrying out research and preparing written manuscripts for publication in peer-reviewed journals. Over a researcher's career it is likely that a specialism will develop and the researcher will become an expert in a narrow field, where they are likely to be involved in attracting grant income to lead the development in the area of specialism.

Applied practitioners are those that work directly with athletes to assist them with psychological factors that have an impact on their sport. These practitioners will often work within national bodies, e.g. the English Institute of Sport (EIS), or as independent practitioners who may well service a range of independent sports clubs and individuals. The work typically involves a combination of one-to-one consultations with group work to enhance psychological skills and build areas such as team cohesion and confidence.

Lecturers are normally found in government-funded higher and further educational environments, and particularly universities. The role of lecturer varies across institutions; however, as a rule of thumb, lecturers are generally expected to spend about a third of their time on teaching-related activities, a third on administration tasks and a final third on research-related activities. Direct teaching with students is perhaps what most people think of as the primary role. Although this forms a substantial part of a lecturer's work, there is also a substantial amount of time spent being involved in committees within the university, ensuring the smooth running of current programmes, developing new programmes, and pushing back the boundaries of knowledge through research (see also Chapter 18, 'The Professional Academic'). This is perhaps the most common way to earn a living through working in sport psychology within the UK.

CASE STUDY

The following case study is presented by the first author and considers an intervention from 2008 with a speedway rider.

The case study will examine an applied example. Before doing so it is important to make clear that in order to maintain confidentiality the name of the individual and a few key details have been changed.

The topic areas that the client can decide to discuss encompass an enormous range of possibilities. The current client was in particular concerned about relationships with key people in his life, and these relationships had a major effect on sport-specific decisions, so that discussion and reflection of these relationships and their effects took up a significant part of the sessions, in addition to the more performance-specific aspects.

Context of the case study

The current case study takes a humanistic approach in the main but also utilises some specific psychological skills and techniques, so that it could be considered *eclectic* by some. The psychological skills are secondary to the main approach, which is a conversation-based reflection between the sport psychologist and client. The case involves a speedway rider from the southern hemisphere who was at the time based in Europe, riding in three leagues across the continent. The rider, for the purposes of this chapter, is referred to as JT. The support offered took place over a four-month period in 2008, through the bulk of the European speedway season. Each session lasted between fifty and one hundred and ten minutes. (The aim was for the sessions to last an hour, but most sessions lasted slightly more than an hour.) There were ten sessions in total over this period and three observations. The client approached the sport psychologist via email before travelling back from his home to race the European season. It was decided that we would meet when he travelled to London from his base in Sweden to race in the south of England.

The initial session

After more than ten years of applied experience in sport psychology the first session now tends to follow a similar process. The main aims of the first session are to get to know the client and how the client has experienced their sport over their career, as well as to begin developing an understanding of the factors that have an impact on their sporting performance. A considerable amount of the initial session is put aside for the client to free associate, and from this discussion, themes emerge. The emerging themes from the client often form the basis of future sessions and, from these, other themes emerge. I also like to gain an understanding of the client's personal situation if possible during this session as well, as I have on a number of occasions found that significant others in the athlete's life (be they a parent, a partner or a friend) are having a significant impact on their decisions and having an impact on the client's sporting life and sporting performances. It is necessary to explain relevant ethical factors to the client. There still remain a variety of connotations or implications to seeing a sport psychologist, many of which can be seen as quite negative. To counter this, putting the client at ease by explaining that all information will remain confidential, describing how any information will be taken and stored, and who the governing bodies are that the client could report to should there be any issues they are unhappy with – these have in my experience placed the client in a more empowered position.

The picture that emerged from the first session was that the rider had been around speedway and motorbikes since he was a young boy aged eight, and that he had always wanted to take part. There was evidence that JT looked up to people on all types of motorbikes and was a motorsport enthusiast. Speedway became progressively more serious as JT progressed through his life and was often deemed a positive influence, in that it was used as an incentive to do well in other areas. For example, 'Do well at school and you get the bike' was apparently a statement used by his parents on more than one occasion. JT reported that whereas others got into trouble, he was not in that environment as he was either involved in or preparing to take part in speedway. Within the first session we also spoke about what JT wanted to get out of the psychology sessions. Most clients tend to come with something that they want to change, and JT reported that he wanted to gain more confidence. The aims of the sessions in my experience tend to emerge or develop as the sessions progress. It was useful to hear what the client wanted to get out of the intervention during the initial session; and many of the future consultations examined where confidence came from for JT, what factors eroded confidence, as well as what confidence means to him. These factors took us into a range of different areas over the time period.

Selected techniques

Throughout the period there were a series of techniques used to enable the client to develop his awareness of where his confidence comes from, what undermines it and how the client can build a confidence that is sustainable over time. In my experience the issue with confidence is not so much about building it up, but is more about having a confidence that is sustained in pressurised environments.

Rogerian-style interviews

The vast majority of this case study involved allowing the client time to free-associate and direct the sessions himself through conversation. A lot of time was spent trying to develop an environment that appropriately balanced support and challenge, with the emphasis being on the supportive at the beginning and more of a challenging environment once the relationship was established. The generic principles of trying to demonstrate the three core qualities of empathy, genuineness and non-judgemental caring were adhered to wherever possible in an attempt to build the therapeutic alliance. The techniques below were secondary to these interviews, which were the main focus of the intervention.

Positive diary

The past decade has seen an increase in usage of positive psychology interventions (see also Chapter 13). With this client I asked him to keep a positive diary. After each meeting he wrote down the positive features from the meeting and was encouraged to ignore the negative factors. In my experience this is rather alien to athletes, who tend to have spent their careers examining how they can improve through addressing the areas in which they did badly. The client came back after the initial entry with a list of good and bad factors, and when asked what the reason was for the bad factors he explained that this is what he does naturally. After several attempts the client was able to write only the positive comments. Bandura (1977) suggests that there are four areas important to building self-efficacy (situation-specific self-confidence), the most important area being performance accomplishments. As a psychologist, I consider perception to be of huge importance, as the way an individual perceives a situation is their reality. The rationale then is to attempt to get JT to perceive his performance in the most positive way possible. The technique has similar aspects to that of appreciative inquiry as described by Watkins and Mohr (2001). In a later session JT was asked to reflect on the usefulness of this very simple technique. He was extremely positive about the technique, which he reported as making him think more positively about the meetings, and feel 'good' about future meetings.

Individualised emotional profiling (IEP)

Individualised emotional profiling (Hanin, 2000) is a technique that is used to facilitate awareness of optimal performance states. The technique in its purist form takes athletes through a series of steps to achieve this awareness. The technique includes getting athletes to reflect on their best and worst performances to give a baseline of emotions that are helpful or unhelpful to performance. These emotions are then rated on a one-to-ten rating scale, and from this there is a baseline from which to investigate how the individual performs at their best. The process then looks to visualisation to enable the process. This case study used an adapted version of IEP. Much of the imagery that followed was based on the information that was discovered through the process of reflection within the IEP process. For confidentiality reasons it is not possible to discuss details of JT's emotional profile here.

Imagery

Throughout my experience in applied sport psychology, the technique that I have utilised the most has been imagery. There are a number of theories for how imagery works with a performer; however, detailed discussion of these are beyond the scope of this chapter. For the purposes of this intervention the black box technique (Syer and Connolly, 1998) was used as a preparatory tool for performance. This technique involves relaxation, a visual image of leaving your issues behind you for the performance and then a performance-based section where JT would imagine using all of the senses while performing in his optimal performance zone. The technique lasts about twenty minutes. The performance section was guided by the IEP section of the intervention so as to enable JT to imagine himself experiencing all of the emotional states necessary to access his individual zone of optimal functioning.

A WORD OF CAUTION

The sport psychology industry has been subject to the criticism that there are a number of individuals working within it without relevant qualifications, and who are not tied to governing bodies and therefore not regulated or required to work within a code of conduct. It can be argued that these people have caused a lot of damage to the reputation of the industry and I am frequently shocked by athletes' poor experiences of those claiming to be sport psychologists. Despite the recent introduction of HPC regulation of the industry in the UK, there has been a long period when the industry was not regulated and as such anyone could use the term 'sport psychologist' without fear of legal reprisals. One example springs to mind of another speedway rider who saw a person that he described as the club sport psychologist. The rider had gained a reputation for being a wild talent who would not follow team instructions. The remit of the sport psychology person appeared to be to sort this out and ensure that the rider's attitude changed to a more positive, team-based one. The sport psychology person began the session by asking the question: 'Do you know why we travel around the track always turning to our left and why we don't go right?' (Speedway races always follow an anticlockwise path around the track.) The rider reports not knowing the definitive answer but came up with a series of technical responses, all of which were apparently wrong (although in practice probably correct). The sport psychologist then replied, 'It is because our heart in on the left!', which was in some way supposed to imply that the athlete did not have a passion for his sport. Although there is some support for the use of metaphor within sport psychology (see Hanin and Stambulova, 2002) there is very little evidence to support beginning a session in this way. This kind of story can travel around the athletic fraternity extremely quickly, generating a cynical attitude and damaging the reputation of the industry. This story was in fact relayed to me by a different speedway rider who wanted help but had had a bad experience of sport psychology previously and knew of others who also had a poor experience, this being an example. Those planning a career in sport psychology should seek full and proper training to avoid such instances occurring in the future. Training for sport psychologists should further assist in building the reputation of the discipline as a whole.

WHERE TO GO IF INTERESTED IN SPORT PSYCHOLOGY

In this section we identify three main areas:

1   for people who are UK based and from a sport science background;
2   for those who are UK based and from a psychology background;
3   for those now based in the UK with qualifications from other countries and interested in working in the UK.

Before starting this section it is important to point out that it is the intention of the authors to provide no biases towards any training system and to simply present the facts at the time of writing. There have been a number of changes within the training of sport psychologists over the past five years and while things appear clear at present there will no doubt be further changes. Readers should use this section as a guide and should follow up through the necessary governing bodies as mentioned below. Should the reader be someone who is not yet committed to any of the three pathways mentioned above, it is down to the individual to make an informed decision on which one they decide to follow. It is anticipated that most readers will have committed to one of the following paths and as such this section gives them clear guidance on how to proceed with their careers.

Those currently studying on a UK-based undergraduate sport science degree programme have three choices to get involved with sport psychology.

- Those wishing to enter into academia as either a lecturer or researcher should follow a postgraduate programme with the aim of completing a PhD. One way to do this would be to follow a relevant master's degree beforehand.

- Those wishing to go into the applied field would need to complete a master's degree in an area relevant to sport psychology and then follow the BASES supervised experience process as discussed earlier in this chapter. Students following the supervised experience process should expect to spend three years training, one year as a full-time postgraduate student and two years as a part-time supervisee/probationary sport and exercise scientist. Successful completion of this process would enable students to use the term 'BASES Accredited Sport and Exercise Scientist'.

- The final option for those studying for an undergraduate degree in a sport and exercise science area, and wishing to enter into the applied domain, is to spend a year completing a psychology conversion degree to a degree with GBC recognition, followed by a BPS-accredited master's degree programme followed by a minimum of two years following the BPS Stage 2 process, the system leading to chartered status as a psychologist. Students entering into this process would have a minimum of a four-year process from the start of the conversion degree programme.

For those studying on a UK-based psychology undergraduate programme with GBC status awarded on successful completion, you would either follow a postgraduate programme with the aim of completing a PhD if you wanted to go into academia, or you would follow a BPS-accredited master's degree in sport psychology followed by the BPS Stage 2 process. Students that are unsure whether they see their future in the applied or academic field would be well advised to follow a BPS-accredited master's degree course as this would provide an excellent grounding to follow either pathway. It could further be argued that there is no reason why potential students could not complete both a PhD and the BPS Stage 2 process at the same time. There are a series of complementary competencies within both systems. For further guidance on the BPS Stage 2 process see the BPS website (www.bps.org.uk). Successful completion of the BPS Stage 2 process enables students to use the letters 'CPsychol' (Chartered Psychologist) after their name. Such students would also be eligible to apply for automatic inclusion on the HPC register, as a Registered Sport and Exercise Psychologist and Practitioner Psychologist.

Students with qualifications from other countries would first need to establish the equivalency of their qualification. This can be done through the worldwide qualification system NARIC. Readers are unlikely to have access to this system so a more practical approach would be to find the course that they think they might want to study and then ask the admissions tutor. There are a number of reciprocal arrangements between organisations, e.g. the American organisation the Association for Applied Sport Psychology (AASP) have an arrangement with BASES that an AASP-certified consultant is automatically awarded BASES-accredited status once they become a member; the reverse is true for BASES accredited practitioners with a specialism in sport psychology, so that BASES accredited practitioners would be awarded certified consultant status through AASP when the practitioner becomes a member. It is beyond the scope of this chapter to discuss all of the possibilities available to students who have qualifications from other countries. The advice from this chapter is that there is a system that compares international qualifications (NARIC) that most UK-based universities have access to and will be able to provide advice on suitability to study further within the UK. Further there are a series of international reciprocal arrangements between governing bodies. The core governing bodies in the UK for sport psychology are the BPS and BASES.

CONCLUSION

The role of the sport psychologist is emerging as one that is valued and has a lot to offer within various fields of sporting endeavour. Although a relatively new specialism, it is now reaching a point where there are clear routes to achieving a credible status as a professional practitioner for those with suitable undergraduate degrees either in sport and exercise science or in psychology. A sport psychologist can offer a number of interventions, working both with groups/teams and individuals. One-to-one work can combine exploratory consultative conversations characterised by the humanistic core conditions of empathy, congruence and non-judgemental acceptance, with more specific psychological techniques, skills and interventions; or it can focus more on one or other of these alternatives.

QUESTIONS FOR REFLECTION AND DISCUSSION

1   Sport psychology has expanded rapidly over the past twenty years. What are the possible reasons for this?

2   What are the key differences between sport psychology and other applied psychology disciplines?

3   The governance of sport psychology has changed radically over the past years. If you decided to undertake training in sport psychology what would be your pathway and why?

4   In this chapter we suggest that the term 'sport psychologist' is an umbrella term. What do we mean by this?

SUGGESTIONS FOR FURTHER READING

Academic texts

Cox, R.H. (2007) *Sport Psychology: Concepts and Applications* (6th edn). New York: McGraw-Hill. A clear and insightful overview of the main theories used in sport psychology. This book is a standard undergraduate text for those looking to enhance their academic understanding of sport psychology.

Weinberg, R.S and Gould, D. (2011) *Foundations of Sport and Exercise Psychology* (5th edn). Champaign, IL: Human Kinetics. The gold-standard academic text for undergraduate students studying sport psychology. This demonstrates a very clear overview of the contemporary theories in sport psychology and has some excellent questions to reflect on throughout.

Practical texts

Orlick, T. (1998) *Embracing Your Potential: Steps to Self-discovery, Balance and Success in Sports, Work and Life*. Champaign, IL: Human Kinetics. This is a practical guide that discusses two areas of growth for individuals in both sport and life. Orlick puts forward the idea of growing in a green (personal) zone and gold (performance) zone. This book offers practical techniques to develop in each of these areas that could be used as a performer, individual or sport psychology consultant.

Seligman, M. (2011) *Flourish: A New Understanding of Happiness and Well-Being – and How to Achieve Them*. Nicholas Brealey Publishing. This book presents a new theory of positive psychology and then examines how to apply this theory in a series of different contexts. Written by the founding father of positive psychology, this is a must read for someone entering into sport psychology. Although this book does not address sport psychology as an independent section, the theory and applications within this book can easily be transferred to a sporting context.

Syer, J. and Connolly, C. (1998) *Sporting Body, Sporting Mind: An Athlete's Guide to Mental Training*. London: Simon and Schuster. This book offers advice to both athletes and practitioners from a humanistic perspective. The book has some very helpful practical tips, not least the chapters on building team synergy and positive attitude change. Although this book was written some time ago it remains one of the most commonly used texts by practitioners looking to enhance athlete performance.

12

COUNSELLING PSYCHOLOGY

Jill Mytton

This chapter discusses:

- the historical and philosophical origins and the identity of counselling psychology;

- whether or not there are differences between counselling psychology and other psychotherapeutic professions;

- where counselling psychologists work and how they work, with some examples;

- the various routes to qualification as a Chartered Counselling Psychologist and the challenges for trainees;

- what the future holds for counselling psychology as the profession reaches its thirtieth birthday in 2012.

INTRODUCTION

This chapter opens by briefly setting the developing profession of counselling psychology in its historical context. The next section describes the nature and philosophy of counselling psychology from a number of different perspectives: historical, official (Division of Counselling Psychology), operational, comparisons with other professions, and philosophical. After reading the relevant chapters in this book, the reader may be feeling somewhat confused by the similarities between counselling psychology, clinical psychology, counselling and psychotherapy. I argue that it is the underlying philosophy that often differentiates one profession from another. The third section seeks to give the reader an impression of what it is like to work as a counselling psychologist, with two contributions from practitioners working in different contexts. A description of the current routes to training and a discussion of a number of issues and tensions faced by the trainee counselling psychologist follows. The final section looks to the future of counselling psychology, especially its evolving identity, using debates about diagnosis and the medicalisation of distress for illustration.

THE HISTORICAL CONTEXT

Human beings have always been fascinated by the search for the causes and treatment of emotional problems and behaviour viewed as abnormal by the society in which an individual lives (Ellenberger, 1994). Hippocrates (460–377 BC), for example, is known to have regarded mental illness as the result of physiological abnormalities, an imbalance of bodily fluids or 'humours'. Other early theories often focused on supernatural causes, including possession by the devil or evil spirits. The cures ranged from drugs, the wearing of charms, massage and diet through to exorcism and confession. In some tribal societies 'abnormal behaviour' was seen as evidence of supernatural gifts, and the person would become the tribal shaman. Throughout history, individuals have received counsel and advice. For example, in a book about chess in therapy, Fadul and Canles (2009) suggest that theoretically based psychotherapy was first developed in the ninth century in the Middle East by Rhazas (AD 852–932) who 'counseled his patients and students according to metaphors and applications of chess game configurations in real life situations' (p. 7). More recently in the nineteenth century the well-known phrase 'talking cures' was thought to have been first coined by one of Josef Breuer's patients known as Anna O, and this phrase was picked up and used by Freud to describe his work in psychoanalyis (Ellenberger, 1994). Since his time a variety of psychotherapeutic professions and approaches have emerged, some of which are described elsewhere in this book.

The profession of counselling psychology began in the USA in the 1940s when Division 17 (Personnel and Guidance Psychologists) was established in the APA. By 1952 the name changed to the Division of Counseling Psychology with the professional goal 'to foster the psychological development of the individual' (Munley et al., 2004: 250).

In the UK, the development of counselling psychology began much later during the 1970s when counselling (not counselling psychology) was expanding rapidly in Britain, focusing largely on providing therapy for problems of living rather than for individuals with mental illness. This development occurred largely separately from the profession of psychology yet there were many psychologists who had taken up training in counselling and psychotherapy, and they played an important role in those early days. They wrote much of the growing literature on counselling and yet they had no 'home' in the BPS; none of the existing divisions were appropriate (Nelson-Jones, 1999).

In 1979 a working party was set up to consider the practice of counselling and its relationship to the professional interests of the BPS. They concluded that there was a need to provide a structure to enable the Society to broaden its interests. A new Section of Counselling Psychology was therefore set up in 1982. By the end of that year it already had two hundred and twenty-five members. Ten years later, in 1992, the society set up a Diploma in Counselling Psychology to provide a route to chartered status for psychologists whose interest lay in counselling.

Two years after this, in 1994, the BPS finally established the Division of Counselling Psychology some forty-two years after its sister division in the USA had been created. For those psychologists already working as counsellors and wanting to join the division there was an 'equivalence' route to chartered status. This option was closed in 1996 and after that anyone seeking to become a Chartered Counselling Psychologist had to undertake formal training either by completing a BPS-accredited course or by completing the Diploma in Counselling Psychology via the independent route.

At the time of writing (May 2011) there are 3,000 members of this division of whom 1303 are Chartered Counselling Psychologists. Chartered Counselling Psychologists are still relatively few in number; however, the profession is now growing fast with about eight hundred and twenty-five students currently on university courses and about seventy-five currently enrolled on the BPS Qualification in Counselling Psychology (QCoP) via the independent route. The division now has a number of regional and national branches including Scotland, Northern Ireland and Wales.

In 2009, when the government required psychologists to be registered by the Health Professions Council (HPC), counselling psychology was recognised as a named specialism. All BPS Chartered Counselling Psychologists (and a small number of others with professional qualifications in psychology and counselling/psychotherapy) have now had the opportunity to become HPC-registered counselling psychologists.

THE NATURE AND PHILOSOPHY OF COUNSELLING PSYCHOLOGY

Since its early beginnings, counselling psychology, as a branch of applied professional psychology, has struggled with its identity. In order for the profession to exist as a distinctive and separate entity there need to be clear statements about its nature and philosophy and how it relates to other areas of psychology. The difficulty for counselling psychology has been in clearly encapsulating its identity in a few words or sentences, a task made more difficult by the fact that the profession has developed and is continuing to develop into a diverse, pluralistic, complex field working with a wide range of approaches and in a variety of contexts.

Attempts to define and describe its activities have been made from a number of different perspectives and here I will describe some of them: the historical, the official Division of Counselling Psychology definition, the operational, by comparison with other similar professions, and the philosophical.

A historical definition

Historically, counselling psychology has been described as a move away from the medical model, from diagnostic categories and from the language of pathology and sickness, to a focus on a more human sciences model. It originated within the humanistic movement and was influenced by the well-established division of counselling psychology in the USA and by European Psychotherapy. Counselling psychology 'positioned itself between the science of psychology and the therapeutic practices of counselling and psychotherapy' (Woolfe et al., 2010: 2). This means that it challenges the natural science model, with its emphasis on the medical model that uses descriptors such as 'psychopathology', 'mental illness' and 'disorders', and focuses instead on a more human sciences model, which sees psychological difficulties not as pathological but as part of the human experience and development. A counselling psychologist's emphasis is thus more on well-being.

The Division of Counselling Psychology definition

In a BPS publication (namely, *Professional Practice Guidelines*, 2005: 1–2), the following statement is made:

> Counselling psychology has developed as a branch of professional psychological practice strongly influenced by human science research as well as the principal psychotherapeutic traditions. Counselling psychology draws upon and seeks to develop phenomenological models of practice and enquiry in addition to that of traditional scientific psychology. It continues to develop models of practice and research which marry the scientific demand for rigorous empirical enquiry with a firm value base grounded in the primacy of the counselling or psychotherapeutic relationship. These models seek:
>
> 1 to engage with subjectivity and intersubjectivity, values and beliefs;
>
> 2 to know empathically and to respect first person accounts as valid in their own terms; to elucidate, interpret and negotiate between perceptions and world views but not to assume the automatic superiority of any one way of experiencing, feeling, valuing and knowing;
>
> 3 to be practice led, with a research base grounded in professional practice values as well as professional artistry;
>
> 4 to recognize social contexts and discrimination and to work always in ways that empower rather than control and also demonstrate the high standards of anti-discriminatory practice appropriate to the pluralistic nature of society today.

Although this statement emphasises our psychological roots and hints at our underlying humanistic philosophy with its emphasis on the therapeutic relationship, it leaves out many aspects of the profession, some of which are mentioned below. An earlier definition provided by the Division of Counselling Psychology (2001: 42) contains the important statement that 'the practice of Counselling Psychology requires a high level of self-awareness and competence in relating the skills and knowledge of personal and interpersonal dynamics to the therapeutic context'.

An operational/competency-based definition

Counselling psychologists are graduate psychologists who have undergone three years of full-time – or part-time equivalent – training in the theory and practice of counselling psychology to a standard recognised by the BPS and also by the HPC. Training emphasises the application of psychology to psychotherapy and the integration of theory, practice and research. With its focus on the trainees' competencies and knowledge acquisition this definition gives a rather limited impression of the nature of counselling psychology – it says little about what actually happens between the counselling psychologist and client.

The competencies outlined by the BPS and the HPC help us gain some understanding of the profession. These are eight broad areas under which the competencies are listed: philosophy, theoretical models, psychological knowledge, research and inquiry, ethics, personal development, professional issues and client work. They form the basis of all training programmes and will be further described later in this chapter.

Using comparisons to define counselling psychology

Comparing counselling psychology with similar professions does not enable us to set up distinct boundaries, as there are clear overlaps. Boundaries are constantly being drawn and redrawn as these professions develop.

Unlike clinical psychology, the philosophical roots of counselling psychology lie in the phenomenological (humanistic) tradition. The phenomenological tradition of valuing the person and their subjective experience and the wider context of the person's cultural and social life provides the links to counselling and psychotherapy. Hammersley (2003) believes that a counselling psychologist, in addition to being practitioner, researcher, scientist and philosopher, also needs to be 'creative and innovative to produce the particular "moments of change" or internal shift which should result from the deep engagement with the client in a therapeutic relationship' (Hammersley, 2003: 638). It is this emphasis on the 'deep engagement with the client' and the therapeutic relationship that is distinctive to this particular branch of applied psychology although again there is an obvious area of overlap with counsellors and psychotherapists (see Chapter 15).

In a discussion of the 'reflective-practitioner model', Schön suggested the need for recognising 'the artistic, intuitive processes which some practitioners do bring to situations of uncertainty, instability, uniqueness, and value conflict' (Schön, 1983: 49). Counselling psychology has been using the reflective-practitioner model for some time in its move away from the more mechanistic approach, towards one in which personal reflection and development play essential roles.

The *Standards of Proficiency for Practitioner Psychologists* from the HPC (2009) indicate that clinical and counselling psychologists engage in very similar professional activities. What differentiates them, as Duffy (1990) suggests, is perhaps not so much 'what' they do but 'how' they approach the therapeutic endeavour and in particular the difference in focus. Counselling psychologists tend to focus less on the medical model and more on the development of the self and on what the presenting psychological issues mean for the individual at that particular moment in life. Clinical psychologists, at least traditionally, tend to focus more on the medical model with its emphasis on assessment, diagnosis and treatment protocols.

The philosophical definition

Briefly, the phenomenological model, as applied to counselling psychology, takes the view that valid knowledge and understanding of what clients bring to the session is best gained by exploring and describing the way they, the clients, are experiencing their world. To achieve this, therapists have to suspend their own assumptions and values – a process that phenomenologists call a 'bracketing off' of any theoretical assumptions the therapist might hold about the clients' experiences.

Traditionally psychologists try to make sense of the workings of the human 'mind' from the outside: we play the role of the scientist who attempts to measure objectively what is and tries to predict what will be. (This is not so true these days with the emergence of so-called 'critical psychology' and the increasing use of qualitative methods of research.) However, when working phenomenologically with clients, we are working from an internal not an external perspective. Valuing the humanistic approach to therapy has led to a distaste for the positivistic approach to working with psychological distress commonly used in the NHS. So by identifying with phenomenology and a humanistic value base, do counselling psychologists struggle to work in the NHS and other settings where the value base is different?

Perhaps it is the value base that defines the profession more clearly. But immediately an important question is raised – are the values of counselling psychology the same for all counselling psychologists? The answer appears to be no. The training courses are attracting people from very diverse backgrounds who come with and develop a breadth of different perspectives on this value base. This is reflected in the theme for the 2011 Counselling Psychology Annual Conference 'Celebrating Pluralism in Counselling Psychology' where a smorgasbord of topics ranging from mindfulness, CBT, medication, bibliotherapy and positive psychology through to the refugee experience, problem drinking, addiction and eating disorders were presented.

What unites us as a profession is that 'we tend to see the uniqueness and complexity of each individual which is not captured by typology or biology or by measuring, atomizing or comparing but only by knowing: getting to know each individual by careful observation, by taking time and by engagement and interaction at many levels' (Frankland and Walsh, 2010). Whether we work with groups, families, couples or individuals the core value is we are always working in relationship with them.

After reading this section on the nature and philosophy of counselling psychology, the reader may feel confused and ask, 'But what do counselling psychologists actually do?' To describe what a good counselling psychologist does when engaged in the 'inner world' of a troubled client is very difficult. So much of a good counselling psychologist's activity (when to remain silent, when to paraphrase, when to mirror back the client's words, when to ask questions, when to challenge, etc.) is based on intuition and instinct and thus the process is difficult to describe. Theory and techniques can be taught but something more is needed above and beyond the knowledge and practice.

I find the following analogy helpful here. Roger Stott (2002, personal communication) described the 'good counsellor' as someone who is like a well-trained and experienced yachtsman or yachtswoman:

all the theory and knowledge is there as a guide but in the immediate turbulence of wind and water something more is needed – a capacity to work on instincts, to improvise, to be able to turn in one's own length, to fail and then immediately to find another way, to maintain steady objectivity even when chaos is threatening ... each counselling psychologist has to find her or his own way through the wind and water and has to do it freshly with each new client.

WORKING AS A COUNSELLING PSYCHOLOGIST

In this section I want to give a taste of what the work of a typical counselling psychologist is like, the problem being that there is probably no 'typical' counselling psychologist. We work in a wide variety of settings, from many different theoretical frameworks and with a very broad range of client issues and problems.

Counselling psychologists can be found working as therapists in many different settings including:

- the NHS:
  - primary care
  - community mental health teams
  - specialist services such as eating disorder clinics, services for older adults, child and family services, services for learning disabilities
  - improving access to psychological services (IAPT);
- prison and probationary services;
- voluntary organisations and charities: for example, the Medical Foundation for the Care of Victims of Torture;
- employee assistance programmes;
- student counselling services (schools, colleges and universities);
- private practice;
- education:
  - further education colleges
  - schools
  - universities.

Counselling psychologists initially train to work with individuals but many go on to work with couples, families and groups. They practise in all the mainstream theoretical orientations including CBT, existential, gestalt, integrative, narrative, person-centred, psychodynamic and family systems therapy. Counselling psychologists work therapeutically with clients of all ages presenting with a wide variety of problems and difficulties. These might include life issues and crises (such as relationship breakdowns, bereavement, domestic violence), mental health problems (for example, depression, anxiety, eating disorders, drug and alcohol addictions, dementias and psychoses), and medical problems (following strokes, HIV and AIDS counselling, cancer).

Counselling psychologists are also employed by universities and colleges as lecturers training future members of the profession and carrying out research. Many have a portfolio of activities. For example, they might work part time for a university, have a small private practice and work part time for the NHS.

In the next section two experienced counselling psychologists provide a glimpse into their work.

A Consultant Counselling Psychologist in the NHS: Dr Yvonne Walsh

The large NHS trust that I work for employs over thirty counselling psychologists in paid positions; in addition we have both university-based and independent-route trainees working on honorary contracts with us. This makes the Trust a good place for counselling psychologists to work, even with the continual cycles of reorganisation and change that seem endemic within the NHS.

There is no easy way to describe the wide range of activities that my post requires: as well as being professional lead for counselling psychology for the Trust, I specialise in working with adult clients who have a combination of complex needs, such as those with dual diagnosis (in which issues of substance misuse are combined with mental health problems), and those who are survivors of complicated childhood abuse.

My client work is the centre of all of my activities, and the reason I became a counselling psychologist. Such work requires me to keep up and continue to develop my psychotherapy skills and it also serves to give me credibility with other staff. I work at the intersection between humanistic and scientific perspectives and focus on an inter-subjective way of relating to clients, respecting their world views as valid in their own right with no agenda to correct their 'erroneous' beliefs and behaviours, or whatever I think is 'wrong' with them. We work together to find a way to resolve their psychological difficulties or problems with living. In other fora this is often viewed as treating psychiatric illness.

I work in groups, with clients on a one-to-one basis and with families or partners as necessary and with my clients' wish and consent, practising cognitive relational therapy in the main. Although I originally trained in systemic family therapy, and cognitive therapy in the past few years, I have worked extensively with a colleague who comes from the person-centred approach, and this has been extremely influential in my psychotherapeutic work.

Sometimes my work, like that of any senior practitioner, is strategic, and I have to take a broad view across the Trust and the various staff groups who work within my speciality. To create a formal strategy for the Trust, research data has to be considered alongside the views of all the stakeholders, and proposals have to be written and reviewed with them, and gradually refined and tested until all the relevant parties (including senior Trust management) believe that we have a document indicating clearly how this issue is to be addressed. We then have a strategy, so the next task is to enable people to understand and operationalise it. After a period of working to the strategy, we have to assess its impact and revise it where necessary. It is a lengthy and sometimes frustrating process; from conceptualising the problem, to putting the strategy into place and then auditing its effectiveness. Activities like this utilise many of my skills as a counselling psychologist such as research, clarification of ideas, communication and feedback, report writing and enabling and evaluating change.

Working with the most demanding cases and strategic work are only part of the job of a consultant counselling psychologist. The rest is made up of consultations with individuals and teams on their complex cases; supervision, both of counselling psychologists and other staff; and both formal and informal aspects of training and teaching.

Another way to understand the range of my job is to think about some of the things that I have done over time.

- I have contributed to a major training development within the Trust; to build capable teams fit for the client work for which a modern NHS trust provides services.

- I have collated and written up a needs analysis for a bid to the Department of Health for a specialist 'detoxification plus' ward for clients with complex needs.

- I was chair of both a support/supervision/training group for staff members who have clients with complex needs on their case-load and a meeting of staff who are employed specifically to work with this client group.

- I set up and ran a centralised placement scheme finding and organising placements for counselling psychology trainees, organising rotations to another placement for those trainees whose placements are coming to an end and who wish to continue their training with us.

- I have participated in the cross-Trust psychological-services managers' team meeting.

- I read the numerous official documents, guidelines and advisories that came to me from the various networks I am a part of, and helped by commenting on some and redrafting others.

- I have written specialist reports for the courts, social services, commissioners and other professionals

- I have done the huge amount of administration that is required when working within the modern NHS. This includes writing up computerised notes, keeping up-to-date a computerised diary of client contacts, processes, outcomes and so forth, taking and making phone calls and of course answering what seems like thousands of emails.

- I have supervised and consulted on the work of a range of colleagues and had case work and professional supervision myself, which is a requirement both of the BPS and the HPC, and essential in a busy schedule like mine – in fact absolutely essential for anyone working psychotherapeutically (and arguably in any demanding relational profession).

Then there is the BPS work that I do … .

I am Lead for promoting counselling psychology for the BPS Division of Counselling Psychology. In this role I spend rather a lot of time responding to queries sent to the Division often via the BPS help desk, and support counselling psychologists who are having difficulties with equal opportunities in their work places. I am also on the executive committee of the Division and as such I have a lot of work put my way by the division committee.

What I find extremely interesting is that all of my roles and tasks complement each other; the knowledge and skills that I develop in one area are useful for the other areas. An example of this is how I can often feed information into the Trust about what is happening nationally (including new ideas and ways of working) that I glean from my involvement in the Division. The networking that I do works both ways in that counselling psychology also benefits because I can promote it as a profession and I get a chance to feed opportunities and information into the Division.

I never thought that I would find myself in this position, but I must say that although my job can be tiring, demanding and sheer hard work – including a huge amount of politics with a small p – and there are times I yearn for a nice 'simple' job in a team, solely seeing clients and supporting the team, I also go home at times thinking ... 'and they are paying me for this!'

A Consultant Counselling Psychologist in Independent Practice: Alan Frankland

I have been in therapeutic practice for almost thirty-five years, initially on a part-time basis alongside an academic career but for the last ten years or so virtually full time in independent practice; that is to say, I work for myself, and the considerable majority of my clients engage with me and pay me on a private contractual basis. Although I have no problem being identified as a counsellor (I have been a member of the British Association for Counselling and Psychotherapy (BACP) for about three decades and am proud to be a Fellow) or a psychotherapist (I am a foundation member of the BPS Register of Psychologists Specialising in Psychotherapy), my core professional identification these days is as a counselling psychologist, since this most completely meets my sense of being an applied psychology professional engaged in relational therapy. Almost every day when I am doing therapy or supervision some information or an attitude derived or developed from my initial training in psychology will come to mind – something from the knowledge I have gained about human development, or sleep or dyslexia to offer some recent examples; or more fundamentally the attitude of informed scepticism and empiricism that gives psychology some claim to being science. At the same time my practice is not enslaved by the mechanistic application of a scientific dogma but is tempered by self-knowledge and my own experiencing (in life and as a client), and from intuition and insights drawn from the phenomenological and humanistic traditions that inform counselling practice (and are also a part of humanistic psychology).

I have put in time within the organisation of the Division and of the BPS, and served as registrar of the independent route for some years. I have made contributions to training and examining and writing in this area (and still do to a lesser extent) but at the centre, indeed the heart, of what I do now is the adventure of working on a regular basis in relationships with troubled people who want to 'sort themselves out' or to find a new way of understanding themselves and to feel differently and act differently in their lives. I also love working in individual supervision to facilitate others doing this work. These two activities fill the majority of my working days.

Because of issues of confidentiality it would be difficult to write in any depth about the people I am actually seeing so the following 'day in the life' is a truthful composite to give a sense of what I do.

It is Tuesday; I am back in my Nottingham practice, which is based in the apartment that my partner and I bought as our town base here when we moved to live in the country. Yesterday I did two or three hours in the evening after travelling up here, and today will be quite a long day as I aim to do a full week's work between Monday afternoon and Thursday evening.

Today I shall start with Zoe, a young client who is confused and unhappy about herself and her future. Part of her difficulty is focusing her attention, as well as overcoming basic shyness and discomfort about talking about herself, so these sessions are hard work for both of us. Next, I shall see a colleague for his monthly ninety minutes of supervision. That work is nearly always a pleasure as Fred is an interesting man and a thoughtful therapist. Before lunch I am to see Jane – whom I previously worked with in couples counselling – who is once again faced with the dilemma of whether her relationship is worth saving. Working with anyone who has a family that is breaking down is technically and emotionally taxing as it draws on a wide range of different skills and knowledge as we consider and explore her pain and responses to it, and try to be clear about what approaches might open up more fruitful discussions at home or might harm the children least and also consider what has to happen next.

After lunch I have a difficult session that usually takes place about once a month with Linda who wants support because she is very frightened about her current health problems but is very resistant to psychological exploration, so we seem very stuck. Then another supervision session.

In the evening I have two clients I have worked with for some months who nevertheless illustrate the range of work that I do quite well. Sinead is in a long and slow self-directed process of self-discovery and self-acceptance as she comes to terms with a difficult past and tries to re-engage with feelings without being overwhelmed. Julian too is engaged in a task of emotional discovery but whereas Sinead needs me to hold back in the most non-directive way, to help her explore with empathy and acceptance but no pressure to change, Julian has opted for a more psycho-educational problem-solving approach that sees us both as very active in structuring, almost engineering, new opportunities for learning and change.

Between clients I do the necessary administration associated with client work and with running my practice (which requires a small business head alongside that of a therapist) and respond to emails and correspondence and so on. But I also take the opportunity to cook lunch and listen to the radio in the middle of the day so that I am refreshed for later work. Even so, on a Tuesday, after seven hours in the consulting room over a twelve-hour period, I feel pretty stretched.

Overall, this work demands of me considerable personal engagement, both in the the thoughts and feelings of my clients and in the lives they live. I have to be able to accept that at the same time I may be really important to them and yet somehow peripheral. I have to maintain a certain professional objectivity and yet enter the subjective world of my clients to create with them an inter-subjective world of relationship which, virtually regardless of technique, is the crucible of therapeutic change. For me this is all part of what being a psychologist and a psychotherapeutic practitioner means and for me it is why I identify as a counselling psychologist.

TRAINING ISSUES FOR COUNSELLING PSYCHOLOGISTS

Counselling psychology training is rigorous and not for the faint hearted. The BPS list eight elements: philosophy, theoretical models, psychological knowledge, research and inquiry, ethics, personal development, professional issues and client work. All these components are compulsory and trainees need to find a way of integrating them in order to become competent professional practitioners – no easy task when also having to run their personal lives, raise their families and earn money. Currently, counselling psychology (and counsellor/psychotherapy) trainees do not receive any funding for their course fees, clinical supervision or personal therapy. Thus, personal and financial pressures are combined with the difficulties of finding placements, beginning work with clients, the tensions experienced when embracing both the scientist-practitioner and phenomenological philosophical perspectives, carrying out research, and meeting the requirements of the BPS and HPC and, for course route trainees, also those of their university.

As with all other applied psychology training leading to chartered status, the first step is to acquire the GBC with the BPS, which is usually gained by having a first degree in psychology. This provides the future counselling psychologist with fundamental knowledge of the various branches of psychology of particular relevance to counselling psychology such as human development, the biological basis of behaviour, personality theory, cognitive and social psychology, along with quantitative and qualitative research methods and skills. The HPC registration does not require GBC although members should have a first degree in psychology.

By the end of their training the counselling psychology trainee is expected to be able to respond appropriately and flexibly to the needs of their clients and contexts. Some will have chosen to work with only one approach such as the psychodynamic; others will be happy working in more than one approach depending on the needs of their client; and yet others will have developed their own integrative approach.

They will have achieved a number of competencies in addition to the therapeutic work with clients; many of these are very similar to those of the clinical psychologist, counsellor and psychotherapist. The key aim of accredited programmes in counselling psychology and of the QCoP is to produce graduates who will:

1   be competent, reflective, ethically sound, resourceful and informed practition-
    ers of counselling psychology able to work in therapeutic and non-therapeutic
    contexts;

2   value the imaginative, interpretative, personal and intimate aspects of the
    practice of counselling psychology;

3   commit themselves to ongoing personal and professional development and
    inquiry;

4   understand, develop and apply models of psychological inquiry for the crea-
    tion of new knowledge that is appropriate to the multidimensional nature of
    relationships between people;

5   appreciate the significance of wider social, cultural and political domans within
    which counselling psychology operates; and

6   adopt a questioning and evaluative approach to the philosophy, practice,
    research and theory that constitutes counselling psychology.

For details on both the HPC and the BPS requirements see the websites listed at the end
of this chapter. The syllabus for any profession encapsulates its identifying philosophy
and defines the knowledge base that underlies the competencies of its practitioners.

Chartered status can be achieved by one of two routes or even a combination
of the two. Trainees can either undertake a BPS-accredited counselling psychology
course at a university or can enrol with the BPS to study for the QCoP independently
under the guidance of a Co-ordinating Supervisor (CS). Sometimes trainees will use a
combination of the two routes, so they might for example complete a course-based
master's degree and then transfer to the independent route to complete their training.

The BPS QCoP is intended for independent trainees who are not attached to accredited postgraduate training programmes. It is designed to be a flexible training option
allowing trainees to develop their own training and learning experiences. Trainees
have to demonstrate the knowledge and skills required for eligibility to apply for
chartered status. For more information on this route see the website listed at the end
of this chapter.

BPS-accredited and HPC-registered university doctoral programmes, which usually award a DPsych or a PsychD, consist of a considerable amount of taught courses
with a variety of assessment components. These courses can either be completed part
time or full time. The research element that is submitted in the final year usually comprises a portfolio of case studies, process reports and a 35,000–40,000-word research
dissertation. Currently there are fourteen institutions offering doctoral programmes
in counselling psychology (see website listings).

Both routes require four hundred and fifty hours of supervised clinical work and a
minimum of forty hours of personal therapy. Both also have a viva at the end of training. The QCoP viva focuses on the trainee's overall competencies, their perceived
strengths and weaknesses and their professional identity as a counselling psychologist.
The course route viva usually focuses mainly on the research component.

Challenges for trainees and trainers

The challenges facing counselling psychology trainees depend to some extent on the route they have chosen: the independent or the course route. One challenge that all trainees have to face regardless of their chosen route is a financial one.

Currently there is no structure providing funding, and the bill for training can run into thousands of pounds. For course route trainees there are the university fees to pay whereas the independent route trainees have to pay their co-ordinators of training and for core therapy training as well as for any short courses they attend. All trainees have to fund their clinical supervision (unless they are fortunate enough to find placements where supervision is provided) as well as personal therapy. Some trainees fund themselves at least partially via career development loans; others manage to persuade organisations they are working for, such as the NHS, to pay their fees; but the majority of trainees obtain part-time employment to cover their costs.

The issue of obtaining funding for counselling psychology trainees, so that they are on parity with clinical psychology trainees, is currently being investigated by the Division of Counselling Psychology. It is likely that in the future at least some trainees will be funded by an NHS scheme although there are some concerns about how this could affect the syllabus. Will the funding body want to have some say in what the trainees are taught?

Trainees choosing to follow the independent route face particular challenges. Their first task is to find a Co-ordinating Supervisor (CS), who needs to be a Chartered Counselling Psychologist. The CS plays a crucial role in guiding trainees through to successful completion. To assist the CS in this task the BPS run regular training workshops. Trainees report that the route can be a very isolating and lonely experience because apart from their CS there is no one to share it with (John, 2010). They feel the lack of support and the opportunity to discuss and debate issues and concerns with other trainees. Both the Division of Counselling Psychology and the BPS have made considerable efforts through the setting-up of induction meetings, workshops and email discussion groups to facilitate networking. Often trainees on this route choose it out of geographical necessity; they live where there are no university courses. This, however, presents other difficulties in that finding suitable workshops and short courses is problematic. The ethos of QCoP is to allow recognition of prior experience and training acquired since obtaining GBC. Although this is a huge advantage for trainees, the paperwork involved can be quite daunting.

Course route trainees face a different set of challenges, though some of these may also be shared by independent route trainees. Szymanska (2002) identified a number of expectations that trainees bring that can lead to disillusionment with the experience of training. Trainees often have the expectation that the course route will provide them with all that they need to know and that once they have finished the course their knowledge base will be complete. The reality is somewhat different: attendance on a course is simply the first step along the pathway of professionalisation. Learning for all trainees, whatever route they choose, is a continuous process that does not end when chartered status is achieved.

Linked to this expectation is the one that trainers will have all the answers, that they are all knowing. In reality trainers on the course route have a number of roles: to provide information, to give guidance and support, and to encourage individualisation thus enhancing the trainee's professional and personal growth (Szymanska, 2002). Although the trainers may be experts in their chosen specialisation(s) and/or area(s) of research, trainers cannot be 'masters of all they purvey'.

Applicants for course route training often minimise the impact that a course will have on their life so it comes as quite a shock when, roughly six months into the course, they realise just how disrupting the course can be. Time pressures as deadlines loom, relationship difficulties as family and friends feel threatened by the trainee's new insights, the demands of the course and financial pressures can all have a serious impact on the trainee's lifestyle. It is not uncommon for serious life events (partnership break-ups/divorce, accidents, serious illness, pregnancy) to occur during the first two years of training.

In recent years the trainers themselves have faced increasing challenges. When designing and running courses not only do the programme leaders have to consider their own institutions' regulations but also the requirements of the BPS, the HPC and sometimes pressures from the NHS too. With universities struggling financially, cutbacks in staffing levels have added to the stresses. In 2005 the BPS requirements for training in counselling psychology were revised. One important change was the shift in standard from master's to doctoral level, which raised a number of interesting challenges particularly with the universities who have yet to fully understand what 'doctoral-level clinical practice' is.

CHALLENGES AND DEVELOPMENTS IN THE PROFESSION

The future for counselling psychology surely lies in its innovative, imaginative and creative ways of working with clients while remaining grounded in empiricism. Yet this very way of being poses challenges for the profession. In this section I briefly mention some of the key challenges and refer the reader to the final chapter in Orlans and Van Scoyoc (2009) for further study.

Counselling psychology's identity

Counselling psychology is still a relatively young discipline in the UK and it is difficult to forecast its future. All evolving professions seek to define their core features and identify the characteristics that distinguish them from other allied professions. This process of professionalisation is still in its early stages in the UK, and the diversity found within its ranks poses quite a challenge to the integrity of counselling psychology. According to Niemeyer and Diamond (2001) this challenge still faces counselling psychology in the USA where the profession can no longer be described as 'young'. They describe calls for counselling psychology to align itself more closely to neuropsychology and clinical psychology and some authors have even predicted that counselling and clinical psychology will merge in some way. As we view clinical and counselling psychology in the UK similar predictions have also been made as both professions have evolved over time. Concern over this led Brammer et al. (1988: 411) to state: 'It is important that counselling psychology be able to define its uniqueness if it is to avoid efforts by some to merge the current applied specialities.'

In a letter to *The Psychologist*, Woolfe (2002) wrote that the answer to questions about the differences between counselling and clinical psychology may lie in the lyrics of the song 'It ain't what you do, it's the way that you do it'. He wrote '[counselling psychology] argues that the most crucial factor in healing is not what we do with clients but how we are with them. In this formulation the emphasis is placed on the power of the therapeutic relationship (being) rather than the application of specific skills or techniques (doing)' (Woolfe, 2002: 168). Some people believe that there are more similarities between clinical and counselling psychology than differences and in recent years moves have been made by both professions that have brought them even closer. For example, the clinical psychologists now recognise the value of the reflective-practitioner model and some programmes include in their training a focus on well-being and therapeutic process. Counselling psychologists now include a greater focus on psychopathology and psychometric testing in their training to make them better equipped to work in the NHS.

Diagnosis, the medicalisation of distress and other debates

Working alongside clinical psychologists and psychiatrists poses a number of challenges for the counselling psychologist. It is easy to be drawn into the framework of the medical model when working within the NHS or within employee assistance programmes (who sometimes use diagnostic categories to market themselves).

For the counselling psychologist this raises a number of questions and concerns. We are more interested in producing psychological formulations about a person's difficulties than in giving them diagnostic labels. We ask: how can we account for this person's actions and experience in a particular biographical and social context? We search for an understanding of the person's psychological difficulties so how can we also be interested in reducing those difficulties to diagnostic constructs?

Many reasons are put forward to support the use of these labels: they are said to facilitate communication between professions, to enable research to be carried out on the specific groupings created, to be essential in the law courts and for insurance and compensation claims. But how do they really help the person who is being diagnosed? The counter-arguments are much more about individual needs. How does the diagnosis of schizophrenia enable the practitioner to help the client, for example? Such a label can unfairly render the communications of individuals invalid, pathological and therefore meaningless.

By using diagnostic categories are we guilty of pathologising normal human experiences? Common human experiences, such as bereavement, childbirth, work stress and difficult living situations can be very distressing but is it appropriate to call this distress depression or even PTSD? Such labels locate the difficulty inside the person involved when in fact it might be more appropriate to regard the problem as a social or cultural one. A young mother living alone with three children in a high-rise flat surrounded by noisy neighbours may well go to her doctor with classic signs of stress. But is this a personal problem, a mental illness or a social problem?

There is little evidence that diagnostic categories have any validity and as yet almost no progress has been made through research into the actual causes of these so-called disorders. The labels used are based on symptom clusters. Psychiatrists have yet to discover any signs linked to mental disorders: there are no blood tests or neurological tests that can verify or validate these constructs. It is possible for two people to have the same diagnosis yet have very few or no symptoms in common. Psychiatrists themselves are now beginning to question the use of pathologising labels. In a debate at the Maudsley in 2002 the following motion was highly supported: 'This house believes that the trauma industry inappropriately medicalises normal suffering' (The Maudsley Debates, 2002).

Another current debate revolves around the use of psychometric testing. Employers including the NHS expect applied psychologists to be trained in their use and this is now included in counselling psychology training. Psychometric tests are typically used to evaluate therapy and to aid the planning of therapeutic interventions. This traditional use of tests ignores the potential for more direct therapeutic usage. Finn (1996) convincingly describes how the Minnesota Multiphasic Personality Inventory-2 (MMPI-2) can be used therapeutically to help clients understand themselves through the use of feedback sessions. Clients become engaged as collaborators, whose ideas are essential to the assessment. Testing is then no longer something being 'done to' the client but 'done with' the client and for their benefit.

CONCLUSION

Counselling psychology can be a very rewarding profession. When asked why they want to train in counselling psychology, many applicants reply that they get personal satisfaction out of helping others overcome difficulties in their lives. During their training, students often comment on how they appreciate the variety offered to them and the choice that they have in deciding their own specialisations and interests. They feel empowered to develop their own pathways to professional status. The fact that students emerge at the end of their training as different from each other in terms of knowledge areas of expertise as 'chalk is from cheese' is seen as one of the strengths of this profession.

In addition to the therapeutic work, there are many other interesting roles open to counselling psychologists. These include providing clinical supervision, carrying out research, developing workshops for Chartered Counselling Psychologists as part of their CPD or for trainees on the independent route, or becoming a training co-ordinator or a university lecturer teaching on counselling psychology courses. Some people even manage to fulfil a number of these roles thus experiencing the richness and variety of tasks that this profession offers.

Finally, a number of writers have described counselling psychologists as mavericks. As Orlans and Van Scoyoc (2009: 19) state: 'in our experience, there is something of the maverick in many counselling psychologists, a quality that is likely to either attract you instantly to the field or send you off looking for something more "mainstream" and less troublesome.'

QUESTIONS FOR REFLECTION AND DISCUSSION

1   Are there any real differences between clinical and counselling psychology?

2   By engaging, even though peripherally, in the medical model, are counselling psychologists supporting the pathologising of normal human misery and distress?

3   Should we be thinking about merging the two professions of counselling and clinical psychology?

4   In what way are counselling psychologists helping/hindering with problems of daily living? Should we perhaps instead be leaving our consulting rooms behind and joining the campaign trail for social and political change?

5   Do any of the three settings described earlier appeal more to you? Why?

SUGGESTIONS FOR FURTHER READING

Bor, R. and Watts, M. (2010) *The Trainee Handbook: A Guide For Counselling and Psychotherapy Trainees* (2nd edn). London: Sage. Anyone thinking of becoming a counselling psychologist, wanting to know what the training involves or a student currently in training, will find this book useful. It covers a wide range of 'how to' chapters on process reports, case studies, essays and research and a useful chapter on training routes for counsellors, psychotherapists and counselling psychologists.

Dryden, W. and Mytton, J. (1999) *Four Approaches to Counselling and Psychotherapy*. London: Routledge. Many students on undergraduate psychology degrees and on the counselling psychology master's degrees have said that they found this book to be an excellent jargon-free introduction to four of the mainstream approaches to counselling and psychotherapy: psychodynamic, person centred, multi-modal and rational emotive behaviour therapy. Each approach is clearly examined in terms of its historical context and development, and its main theoretical concepts, aims and practice. In the final chapter these four approaches are compared.

Orlans, V. and Van Scoyoc, S. (2009) *A Short Introduction to Counselling Psychology*. London: Sage. An enormous amount of information and ideas are packed into this well-written and very accessible book. It is an ideal read for those who are considering entering the profession and also for those who have already embarked on the training.

Wilkinson, J. and Campbell, E. (1997) *Psychology in Counselling and Therapeutic Practice*. Chichester: Wiley. This book explores how psychological knowledge and research can inform counselling psychology practice. Areas of psychology addressed include personality theory, emotion, memory processes, thinking, states of consciousness, lifespan development and the social psychology of self and relationships. Throughout, case material, examples and discussion illustrate the text in a very useful way.

Woolfe, R., Strawbridge, S., Douglas, B. and Dryden, W. (eds) (2009) *Handbook of Counselling Psychology* (3rd edn). London: Sage. For those interested in counselling psychology, this would be a useful textbook to dip into, to obtain a good overview of what this profession is about. It has seven sections covering: what is counselling psychology?; tradition, challenge and change; difference and discrimination; developmental themes; opportunities and tensions in difference contexts; professional and ethical issues; and future opportunities and challenges.

Websites

British Psychological Society: http://www.bps.org.uk
Health Professions Council: http://www.hpc-uk.org

Training courses

For details of training courses accredited by the BPS see: http://tinyurl.com/3d6cgnk
For more information on the QCoP see: http://tinyurl.com/3jlz6h9
For details of training courses registered by the HPC see: http://tinyurl.com/3vguqg9
For details of the aims and competencies required:

- by the BPS see: http://tinyurl.com/3t6lb8f

- by the HPC (see Standards of Proficiency Document): http://tinyurl.com/lxwy4f

13

POSITIVE PSYCHOLOGY

Kate Hefferon and Ilona Boniwell

This chapter discusses:

- major subject areas and research in positive psychology;

- how positive psychology is currently being applied to enhance societal well-being in seven areas;

- how research designs in applied positive psychology (APP) have developed;

- educational training routes and current programmes;

- student and expert experiences;

- current issues and our thoughts on the future of this applied psychological discipline.

INTRODUCTION

What is positive psychology?

Positive psychology was placed at the forefront of the APA agenda in 1998, by its newly appointed president, Martin Seligman. The underlying focus was to shift the direction of psychology to encompass not only pathology and illness, but well-being, happiness, personal strengths, wisdom, creativity as well. Ultimately, positive psychology aims to discover and promote the factors that allow individuals and communities to thrive (Seligman, 1998).

Positive psychology focuses on several aspects of human flourishing including positive experiences and states across past, present and future (e.g. happiness, optimism, well-being); characteristics of the 'good person' (e.g. talent, wisdom, love, courage, creativity) and positive institutions, citizenship and communities (e.g. altruism, tolerance, work ethic).

Today, the field has increased in focus and followers, offering several respected conferences and academic journals, as well as hundreds of well-written books on the subject matter (e.g. Boniwell, 2008).

What is applied positive psychology (APP)?

So what is the difference between positive psychology and APP? As you will have already ascertained from this book, there is a tension between the study of theory and its direct application to the real world ('Ivory tower to the mainland'). Our theoretical assumptions do not always work out the way we planned and, in order to develop this new field, we need a direct and open relationship between practitioner (real world) and researcher (ivory tower).

Applied positive psychology is currently recognised as the application of the topics and theories within the discipline for the betterment of society (individuals–communities–nations–the world) (Donaldson et al., 2011). Therefore, applied positive psychologists attempt to discover what, if anything, works on the ground level.

There are several branches of APP, including the following.

1 **Everyday life**: judging by the international sales figures of self-help books, it is evident that citizens want to be happy or are at least interested. This area of APP looks at what/who makes individuals happy. Mainly focused on subjective well-being (satisfaction with life and experiences of more positive versus negative feelings), APP informs members of the public as to what they can do to enhance their levels of well-being. For example, research has helped us to understand that there are small, but tangible, changes we can make to commuting, social relationships, work and income to enhance our well-being (Donaldson et al., 2011).

2 **Business**: as history would have it, businesses have traditionally focused on evaluating what was going wrong in the workplace. Positive psychology is now being used within organisations (positive organisational behaviour and positive organisational scholarship), applying the theoretical concepts to enhance productivity, success and employee well-being.

3 **Health**: with regards to health, there are several avenues to applying positive psychology (physical/mental) – especially with the new branch of 'positive health' (Seligman, 2008, 2011). We look to research to understand how happiness can influence good physical health as well as the effects of ill health (cancer, etc.) on well-being.

4 **Education**: the education sector is the most rapidly growing area of APP. Several research teams, from around the world, have developed their own well-being programmes (including at UEL, Boniwell and Osin, in preparation), which have been found to significantly enhance resilience among school children. In addition, other researchers have adapted the school curriculum to embed positive psychology theory within teaching practice and the school ethos.

5 **Governments and public policy**: positive psychologists have made progress within the area of public policy, recommending the implementation of subjective well-being measures into a government's assessment of individual and societal quality of life and subjective well-being (Diener et al., 2009; Stiglitz et al.,

2009). Not only can these tools give governments an idea of how 'happy' their people are, it can help distinguish between what projects and schemes actually increase/decrease their citizens' well-being (Hefferon and Boniwell, 2011).

6 **Communities**: several organisations are implementing APP in community/national happiness initiatives such as *Action for Happiness*, a London-based not-for-profit organisation, which encourages and equips community-led happiness groups with information about well-being.

7 **Environment**: positive psychology has also started to look at the applications and integration of environmental care and well-being. For example, researchers at the New Economics Foundation have created the Happy Planet Index (HPI) 2.0, which reviews the 'ecological efficiency with which human well-being is delivered' (New Economics Foundation, 2010). The main focus is highlighting nations that are not necessarily the happiest, but in harmony with their consumption of natural resources.

Research designs within APP

In the beginning, positive psychology took on the 'scientific method' as its primary research design, commencing a decade-long preoccupation with post-positivist, empirical research. This approach was seen as a direct attempt to separate itself from humanistic psychology, which relied heavily on less 'scientific' modes of discovery (Hefferon and Boniwell, 2011).

The vast majority of early research utilised correlational designs, which quickly became the 'Achilles heel' of the discipline area. As positive psychology matures, there are a greater number of longitudinal research designs in place as well as large, multinational studies that aim to ascertain causal links between variables and well-being. A strong emphasis on cross-cultural research has also become popular, especially with the broadening of relevant journals to encompass international perspectives.

At the present time, research designs have become more holistic, including the use of qualitative research in order to achieve a deeper understanding of the phenomenon of interest. Qualitative research has been particularly popular within Europe and the UK, with American researchers slowly adopting a more pragmatic approach to research (Hefferon and Boniwell, 2011).

Current research areas in positive psychology

In addition to criticism regarding methodologies utilised in positive psychology, there have also been complaints surrounding the restricted focus on certain topic areas (e.g. optimism). Researchers have argued that if we are to move APP forward into the next decade, we need to take a broader, cross-disciplinary approach to positive psychology, including social, cognitive, biological, personality and applied perspectives (Sheldon et al., 2011). It is essential that positive psychology findings from these areas feed into each other so that we access a 360-degree view of well-being (Biswas-Diener, 2011). Furthermore, the focus of positive psychology must shift from a narrow concentration on individual well-being, to more research into group, institution and community-based flourishing.

There are currently several new areas of research interests and funding opportunities within APP. The most notable areas include the following.

1   *Positive neuroscience*

In 2009, the University of Pennsylvania Positive Psychology Center received a grant from the John Templeton Foundation to support their new venture, the 'Positive Neuroscience Project'. Fifteen promising researchers were each awarded between $180,000 and US$250,000, to fund research into how the brain effects flourishing. There was great diversity in the range of topics, including altruism, positive parenting, resilience and much more (see www.posneuro-science.org for information). Overall, this new wave of objective research lends further credibility to the area of positive psychology.

2   *Well-being theory (PERMA model)*

In 2011, Seligman proposed a new direction for positive psychology, shifting away from *'authentic happiness'* to a more holistic state of flourishing. 'PERMA' was introduced as a new 'well-being theory', which aims to increase flourishing by enhancing the following elements:

Positive emotions

Engagement

Relationships (positive)

Meaning

Accomplishment.

Research into measuring these elements and their effects on well-being and flourishing are currently underway.

3   *Positive psychological interventions (PPIs)*

Although not a new area of research, PPIs maintain their stronghold on research and grant funding, with the application of theories and interventions across populations as a primary focus for development of the area. Laboratories such as Barbara Frederickson's Positive Emotions and Psychophysiology Laboratory (http://www.unc.edu/peplab/home.html) and Sonja Lyubomirskys' Positive Psychology Laboratory (http://www.faculty.ucr.edu/~sonja/index .html) continue the advancement of real-world applications of the discipline.

4   *Genetics*

The role of genes in the development of well-being has always been of interest for APP with a general consensus of genetics accounting for approximately

50% of a person's happiness (Lykken and Tellegen, 1996). The current developments within epigenetics and differential susceptibility (Belsky and Pluess, 2009) have once again thrust genetic research into the forefront of APP with a new focus on the roles of specific genes and their effects on well-being (e.g. serotonin transporter gene (SLC6A4)).

Box 13.1   APP case studies

Below are two case studies of applied research that we are currently undertaking. The first case study reviews Kate's work in the health sector whereas the second case reflects upon Ilona's work within the education domain.

Health (exercise and mental health patients)

Kate works within the area of health and well-being in clinical populations. A few years ago, the director of a fascinating exercise intervention for people with mental health difficulties approached Kate after she presented a speech on the theoretical links and research behind exercise participation and resilience, growth and exercise. The director was sure he was seeing resilience and growth within his participants, and asked Kate if she would like to join their team. This meeting would create several years of collaboration, research and application of positive psychological theory on the ground level.

   The exercise intervention consisted of six weeks of aerobic 'boxercise' workouts, led by a former world champion. The results of this applied positive psychological study are currently being analysed; however, we have preliminary evidence to show enhanced self-esteem, higher levels of well-being and increased confidence from participation in the exercise programme. This is an excellent example of using positive psychology theory and research for the betterment of health and clinical populations.

Education (resilience curriculum)

Positive education is a rapidly growing area in APP. A few years ago, Ilona and her colleagues won a large contract to create, disseminate and evaluate a twelve-week resilience programme for year-seven students. Developed for and piloted in deprived neighbourhoods of East London, the *SPARK Resilience* programme builds on research findings from four relevant fields of study: CBT, resilience, post-traumatic growth and positive psychology. Organised around the SPARK acronym, it teaches students to break simple or complex situations into manageable components of situation, autopilot, perception, reaction and knowledge. Through the use of hypothetical scenarios informed by consultations with students in pilot schools, students learn how an everyday *situation* can trigger in them an *autopilot* (feelings and emotions). These autopilots vary for different people and different circumstances because of the unique way they *perceive* these situations. People then *react* to the situation and learn something from it, acquiring *knowledge* about the way they are,

(Continued)

(Continued)

or others are, or the way the world is. To help students understand these concepts, they are introduced to 'parrots of perception' – imaginary creatures representing common distortions of human cognition and thinking. The programme teaches students how to challenge their interpretation of any life situation and consider other alternatives by putting their parrots 'on trial', understanding their automatic emotional responses and learning to control their non-constructive behavioural reactions. Alongside, they are introduced to the skills of assertiveness and problem-solving, and are helped to build their 'resilience muscles' through identifying their strengths, social support networks, sources of positive emotions and previous experiences of resilience. The statistical data analysis showed significantly higher resilience, self-esteem and self-efficacy scores in the post-assessment compared with the pre-assessment data. A marginally significant decrease was also observed in depression symptoms (Boniwell et al., in preparation). This is an excellent example of using positive psychology theory for the betterment of education curricula.

APP TRAINING

So how does one become an 'applied positive psychologist'? At present, there is no governing body regulating the term (implications discussed in conclusion); however, the majority take the traditional academic route specialising in the discipline areas.

Bsc-level APP training

At this point in time, there are no undergraduate positive psychology programmes. However, hundreds of positive psychology option modules exist across Britain and the rest of the world. At UEL, we offer one such third-year option, which consists of eleven three-hour lectures per week, introducing the theoretical concepts within positive psychology and some applications. We use a highly comprehensive textbook (Hefferon and Boniwell, 2011), which includes tools, time-out sections, personal development interventions and mock essay questions to help the students gain the most from their educational experience. The Bsc-level assessment consists of two 2,000-word written coursework assignments: one essay and one personal portfolio. On the whole, this option module is very popular with our students and leads to a number of students applying for our postgraduate MSc in APP (a.k.a. MAPP).

Msc-level APP training

In 2007, UEL was the first university in Europe and the second university in the world to offer a postgraduate programme in APP. The programme is housed within the School of Psychology, the largest department of psychology in the UK, with a considerable record in delivering high-quality undergraduate and postgraduate programmes and courses, research of international standing, and consultancy. Knowledge and expertise in the School incorporates positive psychology, coaching, counselling, neuropsychology, organisational development, health, educational, evolutionary and several other domains of psychology. The MAPP enables the use of this multidisciplinary expertise at a postgraduate level, permitting the development of both the positive psychology itself and other relevant fields of knowledge.

The objectives of the programme are to help its students to:

- develop the depth of knowledge and critical understanding of the theory, research and intellectual history of positive psychology;

- become proficient in selecting and using positive psychology assessment methods;

- study a range of positive psychology interventions, be able to apply them within professional settings and develop innovative approaches for new situations;

- gain a thorough knowledge of research methods and data analyses.

The MAPP is taught part time over two years, or it can be taken as a full-time option (one year). It follows an executive education model, in which teaching is delivered once a month over intensive weekends. This model makes the programme accessible not only to London-based students, but also to students from other UK and European destinations. It also enables those in full-time employment to combine work and educational demands. From 2012 the MAPP is also offered in a distance-learning format, offering first-class positive psychology tuition to those unable to attend on-campus lectures.

Completing the programme enables students to be among the first positive psychology specialists in the UK and in Europe. As the field is still young and is constantly in the process of developing, students often become co-creators of knowledge, shaping the emergence of new ideas and connections.

Leading to the award of an MSc (Master in Science), the programme reasonably places a lot of emphasis on the development of research skills, with a proportion of MAPP dissertation projects reaching publishable quality. As all of the programme team is research active, with ongoing projects on well-being, resilience and evaluation of interventions, students also have additional opportunities to participate in these research projects, and develop and test new positive psychology interventions. However, research and science are not everything. The programme also fosters experiential opportunities for participants to become more reflective, self-aware, and to practise and experiment with new skills. The MAPP requires its students to submit both an experiential portfolio and a consultancy project, applying the learnt skills both to themselves and to real-world client needs.

In addition to the full MSc (one hundred and eighty credits), the programme offers two intermediate awards. A Postgraduate Certificate in APP is awarded following successful completion of sixty credits (Foundations of Positive Psychology). A Postgraduate Diploma in APP is awarded for achieving one hundred and twenty credits for the following two double modules: Foundations of Positive Psychology, and Advanced Positive Psychology: Theory and Practice. The awards enable students to exit the programme earlier, but still acquire a qualification for the work undertaken.

Entry qualifications

An undergraduate honours degree (or equivalent) in psychology, sociology, health and social welfare, counselling, education studies, human resources, business or social enterprise studies or other related disciplines with a minimum lower second-class honours classification is usually required to enter the programme. However, given the high competition for places, preference is often given to applicants with excellent first degrees or those with existing postgraduate qualifications. In addition, a written application outlining academic and professional background, career objectives and reasons for choosing the MAPP programme at UEL is necessary. Students whose academic background is outside of the above-mentioned disciplines are further requested to explain (in no more than 2,000 words) how their professional or life experience has prepared them for studying positive psychology. Potential students whose first language is not English have to demonstrate their competence through established routes (i.e. International English Language Testing System). In addition, all applicants need to provide two references, one of which has to be academic.

MAPP delivery style

The programme provides a blend of teaching and learning approaches, including traditional lectures, seminars and workshop activities; Skype and email support; group and individual tutorial sessions; group exercises and peer study groups/action-learning sets.

Student profiles

The culture that surrounds the MAPP is not the normal image of a postgraduate programme. The students are extremely diverse in both cultural backgrounds and age, with most students formally falling into the 'mature' category. Often they are high achievers in their own professional life, and come to the MAPP to consolidate and choose the next steps in life that are highly meaningful for them personally. This also makes them highly self-motivated and fully engaged in the learning process. Extrinsic motivation is not usually a significant part of undertaking the programme.

Applications of the MAPP

First, a MAPP is an attractive option for psychology graduates unwilling to take a much longer route towards BPS chartered status and wishing to combine postgraduate studies with employment. Second, a large number of applications are from mature candidates already in professional employment (within business or public sectors), wishing to enhance their personal development and career progression opportunities. The programme leads to a wide range of employment opportunities. Graduates develop careers in organisational or business consultancies through their knowledge of tools for transforming business, institutions and social practices. Business executives, human resource personnel and managers can enhance their career prospects, although self-employment is another possible pathway for the programme graduates.

Skills and knowledge obtained are being usefully applied in the charity, voluntary and social enterprise sectors, as the programme educates for co-operative systems and sustainable well-being and development. The MAPP is useful for qualified clinical psychologists, counsellors, psychotherapists, nurses and doctors who intend to use positive psychology theory, research and applications in their clinical work. Teachers often use positive psychology expertise to inform their practice. The programme can be of benefit to other existing and aspiring youth workers and educators, from primary school through to university level. Importantly, a number of graduates go on to develop specialisation in positive psychology within a research career, and thus use their programme as a stepping stone towards a doctorate or PhD.

Past student achievements

Out of the first MSc graduates, several entered a career pathway in positive psychology (employed or self-employed), some utilised their MSc to secure positions in local or central government, some progressed onto further studies (MA in counselling or PhD in positive psychology), some are now using elements of positive psychology in their existing careers (employed or self-employed) and some have been commissioned to write books. As the number of graduates increases year on year, our students continue to make an impact within these areas and trail-blaze for APP.

Box 13.2   Past students on the MAPP programme*

Denise

Before graduating with a MAPP in 2009, Denise worked in the public sector for fifteen years. On the MAPP, Denise learnt to question how and why we choose how we make a living. Today, Denise is about to embark on a career more aligned to what she is passionate about, a career that gives her a greater sense of contribution. Ultimately, a MAPP has been a gift that Denise feels keeps giving her endless possibilities in her personal and professional life. Furthermore, in 2011 Denise launched a successful 'In-Tents Happiness' project at a London festival where participants were invited to create a work of art that represented 'happiness' for them. In her own words, '*MAPP needs to come with a warning: "This course may improve your life and that of those around you". You've been warned!*'

Miriam

Miriam first came across positive psychology when she was producing a programme on happiness for BBC Radio 4. After trying out the interventions for herself and finding that they really did work, she trained as a coach and later completed her career transition by becoming one of the first people to graduate from the UK MAPP. Miriam found that the MAPP exposed her to other important ingredients in well-being besides happiness, such as the strengths approach. Miriam has specialised in positive psychology interventions, developing programmes, running workshops, working one-to-one and writing a self-help coaching book – *Positive Psychology for Overcoming Depression* (Duncan Baird Publishers).

*Thank-you to the featured students for their contribution to this section.

PhD/Doctorate-level APP training

There are, unfortunately, limited options with regards to PhD programmes specifically within the domain of positive psychology. Claremont University, located in the USA, was and to our knowledge remains the only university in the world to offer a PhD in positive psychology. The programme is run by one of positive psychology's 'founding fathers', Mihaly Csikszentmihalyi, Director of the Quality of Life Research Center.

At the University of East London, the MAPP team supervises one PhD student who won a departmental studentship for her research on 'Eudaimonia'. Unfortunately, such opportunities do not come around often. Members of the MAPP team also supervise the research of another PhD student on 'Flourishing within Higher Education', although this again is not an ongoing studentship.

Students who wish to continue their academic career are advised to search for PhD studentships although these may not be specifically labelled under the discipline 'positive psychology'. For example, our former students have gone on to study PhDs in the areas of emotional intelligence, flourishing and quality of life in women's well-being, and neuro-aesthetics.

Furthermore, at the present time, there are no doctorate courses (an applied route to chartership) within the area of positive psychology, although this may be an organic evolution given the emphasis on applications and training in APP.

APP and coaching

There are alternatives to the academic route when deciding on your positive psychology future. If you simply want to learn the concepts through an MSc in order to work on an individual basis with others, we recommend that our students undertake a recognised qualification in coaching. This, of course, is not a short cut – there are several limitations as to what you can do and how you publicise yourself; however we recognise that not everyone wants to dedicate six to ten years to becoming a university lecturer.

WORKING IN THE AREA OF POSITIVE PSYCHOLOGY: A DAY IN THE LIFE OF AN APPLIED POSITIVE PSYCHOLOGIST (KATE)

I can safely say that no two days are ever the same. The exciting work of applied academia ensures a variety of demands and experiences that make our lives very, very interesting. I continually shift between research, teaching, consultancy and applied evaluations in order to make sure I stay on top of positive psychology in practice. Below is a taster to see what I might get up to on any given day.

Box 13.3   A day in the life

8:00	Set up office and log on to computer. Find fifty emails. Answer throughout the day.
8:00–9:00	Supervision meeting with two students.
9:00–13.00	Finalisation of the qualitative section for SPARK resilience programme report for Newham Council.
Lunch	At desk.
13:00–15:00	Create two ethics proposals for two new research projects in Uganda and London. These are looking at health and well-being across cultures. Write case report for change in assessment on the MAPP for quality assurance enhancement review.
15:00–16:00	Research development meeting with fellow colleague.
16:00– 17:00	Review assignment for student as per supervision requirements.
17:00–17:30	Meeting with said student and discussion.
17:30–20:30	Finish examination of a counselling doctorate thesis for student's upcoming viva. Finalise a twenty-page report for external examining body.

CONTINUING PROFESSIONAL DEVELOPMENT (CPD)

In order to maintain an up-to-date perspective on the discipline, students and lecturers/researchers are expected to engage in CPD activities. These are typically the attendance of training courses, conferences and group peer meetings/discussions, the implementation and dissemination of research, with some collaborative publications, and personal/professional reading.

For example, the International Positive Psychology Association (IPPA) and European Network of Positive Psychology (ENPP) offer bi-annual conferences that draw the leading experts from around the world to showcase their latest research and developments. Attending and presenting at these conferences is important for us to continue our own personal development, as well as inform students of the latest research.

ISSUES IN POSITIVE PSYCHOLOGY

There are currently several issues within the field of positive psychology. We will discuss three of the most pertinent to understanding positive psychology as an applied field.

Regulation

The first issue pertains to the fact that positive psychology is not governed by any external body, such as the BPS or HPC. This means that the title 'positive psychologist' is not legally protected, allowing inappropriate use of this highly recognised term. We see this issue as similar to the problem the BPS Division of Sport and Exercise Psychology had up until seven years ago, when it was formalised as a separate discipline within psychology itself. Until this happens, we fear that some individuals without the accepted qualifications (PhD, professional doctorate) will make false claims.

Cohesiveness

Second, the APP discipline has not yet decided on a cohesive theoretical link between the vast number of subjects that fall under the positive psychology tree. Thus, many professionals find an illogical connection to fellow researchers (cancer research versus morality research), perpetuating the criticism of a lack of cohesive guiding theory (Lazarus, 2003).

Longevity

The last issue with positive psychology that we will cover here (there are of course more) is the issue of staying power. Does positive psychology have a future and, if so, what does that look like? The initial aim of positive psychology was to remind psychologists to redirect their attention to what makes things work, rather than fixing what does not. Today, we see a dramatic shift in the psychology world's attention, with several branches, from developmental to neuroscience, adopting this approach. Thus, the major dilemma is whether positive psychology has completed its aim, or whether it can continue to stand alone as a separate discipline.

The discipline of APP is clear on its aims for the future: positive psychology would like to branch out into more biological and psychosocial areas, such as positive health, positive neuroscience, positive social science and positive education (Seligman, 2011). We feel that these are worthy areas of research that will enable positive psychology to add experimental evidence and objective markers to the breadth of existing research findings.

CONCLUSION

Applied positive psychology is a fairly new branch of the discipline of applied psychology and it contains several sub-branches (everyday life, business, health, education, government and public policy, communities, and environment). There are several training opportunities (BSc options; MAPP); however the PhD/professional doctorate is the only recognised route to becoming a 'positive psychologist'. A day in the life of a positive psychologist consists of report writing, research, lecturing, development of materials, onsite work and much more. There remain some issues within APP (regulation, cohesiveness, longevity) – although these are being continuously assessed throughout the field.

QUESTIONS FOR REFLECTION AND DISCUSSION

1   How could positive psychology ensure proper regulation? Should the title of 'positive psychologist' be a protected title? If not, what implications does this have?

2   If positive psychology continues to grow at its current rapid rate, does it seem plausible that it will eventually integrate and disappear as a separate discipline?

3   How can positive psychologists better 'walk the tightrope' of academia and application?

4   List the ways in which governments and public policy have, and could further, adopt a positive psychological approach to societal well-being.

SUGGESTIONS FOR FURTHER READING

Boniwell, I. (2008) *Positive Psychology in a Nutshell* (2nd edn). London: PWBC. This brief book combines a breadth of information about positive psychology with a pinch of critical commentary. It is written in an accessible and engaging style with light-hearted illustrations.

Diener, E., Lucas, R., Schimmack, U. and Helliwell, J. (2009) *Well-Being for Public Policy.* Oxford: Oxford University Press. Written by some of the founders of positive psychology, this book is the first to address the practical application of positive psychology, well-being and public policy.

Donaldson, S., Csikszentmihalyi, M. and Nakamura, J. (eds) (2011) *Applied Positive Psychology: Improving Everyday Life, Health, Schools, Work and Society.* New York: Routledge. Part of the applied psychology series, this edited book covers the current applied areas of positive psychology, written by the experts in the field. An easy-to-read and relevant book.

Hefferon, K. and Boniwell, I. (2011) *Positive Psychology: Theory, Research and Applications.* Maidenhead: McGraw-Hill. This is the first comprehensive undergraduate textbook on positive psychology, written by the leaders of the UK MSc in Applied Positive Psychology.

Linley, P.A. and Joseph, S. (eds) (2004) *Positive Psychology in Practice.* Hoboken, NJ: John Wiley. Still the 'go-to' book in terms of breadth and depth of applications of positive psychology. A reference book that has stood the test of time.

14

COGNITIVE PSYCHOLOGY

Volker Thoma

This chapter discusses:

- how we can study the mind and its inner workings;

- how cognitive psychology emerged as one of the main disciplines in psychology;

- how the mind represents the world, and how we think – the relationship between mental processes (such as judgements, actions or decisions) and their results in the real world;

- application – how we can design our environment to better suit our perception, memory and decision-making processes;

- how researchers can help practitioners and people outside psychology to use the knowledge gathered in cognitive psychology.

INTRODUCTION

While reading this text you are probably not far from a mobile phone or a computer hooked up to the internet. If this is the case you are familiar with being alerted to a new message (such as a text or an incoming email). You would normally see the notification and then read the related text, and probably respond to the sender. Your response would involve sharing a memory of a recent event (for example, describing that film you saw recently), which you describe (not that great). Alternatively, you could simply write back suggesting a plan to do something that might interest the sender (what about seeing a different film?).

This example, in a nutshell, covers many activities of the human mind that cognitive psychology is interested in: how we pay attention to things or events (like the notifications on a mobile phone), how we perceive and understand information provided by our environment (seeing or reading a message), how we memorise previous events so we can recall and share them later (such as personal memories or general knowledge), and how we judge situations – or people – and make decisions, thereby trying to solve problems (such as 'What's the best film to watch together?'). But why should we investigate these activities of the mind anyway? How should we study them, and can we practically apply what we may learn about the mind? This chapter will introduce cognitive psychology by way of examples, and hopefully reveal the inherent creativity and elegance of this young science – but most of all demonstrate how deeply relevant an understanding of the human mind is. You may discover along the way that you are already a bit of a cognitive psychologist.

BEGINNINGS OF COGNITIVE PSYCHOLOGY

Why study the activities of the mind? First, we perceive ourselves as active agents in the world – we want to make a difference. Knowing more about how we think gives us an advantage in influencing our environment, and helps us to better respond to problems and decisions we face in our lives. Second, there is also the natural curiosity we have about ourselves as human beings, or in other words, the question of what makes us – and others – 'tick'. Indeed, the beginnings of cognitive psychology can be traced back to the ancient Greek philosophers. Plato for example was concerned with how we actually learn things and form ideas, and was convinced that all knowledge comes from within the mind by thinking hard and logically (this led him to propose that societies should be ruled by wise leaders). His student Aristotle, however, argued that our mind learns from experience, and that our thinking and ideas (or 'souls') are connected to the environment, which must therefore be studied empirically through structured observation and measurement. This is an important notion, because it is still the main framework (or 'scientific method') for research in cognitive psychology and science in general. Thus, ever since Plato and Aristotle, people have been grappling with the question of how best to think about the faculties of the mind – which were then called 'perception', 'imagination', and 'desire' – and how to study them. Should we rely on reason and critical thinking alone, or should we mainly observe and measure things? How do we learn, how do we know about things – and how certain can we be about our thoughts and experiences? Questions such as these led Aristotle and others to investigate fundamental issues and complex problems, such as: is the soul (the mind) the same as the body (the brain) or are they separate? This mind–body problem is, of course, still discussed by cognitive scientists and philosophers nowadays (although most agree after a night out drinking that the mind is indeed painfully connected to the body). But if we do not want to rely on philosophical thinking alone, how can we study these questions?

Try for a moment to remember a situation in which you thought hard about a previous experience and picked it apart into its elements. Take a movie, for example: just like a film critic, you could give different marks for music, acting, photography, script, etc. People vary in how they experience these elements and may consequently find a film either bad or a 'must-see'. Another example would be when you are looking at a flat and you are wondering what colour the wall paint is: you say it's cream, but your partner is adamant that it is eggshell. This sort of appraisal or 'introspection' was the method of Wilhelm Wundt, credited as one of the first modern psychologists. At the end of the nineteenth century, Wundt had established an experimental psychology laboratory in Leipzig, where he and his students tried to learn about perception by way of 'self-observation' of their inner experiences, or sensations. Of course they realised that all sorts of influences could have an impact on introspection (take alcohol for example, or tiredness), so Wundt and his students trained themselves to be disciplined and systematic in their observation of their experiences (e.g. colours and shapes) when perceiving an object (such as an apple). That is why Wundt insisted on replicating these investigations time and time again, best done in a laboratory, so one could be sure that what was introspectively observed was a relatively stable experience and not influenced by random events. Today not everyone still shares Wundt's idea that sensations can be unpacked into different elements or 'structures' that way. But Wundt's insistence on systematic investigations, varying the objects of study slightly, and making repeated observations in controlled conditions remained one of the core research principles in psychology.

Wundt, together with memory researcher Hermann Ebbinghaus and others, established psychology as an experimental discipline, but his approach of self-observation was still not scientific enough for some people. In America, psychologists such as John B. Watson were dissatisfied with the idea of introspection, because this method was dependent on the observer, and often not quantifiable, i.e. measurable in a numeric way. According to Watson, psychological phenomena should be made equally observable to everyone, which meant that only overt behaviour was deemed as worth studying: what people actually do can be seen, counted and thus verified by most observers, unlike sensations and thoughts. Watson's programme was therefore termed 'behaviourism' and it was influenced by more established scientific endeavours, such as biology and physiology. For example, at the beginning of the twentieth century Ivan Pavlov had shown that dogs can learn to associate the sight of food with the sound of a bell, such that eventually hearing the ring of the bell alone causes the dog to salivate. This experiment showed that one does not need to rely on describing inner mental activities to explain a psychological process such as learning. The mind may as well be a 'black box' – what goes on inside it cannot be measured. Rather, it is enough to observe animals or humans under different conditions, and investigate learning by looking at which stimuli and what sorts of reward are associated with a change in behaviour. Behaviourism was taken to such an extreme by psychologists (most famously, Burrhus F. Skinner) that it led to the claim that even language was nothing more than learnt verbal behaviour.

THE COGNITIVE REVOLUTION

Although behaviourism with its scientific rigour was hugely influential for over half a century, things were changing by the 1950s. A brilliant young, linguist, Noam Chomsky, challenged the behaviourist idea that higher mental functions – such as language – could be acquired by simple associationistic learning mechanisms. According to Chomsky (1957, 1959), behaviourists could not explain why people were able to construct new sentences that they had never heard before. Language was such a creative and powerful faculty that its acquisition could not be explained by pure instruction – children would take far too long to learn words and grammar that way. Rather, Chomsky suggested, we are born with a mind that already has certain rules and structures allowing us not only to learn words and sentences very quickly, but also to use what we have learnt in completely new ways. Let us take a simple example – the plural form in English. In behaviourist thinking you would have to learn separately that 'dogs' is the plural form of 'dog' and that 'cats' is the plural of 'cat' – which means a lot of learning has to happen before you master a fairly simple linguistic task. But a mind born with a rule that allows us to use a word stem and the plural extension separately (in English it is, of course, 's') means that you do not have to learn both singular and plural separately – you can just add 's' to a singular word. Of course, there are a few exceptions, and that is why young children often first say 'sheeps' – again something behaviourists would not predict if learning happens only by listening to adults.

Other work, too, showed that behaviour can have innate roots, such as instincts in animals. But even behaviour that is acquired through learning seems to contain more than just learnt responses to certain stimuli. For example, rats are able to find food in a maze even though the route they had previously learnt (e.g. 'first right, then second left to get to food') was suddenly blocked off (Tolman, 1948). The conclusion is that if rats can find a location without resorting to simple stimuli–response learning, then their brains must have the ability to form something like a 'mental map' (i.e. a type of memory content that helps to find a route like a real map). This idea of mental representations – i.e. manifestations of objects or events in the mind – was a crucial step away from behaviourism to a science that is interested in what goes on inside the mind. Other developments also contributed to the idea that scientists may – after all – actually be able to describe what goes on in the mind if we think of mental representations as being similar to symbols used in other domains. Many machines and new applications at that time, such as the radio and keyboard (invented in the 1940s) have 'internal states' (i.e. representations) that transform an input (a signal) into an output (e.g. another signal, or a mechanical effect). The notion of representations and processing stages gave psychologists a model for how mental phenomena such as memory could be conceptualised. For example, a computer uses different memory banks: what you type into the keyboard is stored in a temporary memory system until you 'save' it as a document or message. Similarly, we can think of human memory as being divided into short-term memory and long-term memory. This distinction has been tested with experiments on humans (and animals) and can be famously seen in patients with amnesia, a condition which renders people unable to remember past events while they are still able to repeat a phone number they heard seconds earlier. Similar attempts to 'model' the mind in order to better understand it also occurred in other research areas – including mathematics, economics, engineering, anthropology, clinical psychology – and the related methods and outcomes were discussed in important scientific gatherings in the 1940s and 1950s. The resulting discussions and related publications led to the so-called 'cognitive revolution'– an understanding that the mind would no longer be treated like a 'black box', as behaviourism had demanded, because now there were ways in which to describe mental processes without relying on subjective introspection. The mind could now be explored scientifically.

The rise of modern cognitive psychology

The term 'cognitive psychology' came into use with the publication of a book of that name by Ulric Neisser in 1967. Since then cognitive psychology has been called the 'science of the mind' and revolves around the idea that if one wants to know how people experience the world and how they think, then you need to figure out what processes are actually going on in their minds. In central Europe, the term cognitive psychology is often substituted with 'general' or 'common psychology' – reflecting the idea that what you learn about cognitive psychology will be an important 'common' knowledge basis for other branches of psychology and in particular for a range of applied psychology disciplines. For example, forensic psychologists are interested in face recognition and memory, to assess whether eye witnesses were likely to have had a chance of accurately recognising a perpetrator, and whether witnesses are likely to recall events as they really happened. Occupational psychologists may want to know whether too much demand on the mind – too many distracting emails, too much negative feedback from colleagues – can cause stress and decrease performance. Developmental and educational psychologists may be interested in how language develops in a child, how it learns numeracy, develops problem-solving skills, etc. This knowledge can be used to design early intervention methods, e.g. by helping children from disadvantaged backgrounds to achieve their full potential. Thus, an interesting aspect of cognitive psychology is that questions regarding the human mind – which may at first seem very abstract and philosophical – have actually very practical implications. Still, it is not always immediately clear how the study of mental processes can be translated into practical applications. Therefore, let us look at an example of how laboratory experiments can help solve problems in the real world.

REPRESENTATIONS IN THE BRAIN

One of the continuing debates in cognitive psychology is around mental representations: because our mind has to deal with the environment and must react to events around us it first needs to symbolise or represent aspects of the environment. For example, when you look for your red car in the parking lot, something in your mind that corresponds to its colour and its shape is activated. But what do representations of objects look like in the brain? We know that if you see a car, the shape of the car will form a two-dimensional (2D) picture at the back of your eye (which is full of sensors and nerve cells, called the retina). This 2D 'image' of the car is then projected from the eyes into the back of the brain. But what then – does our mind store a picture-like memory of the car to help us search for it next time? And if so, what about recognising other objects, such as houses, cups, dogs or even faces? Somehow our brain would have to store all these things and their corresponding pictures in memory – because otherwise we would not be able to recognise what we are looking for. So the question is: what are the attributes of mental representations of objects, and in particular, are they like 2D pictures similar to photographs, or are they more abstract like symbols we use in language?

We studied this question with experiments in which we showed participants images of objects on a computer screen. People saw pictures of objects – such as a car, a dog, etc. – and had to name them, and these pictures were sometimes shown again a second time (Thoma et al., 2007). We found that people recognise objects faster when they were presented in a familiar view (e.g. a picture of a car shown as you would see it parked in the street) than when they were presented in an unfamiliar orientation (e.g. a car shown upside down, with the wheels on top). This seems to support the idea that we store objects preferably in a picture-like form – but then why do we still recognise an upside down car at all, if we have never seen it like that before.

It turns out that attention is the key to understanding how the mind represents things and enables us to recognise objects. First, if people see an object but are prevented from paying attention to it, they will recognise it faster when they see it a second time compared to an object they have not seen before. However, this improved recognition for an unattended object only works when it was seen in a familiar view – not when it was shown upside down. This is evidence that the human mind uses representations that are very similar to 2D images, in particular when there is no opportunity to pay attention to a stimulus. Second, if people see an object and do pay attention to it, they are subsequently faster in recognising that object later even when it had previously been seen in an unfamiliar view. In this case, with attention, the brain uses a more general type of representation that can recognise objects even in unfamiliar views probably because it extrats the parts of an object rather than the whole 2D image. Attention allows us to construct a part-based form of representation – just as using ':' and '-)' together form the parts of a smiley face ':-)'. It seems that the mind has a double strategy – objects are not only stored as 2D images or views, but also as part-based descriptions which have the advantage that they give the mind more flexibility: as long as you can identify vital parts of an object – such as the wheels and body of a car – you will be able to recognise it as a car, even if its seen in an unusual view (see Figure 14.1). Because of this flexibility our minds do not need to store multiple image versions of each object. Indeed, people are still very good in recognising images in which parts of objects are disconnected (Thoma et al., 2004). These and other experiments provide us with a clearer picture of how the brain represents the environment: objects are stored in typical views for quick recognition – even if we do not pay much attention to them or their location – and at the same time they are stored in more abstract form based on crucial parts, so that we can recognise them in novel situations.

Evidence for two different types of representations also comes from studies with brain-damaged patients – depending on the location of the brain damage, they either

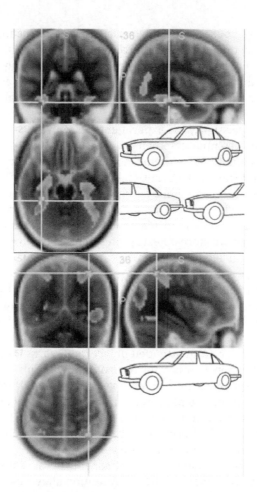

Figure 14.1   Brain areas that respond to repeated images that had either been attended or unattended in a previous presentation. The top panel shows an area in the left temporal lobe that responds to attended objects that were presented in a scrambled (split) or intact configuration. The bottom panel shows an area in the right parietal lobe that responds only to intact images, independent of whether they had been attended or not during their first presentation

Source: Thoma, V. and Henson, R.N. (2011) 'Object representations in ventral and dorsal visual streams: fMRI repetition effects depend on attention and part-whole configuration', *NeuroImage*, 57 (2): 513–25.

have problems with recognising parts of objects (Davidoff and Warrington, 1999), or with familiar views (Warrington and Taylor, 1978). Obviously, knowing what these patients are able to recognise has implications for their rehabilitation and daily care.

Recently, studies using brain imaging techniques have found that objects in familiar views may be recognised by parietal brain areas (that is, the parts of the cortex above your ears) – which are commonly known to prepare the body for actions, such as grasping. Interestingly, this brain area responded to common views of an object even if the participants saw it for a very brief time and did not pay attention to the location where it was shown (Thoma and Henson, 2011) (see Figure 14.1). This result again demonstrates that the brain can still process stimuli even without attention – as long as images are shown in a familiar view.

It can be very important to know how images are recognised, e.g. in places where it is necessary to effectively communicate information visually. Imagine people who have to perform split-second judgements and fast actions in stressful jobs, such as air traffic controllers, pilots or nuclear power-plant operators. People in these situations need to be able to recognise symbols on screens and consoles very quickly and accurately, which makes the systematic, informed design and arrangement of interfaces at workplaces very important. Similarly, if you create a piece of advertising or a webpage, you want to make sure that people have a good chance of finding and recognising the information that you created or placed there – even in situations in which they may be distracted otherwise. Of course, the whole idea of 'branding' in marketing and sales relies on this principle, because the more often people see an image (such as a company logo or a product) the more they tend to like it and prefer it over other brands. Indeed, a number of psychologists find themselves working in advertising or marketing departments of companies, often also because of what they had learnt studying research methods at university. Cognitive psychology also contributed to the emergence of a whole new area of applying knowledge about the human mind to real-world problems – 'human machine interaction', which is described in the next section.

APPLIED COGNITIVE PSYCHOLOGY IN THE REAL WORLD

Have you ever cursed your mobile phone or your computer because it would not let you do what you wanted? I thought so. In 1988 the cognitive psychologist Donald Norman published a very popular book called *The Psychology of Everyday Things*. In it Norman (1988) describes how many everyday products, such as cooking stoves, door handles, telephones, etc. are badly designed and cause unnecessary frustrations or problems. Electric switches are arranged in a confusing way so that we often use the wrong one, and doors have handles that look like they have to be pulled to open them when in fact they have to be pushed. And modern gadgets such as navigation systems and smart phones are often too complicated to use because of the many – often hidden – functions they now have. But Norman did more than just complain about annoying products and their interfaces: as a trained cognitive psychologist he was able to explain why so many products are badly designed, and these explanations were based on the principles of how the mind works. For example, products should convey perceptually how they are meant to be used: if there is a handle that looks like a grip on the door, our mind automatically assumes that we have to pull the handle; if the door handle is designed in the shape of a flat surface, we automatically put our palms on it to push it open. (Have you ever wondered why something as common as a door should need a 'push' or 'pull' sign to be operated?) Another important principle for good design according to Norman is that the product helps to establish which sequence of actions is expected – or in other words, design has to take into account that users often already have a preconceived idea about how to use a product. These implicit expectations are often called 'mental models' or 'scripts' – they are memorised information structures that help us to deal with the environment and predict future events. But if a designer does not take people's mental models into account, the experience of using a product is often worse than it should be. For example, for years you may have used word processor software in which you had to select the menu item 'File' to find the 'Print' option. However, in the new version of the software the 'File' menu item is suddenly gone – your mental model of how to find and select the print menu does not work anymore, and you have to learn the hard way that the 'Print' option is now only available if you click on a squiggly logo. Presumably the software designers thought that users already have an expectation (i.e. a mental model) to look for the 'Print' option there because the logo is placed close to where the 'File' menu had been located previously. However, many people apparently have a different mental model – such as 'Logos are not interactive elements but decorations' – which makes them less likely to click on it and consequently do not manage to print.

In the 1970s and 1980s, personal computers arrived and became a mass medium with the rise of the internet in the 1990s. But it also became clear that many people were complaining about the software they had to use: programs or applications were often hard to learn or understand (as one regularly encounters after a new software update). When software and web applications became big business, computer scientists and cognitive psychologists began working together to make these products easier to learn and more intuitive to use. Previously cognitive psychologists had already improved information design (e.g. by testing the best way to display traffic information), organised work processes and helped to devise training materials for a variety of learning environments. But the work of cognitive psychologists on 'human machine interaction' or 'human factors' took on a new dimension with the proliferation of computers. It became important for companies and organisations to make sure users did not get frustrated when using their software, to save costs in training staff, increase productivity, and avoid having to 'fix' issues in software applications after a release because there were too many complaints from customers. Psychologists were in a good position to do this, because they knew how to study people's behaviour and thoughts, and could give recommendations on how to design products (see Box 14.1).

Box 14.1   The work of a user-experience researcher

Over the past twenty years, cognitive psychology has increasingly informed 'user-centred design' or 'user experience' research (previously subsumed under the more general term 'ergonomics').

In my first full-time job as a psychologist I was conducting 'user tests' on interactive products – anything from vending machines, financial software, online catalogues, programming panels of hot-water boilers, to online shopping platforms and interactive TVs. Potential users of a product are often invited into a 'usability lab' to test a new prototype, in order to see whether people would actually get to grips with handling a new product through its interface.

The 'usability lab' consists basically of two rooms connected by a one-way mirror. The usability team typically observes what users are doing in the main testing room while recording all actions and comments. Participants in user-tests are usually asked to 'think aloud' when performing certain tasks: while they may be searching for a certain function, they describe at the same time what they are currently thinking and planning to do. This way the researchers not only find out where users have problems performing a task, but also gain valuable insight into the reasons for poor performance and frustration. When users are asked to 'test' a website, they very often have problems understanding the labels that are used (for example, they may say something like 'I have no idea what the link "Basics" means here'), the navigation structure of the website ('Is this now the home page?'), or are uncertain whether their actions have the effect expected ('I really do not know now whether my payment has gone through').

User experience evaluations are just one way cognitive psychologists help to design user-friendly interfaces. Other work includes conducting interviews and design questionnaires to find out what prospective users want from a certain service, comparing competitor products, analysing the types and sequences of tasks that typical users have to perform, profiling types of users that are interested in a given product.

These activities involve not only doing research, analysing and reporting results, but also planning, project management, as well as communication with all parties involved – the so-called 'stakeholders' (users, designers, management, etc.). On the research side, data-gathering in human factors work involves both quantitative and qualitative techniques. Although, for example, people's performance in user tests and ratings from questionnaires are analysed using quantitative methods, interviews and diary studies are also employed to elicit qualitative aspects of users' experiences. In much of the academic environment one encounters epistemological schisms (i.e. quarrels) between proponents of these two approaches, but for the pragmatic researcher in human factors it is fairly straightforward: both methodologies are recognised as valid and necessary, and stakeholders such as users and clients hardly ever question the usefulness of either approach. In fact, there is evidence that both quantitative and qualitative methods complement each other in human factors research and can lead to similar results in categorising user types (Thoma and Williams, 2009).

COGNITIVE PSYCHOLOGY AND DECISION-MAKING

The example of user-experience research shows that applied cognitive psychology is already part of our lives, in the form of the many products and services that have benefited from the insights of cognitive psychology during their development. But cognitive psychology's biggest impact may yet be in another area. In 2002, the Israeli-American psychologist Daniel Kahneman received the Nobel Prize in Economics for his work on human judgement and decision-making (sadly, there is no Nobel Prize for psychology). Kahneman and his late co-worker Amos Tversky had investigated how our judgements of events and their prospective outcomes diverge from rationality. For example, in a famous study Tversky and Kahneman (1981) described the following scenario to participants:

> Imagine that the US is preparing for the outbreak of an unusual Asian disease, which is expected to kill 600 people. Two alternative programs to combat the disease have been proposed. Assume the exact scientific estimate of the consequences of the programs are as follows: In a group of 600 people, if Program A is adopted: 200 people will be saved; if Program B is adopted, there is a one-third probability that 600 people will be saved, and a two-thirds probability that no people will be saved. Which program would you choose?

A majority of 72% of participants preferred programme A, which would imply that people are risk-aversive and go for the 'sure' outcome of saving two hundred people. Of course, from a strict rational point of view programme B is just as good, because a 'one-third probability that 600 people will be saved' equals the outcome of option A. But consider what happened when a second group of people was given the problem with the same description, except that 'Program C: 400 people will die; Program D: there is a one-third probability that nobody will die, and a two-thirds probability that 600 people will die'.

Which option would you choose? After this last description of the disease problem, 78% preferred programme D, with the remaining 22% opting for programme C. But as is probably obvious to the reader, programmes A and C are describing the same outcomes, as are programmes B and D. Nevertheless, the observed preferences, however, were reversed – by simply rephrasing the outcomes from '200 will be saved' to '400 will die' (which amounts to the same outcome for six hundred people), participants make dramatically different decisions. On the face of it, this means that the wording (or 'framing' as the authors called it) of a choice problem can dramatically affect judgements and decisions. But even more interesting is that in the second description, people became risk-seeking: if people are confronted with a sure loss versus an opportunity to gamble and have a chance to avoid the loss (but equally of course risk increasing their losses), people choose to gamble – they become risk-seeking. This notion seems counter-intuitive but ask yourself: If you are offered to lose £100 for sure or have the opportunity of a gamble with a

50% chance of losing nothing and a 50% chance of losing £200 – which option would you take?

You can see from the cover story used by Kahneman and Tversky for the 'Asian disease' problem that these findings have important practical implications for decision-makers in government and organisations. Concrete health messages, too, have been found to reveal framing effects. In a study by Banks and colleagues (1995) women were encouraged to take part in regular screenings for breast cancer by showing them different information videos. Videos were more effective when they emphasised a potential loss, i.e. when they presented the dangerous consequences when breast cancer was not spotted early.

But surely, one may say, experts such as policy-makers, doctors and politicians would not be easily influenced in their decisions by the way information is put to them? Unfortunately, experts are far from immune to framing effects (for a review, see Hardman, 2009). For example, Camerer (2000) described a number of studies showing that even professional investors hold on to stocks too long when their price is falling, but sell stocks too early when they have risen in value. This phenomenon is explained by Kahneman and Tversky's observations that people are more sensitive to losses than they are to potential gains and that investors therefore gamble when they are confronted with losses (they hold on to stocks in the hope to recoup the 'losses' after a previous drop in price). The desire to avoid a loss at all costs is very strong – individual people and whole societies invest resources in certain projects (from small ones such as buying a cinema ticket up to whole countries engaging in a conflict) but when they find out that the project does not turn out so well (the film is bad, initial battles in the conflict are lost) they often do not do the reasonable thing and stop their actions to cut their losses, but instead invest more time and resources in the hope that all will get better.

There is a wealth of findings now on how people form judgements and make decisions in domains such as economics, politics, health, education and many more. For example, it is well known that people are reluctant to indicate in an official document (such as when applying for a driver's licence) their consent to becoming an organ donor (Johnson and Goldstein, 2003). But this apparent unwillingness to donate organs seems to depend not so much on strong convictions, but rather on an unwillingness to change a perceived default situation. Evidence for this 'status-quo' bias comes from a striking difference in consent rates between two countries with similar backgrounds, Austria and Germany. In Germany an opt-in system is used, that is, you have to tick a box to become an organ donor. Only 12% give their consent. In Austria, which uses an opt-out system (you have to tick a box to *not* become a donor), nearly everyone (99%) agrees to donate their organs in case of a fatal accident (see Figure 14.2). Similar effects were found for opting-in or -out regarding insurances and pension schemes.

These findings – like Kahneman and Tversky's results in the 'Asian disease study' described above – are dramatic demonstrations that many choices are less dependent on our (assumed) personal preferences but influenced by the context and the way in which choices are presented. But if you know what factors can influence people's

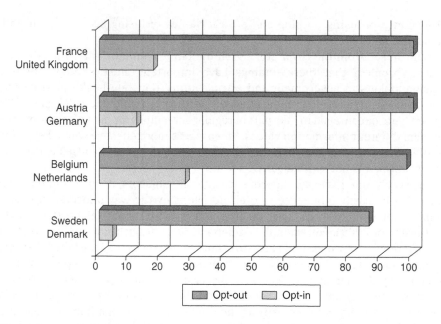

Figure 14.2   Organ donation rates (in percent) in Europe across similar countries (language, culture, size); countries with a light bar graph have an 'opt-in' system (people have to give explicit consent by ticking a box), whereas countries with a dark bar graph have an 'opt-out' system (people 'implicitly' consent unless they tick a box)

Source: Adapted from Johnson, E.J. and Goldstein, D. (2003) 'Medicine: do defaults save lives?', *Science*, 302: 1338–9.

decisions, you can use this to your advantage – or the general advantage of society. That is why a growing number of academics and policy-makers suggest designing choice contexts in a manner that benefits society (such as having more people sign up as organ donors, or preventing people from smoking or eating unhealthily). This idea is called 'choice architecture' and is reminiscent of a 'human factors' approach: people are induced by design to make better choices. Richard Thaler and Cass Sunstein (2008) suggested 'nudging' people to choices that benefit society and optimise outcomes. This idea is not without its critics, because one may ask who is to decide what is beneficial for society. Thaler and Sunstein acknowledge this but argue that research such as the one on organ donorship shows that there is no 'neutral' design anyway, and therefore 'nudging' can simply not be avoided.

Box 14.2   Careers in cognitive psychology

Many cognitive psychologists are employed in teaching and research positions by colleges and universities. Other areas of employment have emerged over the last decades, including human–computer interaction, marketing, software development, and industrial and organisational psychology. Because of this broad range, career information given elsewhere in this book may be helpful in determining the next steps for education and training.

There are now dedicated courses in a number of universities that provide training (often at master's level) in human–computer interaction (HCI). For further information about careers, visit the websites of the Usability Professionals' Association (www.ukupa.org. uk), or a list of HCI organisations (www.upassoc.org). Another area in which cognitive psychologists find employment is in the area of judgement and decision-making, which encompasses behavioural finance (or behavioural economics), policy-making and sustainability. Many major universities offer courses, sometimes associated with business schools (see also http://www.sjdm.org/).

It is worth reflecting on the substantial contribution cognitive psychologists have made to knowledge in the area of judgement and decision-making. Despite appearances from our examples, research in this area does not necessarily indicate that people are completely irrational or easily fooled. Just as object recognition seems to rely on two different ways of representing objects depending on the task at hand, there are probably different processes in decision-making. Some processes are more abstract and 'rational' (in the sense that they are based on logic and involve analytic thinking that can be used across different problem areas), whereas others are more automatic ('intuitive') and purpose-specific. Much of the research and application work is currently directed at disentangling in which situations these different processes work best for decision-makers.

CONCLUSION

Cognitive psychology is rightly called the 'science of the mind' and its reach is far beyond the research laboratory. Contrary to common belief – even within the psychology community – cognitive psychology is not just a 'base' science for applied fields such as forensic, neurocognitive, occupational and educational psychology. It has many direct applications in such areas as human factors, policy-making, economics, health and well-being, engineering and many more. Cognitive psychologists use a range of techniques to investigate the human mind and its experiences, and increasingly engage with many other disciplines and professions not only to find out what makes us 'tick', but also how to improve our lives.

QUESTIONS FOR REFLECTION AND DISCUSSION

1 What developments and events in the first half of the twentieth century were important for the emergence of cognitive psychology?

2 Would Chomsky agree more with Aristotle or Plato on how we should engage in research?

3 How can the study of attention, perception, memory and thinking improve daily life? Think of an experience with a product with an interface (websites, smart phones, software application) that is sometimes frustrating to use. What is the reason for this, and how would you find a way to improve its design?

4 How should policy-makers take into account what research in decision-making discovered about people's susceptibility to framing effects and loss-aversion?

SUGGESTIONS FOR FURTHER READING

Eysenck, M.W. and Keane, M.T. (2010) *Cognitive Psychology: A Student's Handbook* (6th edn). Hove: Psychology Press. This is an excellent textbook used widely in the UK and beyond, and is regularly updated with the latest research. Its particular strength is to look at the main research areas and critically evaluate the contribution from different research methodologies, such as experiments, neuropsychology, neuroscience or modelling.

Hardman, D. (2009) *Judgment and Decision Making: Psychological Perspectives.* Chichester: Wiley-Blackwell. Another textbook that manages to explain a complex research area in an illustrative way, and describes the major debates and challenges in the field. It covers many relevant topics and is very readable as an introduction to the field.

Kahneman, D. (2011) *Thinking Fast and Slow.* London. Penguin. Nobel prize laureate Kahneman summarises his and other people's influential research on decision-making, and includes two famous papers. Has to be recommended.

Rogers, Y., Sharp, H. and Preece, J. (2011) *Interaction Design: Beyond Human–Computer Interaction.* Chichester: Wiley. This book covers a broad area of topics in the field of human–computer interaction, but discusses them from a psychological background. It is therefore an excellent introduction to the field for psychology students.

15

COUNSELLING AND PSYCHOTHERAPY

Gordon Jinks

This chapter discusses:

- what is counselling and psychotherapy?

- training in counselling and psychotherapy;

- contexts in which counsellors and psychotherapists work;

- a day in the life;

- the range of approaches and integration;

- regulation of counselling and psychotherapy;

- research and evidence-based practice in counselling and psychotherapy.

INTRODUCTION

Counselling and psychotherapy have developed from separate traditions, but are both concerned with helping clients move in the direction of increasing some or all of a range of attributes such as self-awareness, self-acceptance, autonomy, self-efficacy, choice and empowerment; and both are also concerned with helping clients towards more positive emotional, psychological, social and indeed physical well-being. The primary tool is considered to be the therapeutic relationship, although research indicates that in fact the most important factors in determining therapeutic outcome are what the client brings with them (Duncan et al., 2010). Counsellors and psychotherapists work mainly with individuals, but also with couples and sometimes groups.

WHAT IS COUNSELLING AND PSYCHOTHERAPY?

The British Association for Counselling and Psychotherapy (BACP) define counselling and psychotherapy initially in terms of *what happens* in a therapy session:

> This might include talking about life events (past and present), feelings, emotions, relationships, ways of thinking and patterns of behaviour. The therapist will do their best to help you to look at your issues, and to identify the right course of action for you, either to help you resolve your difficulties or help you find ways of coping. (O'Driscoll, 2010: 1)

The BACP information sheet goes on to describe 'types' of therapy (one to one, couples, group, etc.) and outlines the relevant contracting and boundary issues, but interestingly does not attempt to distinguish between counselling and psychotherapy as distinct activities, using the generic term 'therapy' throughout. This issue will be discussed further below.

In essence counselling and psychotherapy are terms that are used to describe an approach to therapy based on regular meetings between the therapist and client (or clients) in which the client is enabled to explore and work on an issue or issues of their choosing within a therapeutic relationship that has certain key characteristics. These characteristics are described in different ways, but importantly include both the qualities and the boundaries of the relationship. The ideal therapeutic relationship is one in which the client feels *understood* by the therapist in terms of their experiences, views of themselves and the world, and feelings; *accepted* by the therapist as a person of value, without judgement or conditions; and engaged in a *genuine relationship* with the therapist that is collaborative, open, honest and transparent. The boundaries of the counselling and psychotherapy relationship usually include an agreement on confidentiality that is limited only if there is significant risk to the client or others; a clear understanding that the therapy relationship is not a social relationship and takes place within the limits of regular and contracted sessions (usually but not essentially weekly); that the relationship is collaborative and non-exploitative; and that its purpose is to enable the client to develop a deeper understanding of themselves or their issues and/or to develop ways forward in terms of goals, strategies, decisions, resources, coping, etc. Counselling and psychotherapy do not usually include the provision of advice by the therapist, but rather the emphasis is on helping the client to help themselves, based on the assumption that people have the resources to develop the insight they need and determine the best course of action for themselves if enabled to explore their situations and their options within an appropriate environment. Counselling and psychotherapy are usually defined as *voluntary* activities. Clients choose to come for therapy, sometimes at the suggestion of another professional (such as a GP) or a friend/colleague, but are not sent or coerced. Usually an initial number of sessions are agreed, though some therapists work in an open-ended way, and the progress of therapy should be reviewed at regular intervals. The client can choose to end therapy whenever they wish to.

The issues that clients bring to counselling and psychotherapy are many and varied, but typically include coping with life events or transitions such as bereavement, loss of job, new relationships or the loss of relationships, role change or injury/illness; problems with for example low mood, anxiety, self-esteem or addictive behaviours; past or present traumatic experiences; social, financial or relationship problems; traits such as a tendency to anger, aggression, insecurity or jealousy; difficulties with social situations, time management or stress; development or identity issues such as identity, self-concept, sexuality or role in family, community, society; or more general issues like a sense of lack of fulfilment and satisfaction, a sense of not meeting one's potential or aspirations or making the best of one's opportunities, or indeed existential issues such as the meaning and purpose of one's life.

The way counselling and psychotherapy are now understood owes a considerable debt to the work of Carl Rogers (see for example Rogers, 2004) who wrote a number of texts in the 1950s and 1960s that presented a radical shift in the role of the therapist from *expert* to *collaborator*. Where psychoanalysis and behaviour therapy had emphasised the expert knowledge of the therapist and seen their role as one that could still be understood in terms of diagnosis and treatment, Rogers' view places the client at the centre of the process and casts them as the expert in their own lives, with the therapist taking a more facilitative role. (See Chapter 12 for discussion of the relationship and tensions between the medical model and the phenomenological philosophy commonly espoused by counsellors.) Although the range of contemporary approaches to counselling and psychotherapy take varying views on the issue of the amount of *direction* offered by the therapist, Rogers' conceptualisation of therapy as a consultative relationship has been influential across the board, and his emphasis on the therapeutic relationship as opposed to theoretical frameworks and technical knowledge has been borne out in research (see later.)

Reference to Chapter 12, on counselling psychology, will indicate that there is a considerable overlap between the work of counsellors and psychotherapists and that of counselling psychologists. The key differences lie in the training routes (see below and Chapter 12), the emphasis placed on the application of specific psychological knowledge, and the contexts in which practitioners are most likely to work.

TRAINING IN COUNSELLING AND PSYCHOTHERAPY

Unusually in the context of this book, not all counsellors and psychotherapists have a background or first degree in psychology. In the UK particularly, the counselling movement took root most vigorously in other areas such as education, health and social work in the latter part of the twentieth century. For many now practising, counselling and psychotherapy is a second career developed after training and working in another profession such as teaching, social work, nursing, or indeed psychology; or as a result of voluntary work in schools, hospitals or the social care sector. Although there exists the specific discipline of counselling psychology (Chapter 12), some psychology graduates still choose to pursue training in counselling and psychotherapy in the more diverse context of the range of diplomas and other courses available. This has some advantages as well as some disadvantages. In general one can train and become qualified more quickly; competition for places may be less fierce – though not for all courses – and less based on academic criteria; and the experience is (for most) enriched by the diversity of the training group. Counselling and psychotherapy training also takes account of a wider range of practice in different contexts and should prepare you to see clients in the voluntary sector, within organisations and statutory services and in private practice. On the down side, counselling and psychotherapy lack the clear career structure available to the counselling psychologist. For most, developing a career as a counsellor or psychotherapist is a gradual process that begins with the placement on a training course, develops through voluntary and sessional work while earning one's keep through another role; and may proceed to part- or full-time employment as a therapist, to self-employment in private practice or to 'portfolio' working where therapy is practised alongside some other activities such as training, coaching, consultancy, etc.

The range of opportunities to pursue training in counselling and psychotherapy is initially bewildering. Courses are offered in further education colleges, at universities and by private training organisations, and may be at a range of academic levels including undergraduate or postgraduate qualifications, but indeed sometimes without clear academic validation. Choosing a suitable course is important in terms of your aspirations, the level of qualification and the focus and approach of the training offered (see Bayne and Jinks, 2010, for further information and guidance.)

Most reputable training courses end with an award of at least a diploma, and involve studying for a minimum of two years part time. Some courses require previous study perhaps in the form of an introductory certificate programme. Usually 'certificate' courses are aimed at equipping students to use counselling skills within another role (such as nursing, social work or voluntary befriending, etc.) whereas diploma courses and above are aimed at preparing students for professional practice as counsellors and/or psychotherapists. For those with a first degree, a postgraduate diploma may be seen as having greater weight at least from an academic perspective, though excellent training courses exist across the range of academic levels. BACP accreditation of a training course may be seen as a valuable 'kite mark' of quality. The BACP course accreditation scheme has been running for approximately twenty-five years now, and assesses courses against a range of professional and practice criteria rather than by academic criteria. As a result BACP-accredited training courses can be found in the further education, higher education and private sectors (see http://www.bacp.co.uk/accreditation/Accredited%20Course%20Search/index.php).

Most training courses will offer a range of experiences and will aim to prepare you by focusing on personal development, theory and practice and professional issues. Personal development includes working on self-awareness and development of the qualities needed by a counsellor/psychotherapist, which include resilience, personal and professional ethics, and an ability to engage in relationships characterised by empathy, acceptance and genuineness. Experiential activities, group discussion, reflective journals and personal therapy are typically used to facilitate such development. Practice will include work on specific skills or 'ways of being' (depending on the orientation of the course) and will typically include skills-training groups with peers as well as supervised practice on an external placement with real clients. Supervision with an experienced practitioner; the keeping of a professional log and the development of reflective practice through careful evaluation of your work; feedback from peers, tutors and clients; and structured reflection on your strengths and areas for development will all be important aspects of training. Theory will be determined by the orientation of the course and it is important to recognise that the theoretical content of counsellor and psychotherapy training varies dramatically. Typically training courses will either have an identified specific orientation, such as person centred, psychodynamic or cognitive behavioural, or will be 'integrative' and cover a range of conceptual frameworks (see below for further discussion.) In either case it is likely that a framework that addresses some or all of how people can be understood, how they develop, how difficulties arise and are maintained, how change can occur and how therapy works will be offered and explored via lecture and workshop sessions, seminars and in essays. Professional issues include the development of an appropriate ethical framework, managing the boundaries of therapy effectively, the contexts in which therapy is offered and issues such as accessibility, diversity and non-discriminatory practice.

The issue of the terms 'counselling' and 'psychotherapy' perhaps needs to be further explored at this point, and the question of whether or not they represent the same thing is a source of some dissent within the profession(s). Thorne referred to the search for a clear distinction between the two terms as a 'dismal quest' as long ago as 1992 (Thorne, 1992: 246), and this author has previously espoused the view that it is not possible to arrive at a generally accepted distinction that takes account of the range of definitions offered and of what practitioners who use the two terms actually do (Bayne et al., 2008). This view seems to be supported at least implicitly in much of what is published by the BACP where care is usually taken either to use both terms, to use a generic term such as 'therapist' or to express things in ways that can apply to either. The BACP criteria for accreditation of training courses do not differentiate between counselling and psychotherapy. However, other views exist (see for example McLeod, 2009: 25–41 for an interesting overview of the separate historical development of the two terms.) In general, however, attempts to distinguish psychotherapy from counselling do so on the basis of greater length or depth of therapy, longer or more intensive training, a focus on working with more fundamental issues, or more training in issues of mental health and assessment. Other professional bodies exist, such as the United Kingdom Council for Psychotherapy (UKCP) who operate different criteria for approval of training courses and for registration of individual practitioners. The UKCP see four years as the minimum period for training and place greater emphasis on personal therapy as a central element of the process – the trainee needs to be engaged in therapy while training – whereas the BACP criteria see this as one way, but not the only way, of demonstrating a commitment to personal development. Depending on your aspirations in terms of career or the context in which you hope to work, these issues may be important in choosing a training course and in choosing how to describe and market yourself as a practitioner.

CONTEXTS IN WHICH COUNSELLORS AND PSYCHOTHERAPISTS WORK

Counselling and psychotherapy are practised in a wide variety of contexts with a wide variety of client groups and issues, but some broad categories can be identified. To some extent the range and diversity of practice can be seen as arising from the parallel historical developments of psychotherapy – initially as an offshoot of the medical profession, attending to specific 'neurotic' conditions and issues such as traumatised returning soldiers from both world wars; and counselling – as a response to social change, specific perceived 'crises' such as an increase in marital breakdown, and the erosion of the supportive role and opportunities for therapeutic communication in professions like nursing and social work (McLeod, 2009). It can be argued that the two terms have evolved and broadened their application to the point where distinctions have ceased to be useful except perhaps to understand the historical context and some of the varying traditions that have developed and are still apparent in certain contexts.

Broadly speaking, counselling and psychotherapy take place in four – inevitably somewhat overlapping – contexts.

- *The voluntary and charitable sector.* Organisations such as MIND, Relate and other national and local groups have for a long time provided counselling and psychotherapy services. Sometimes these will be targeted towards specific issues (e.g. mental health problems, relationship difficulties, drug or alcohol problems, etc.); or sometimes specific, often marginalised or 'hard to reach' groups will be targeted (e.g. unemployed, homeless, specific cultural or ethnic groups, gender or sexual minorities, etc.). Often such services will rely heavily on volunteer counsellors in order to provide a low-cost or economically viable service. These may be counsellors in training, those who are continuing to work voluntarily in order to accumulate experience for professional accreditation or to improve their CVs, or those whose values direct them to work a certain proportion of their time 'pro bono'. Sometimes a proportion of the service will be delivered by paid counsellors, including assessment and allocation of clients, and professional standards of supervision are still applied.

- *Statutory, health and social care services.* Counselling and psychotherapy are now fairly well established as part of the range of services offered by the NHS in the UK and other statutory services such as social work and probation services. In these cases publicly funded services exist in order to provide for client groups who are in a sense defined by having a particular 'problem'. Often clients are referred for counselling or psychotherapy by another professional, such as their GP or probation officer. Referral is likely to be as a result of a specific identified issue, such as depression, stress, drug or alcohol dependence, etc. and is often subject to guidelines such as those provided by NICE (www.nice.org.uk). Counselling or psychotherapy may also be provided as an adjunct to other therapeutic interventions or treatments, for example in cancer care or pain management. In this category, the therapy is more likely to be provided by a practitioner who is employed by the service, though trainees will also carry out some of the work when on placement. Overlap with the charitable and voluntary sector has increased in recent years as services have been contracted out to external providers and charitable groups have bid for contracts, while pressure to maintain services in the face of cuts in funding continues to grow.

- *Services offered within particular organisations.* In this case counselling and/or psychotherapy is made available to the members of an organisation or institution that exists for a different purpose. These might be the employees of a business or service, or the students (and staff) of a university, college or school. The provision of employee counselling saw a significant boost in the 1980s and 1990s as a result of accumulating evidence that indicated that gains could be made in terms of sickness and absence rates and productivity (Carroll and Walton, 1997); and pioneering services were introduced in organisations like the Post Office, British Airways, police and fire services. Similarly, universities and colleges were persuaded that retention rates and student achievement could benefit from the provision of counselling services. More recently organisations like ThePlace2Be have expanded widespread provision of counselling in schools, as a distinct and professional service rather than adjunct to a generic pastoral care system. Counselling in organisations may be provided by a service or department within the organisation such as occupational health or human resources, or may be contracted out to an external provider (often as part of a broader employee assistance programme). Issues sometimes arise around trust in confidentiality by potential users of the service when their counselling is being paid for by their employer or their educational institution, or around the particular issues clients can bring – such as to what extent does it have to be work related?

- *Private practice.* Individual counsellors/psychotherapists or groups working together as a business venture provide therapy to those individuals who can and are willing to pay. Rates vary according to demand and the qualifications and experience of the therapist, and many operate a sliding scale or provide some 'low-cost' services as part of their package. In the case of a group practice, it is fairly common to offer practice placement opportunities to trainees in order to enable the provision of a low-cost service. Private practice therapists are usually generic, in that they will see clients with a wide range of presenting issues, though some do develop specialisms in particular areas, either consciously and deliberately or as a result of word-of-mouth referral and recommendation. Relying purely on private practice for one's income is potentially risky for a therapist as demand tends to fluctuate across the annual cycle, in response to economic conditions and somewhat at random, so often such therapists will be portfolio workers who also engage in sessional or part-time work, training, supervision or other activities.

Economic and time pressures have meant that time-limited therapy has become the norm in our society, as opposed to open-ended or unlimited therapy. At the private practice end of the spectrum, relatively few people have the financial resources to engage in long-term or unlimited therapy or would see it as a priority in the face of competing priorities; and in all of the other sectors the resources available generally mean that pressure from demand and waiting lists have led to the adoption of a time-limited approach in order to ration the available service. In the UK, open-ended counselling or psychotherapy tends only to be available at the extreme ends of the spectrum – for particularly well-to-do clients or from particular charitable/voluntary providers who see that as their particular contribution, usually to a specific client group with specific needs. The norm for contemporary counselling and psychotherapy is an initial contract for a specified number of sessions (usually between six and twenty-four depending on context) with sometimes (though not always) the possibility of re-contracting for more as the initial sessions draw to a close. This has probably led to increased interest in more action-oriented or goal-focused approaches to therapy, or at least to the 'rebranding' of traditionally more open-ended approaches such as person-centred therapy or psychodynamic therapy in 'brief' or time-limited forms.

A DAY IN THE LIFE OF A UNIVERSITY COUNSELLOR

Drawing on my own experience, I offer the role of a counsellor employed within the student services department of a large modern university as an example of how a full-time counsellor might be occupied. A typical day could be something like Box 15.1.

Box 15.1   A day in the life

9:00   Arrive and check mail, email, notes under door, left at reception, etc. Typically these will include new referrals, cancelled appointments, requests to re-schedule, requests for letters to tutors, requests for advice from tutors, invitations to training and CPD events, requests for practice placements from trainees and many things circulated to 'all staff'. Respond to as many of these as possible.

9:50   Prepare for first client – draw case notes, remind self of last session, goals, progress, evaluate how we have been working, intentions for this session, any agreed home-work tasks, etc.

10:00   First client of day – students tend not to be too keen on 9:00 am sessions!

10:50   Write up notes of first client and prepare for second client.

11:00   Second client.

11:50   Write up notes, probably finish notes from first client, check emails and do a few more responses, plan afternoon session and prepare for next client.

12:30   Lunch.

1:00   Third client – lunch times and other times when lectures are not always happening tend to be popular.

1:50   Write up notes.

2:00   Often there will be a group session or presentation here. Maybe a stress management group, exam preparation group, social anxiety or eating disorders group, etc. or a presentation to a group of students or tutors about what the counselling service offers, how to access it, etc. or there may have been a request from a particular department for some guidance on supporting students with mental health problems, or to be present when the education students have a session on child abuse, etc.

3:00   Coffee and catch up with some more admin stuff or with colleagues.

3:30   Fourth client of the day – that is about average (eighteen to twenty client hours per week is the maximum recommended by BACP for a full-time counsellor).

4:30   Drop-in session – available for any students who need some urgent time or support in a crisis.

5:00   Go home unless there is an evening session – sometimes keep an 'out of hours' slot for students on particular courses who cannot attend in 'office hours', or there might be an evening group, or a supervision group for the trainees on placement with the service.

The four clients on an average day might typically include the following.

Box 15.2   Types of clients

- A student who is preparing for a presentation and has a lot of anxiety connected with public speaking – maybe including panic attacks.

- An overseas student who has a history of trauma either in their country of origin – they might be a refugee, victim of torture or oppression – or since arriving in the UK, where they might have been discriminated against, bullied, threatened or be struggling to make sense of the expectations of the UK educational system.

- A student who is not coping well with their course and considering withdrawal – they may be depressed or suffering from low self-esteem; they are probably behind with work and feeling overwhelmed. They will be struggling to prioritise and see a way

(Continued)

(Continued)

forward, and may also have financial problems. They probably have a part-time job as well as a full-time course. They may hope a letter from a counsellor to their tutor will help in some way.

- A student who came to university with an existing problem – maybe depressive episodes, panic attacks, a survivor of abuse, a tendency to substance abuse, a relationship problem, isolation, loneliness, etc. They may have been able to get to some kind of coping/equilibrium previously, but coming to university and entering a new phase of life has de-stabilised things

These are of course just examples, and almost any generic counselling service will involve working with a huge range of clients and issues. It is challenging, sometimes depressing, frustrating or upsetting, and needs concentration, commitment, resilience and careful attention to your own well-being; but is also fulfilling and sometimes joyful and uplifting.

THE RANGE OF APPROACHES AND INTEGRATION

There are many (literally hundreds) of identifiable approaches to counselling and psychotherapy. It is beyond the scope of this chapter to address specific approaches in any depth. For an overview see McLeod (2009) or Feltham and Horton (2012). A frequent attempt to make sense of the field is to classify the approaches according to three broad groups.

Box 15.3   Psychodynamic approaches

The psychodynamic approaches have their roots in the psychoanalysis movement beginning with Freud, and place an emphasis on the importance of unconscious processes in understanding human behaviour and emotion. Early experiences, often going back to infancy, are seen as important, laying the foundations for patterns of relating to oneself and others that will be repeated throughout life unless brought into awareness. The individual will be defended by unconscious mechanisms and will rarely be fully aware of their motivations. The therapy relationship is seen as a venue for the exploration of these patterns, which will often play out via the medium of transference. The client will respond to the therapist on the basis of past patterns and will respond as if they were some past figure or a representative of some role or group. By engaging with this process the therapist can help the client to raise their awareness, challenge established patterns and experiment with new behaviours and experiences. Hopefully new insights and learning can then be taken out into the client's life beyond therapy.

Box 15.4   Cognitive–behavioural approaches

The cognitive–behavioural approaches are based on a model for the inter-relationship of experience with thinking, feeling and behaving. 'Cognitive appraisal' – how an individual makes sense of and thinks about a particular experience – is seen as central. *If I believe that dogs are dangerous, then I will feel scared when I see a dog.* In this way cognitive appraisal influences emotion, and both thinking and feeling influence behaviour. *If I feel scared, and I think this dog is dangerous I am less likely to act confidently and more likely to run away.* In turn, thinking, feeling and behaviour influence how the experience unfolds. *Running away may encourage the dog to run after me, reinforcing the fear and belief and so on.* Cognitive-behavioural approaches usually involve helping the client to analyse their experience in these terms in order to establish a causal chain of connections between experience, thinking, feeling and behaving. This chain is then examined to find a target for change – usually at the level of cognitive appraisal or behaviour – which will lead to a different (and better) outcome. *If I can believe the dog is friendly, I can approach it confidently and it will sit down submissively... etc.*

Box 15.5   Humanistic approaches

The humanistic approaches are characterised by a positive view of human potential and the emphasis on the client as the expert in their own life. The function of therapy is to expose the client to the right conditions for growth and positive change to occur, usually based on Rogers' concepts of empathy, unconditional positive regard and congruence (Rogers, 2004). In such an environment the client will feel understood, accepted and valued, and will learn to understand, accept and value themselves more, which will in turn liberate their inherent potential to grow and develop in a positive direction.

The history of counselling and psychotherapy includes two opposing tendencies in relation to the spectrum of approaches. On the one hand there has been a positive tendency to try to respect and understand what other approaches have to offer, and recognise that each 'school of thought' can make a contribution to the practice of therapy. It is also helpful to explore what the approaches have in common and to recognise that when we get to the level of what therapists actually *do* there is a great deal of convergence. Often different approaches will describe what are essentially similar phenomena in different terms. On the other hand there has also been a tendency towards competition between the approaches, with particular adherents proclaiming the wisdom of one approach over all others.

In reality, most practising counsellors and psychotherapists describe themselves as integrative or eclectic practitioners (Horton, 2012). This means that they make use of a range of perspectives, conceptual frameworks and techniques in order to meet the needs or preferences of the client, generally guided by some overarching theoretical model or an integrating framework. Some integrative practitioners attempt to work on the basis of a specified *theoretical* framework that brings together elements of, for example, humanistic and cognitive–behavioural theory, whereas others use an a-theoretical framework such as Egan's skilled helper model (Egan, 2010) that describes the *process* of therapy in a way that enables many different explanatory concepts and techniques to be drawn on when appropriate. The former is sometimes referred to as 'theoretical integration', whereas the latter can be described as 'open-system integration'.

No approach has yet been developed that seems to provide all the answers, and few therapists find a 'one size fits all' approach meets the needs of their diverse clients. In the examples quoted in Box 15.2 above for example, the first client would probably benefit from some fairly structured cognitive–behavioural work on the specific experience they are facing that is causing them anxiety. They are likely to benefit from challenging their existing beliefs about their abilities and the experience of presentation, rehearsing alternative thoughts and practising their desired behaviours both in their imagination and if possible in reality. The second client on the other hand may need space to talk about their past experiences, be listened to and understood in a supportive environment and have someone who understands and cares ('bears witness') to what has happened before they are able to move on. The third client seems more immediately in need of some help with identifying and prioritising specific issues and problems, identifying realistic goals and developing positive strategies that are within their control to begin to get to grips with their situation. The fourth client may need to explore their past experience in the light of their development through the stages of life, reflect on patterns and transitions and the influence of early experiences on how they are now, and develop ways to discard unhelpful patterns and develop new and healthier ways of coping. Therapy should provide a venue in which issues can be explored, but also in which the client can experience themselves, the impact they have on another and the impact the other has on them within a relationship that is genuine, non-judgemental and empathic.

Although most therapists describe their practice as integrative or eclectic there remains some discussion about the orientation of training courses. A quick scan of the BACP directory of accredited training programmes suggests that a majority have a core orientation to one approach/theoretical model, and relatively few are integrative. Some argue that a core training in one approach provides practitioners with a depth of understanding and application in that approach, and that other approaches, techniques or frameworks can then be integrated post-qualification. The implication is that such depth in one approach is preferable to the breadth that might be available from an integrative training. On the other hand, proponents of an integrative approach to training would argue that integrative models can and do include the depth needed in terms of understanding and working with the core therapeutic relationship, while also offering some breadth in covering a range of perspectives, conceptual frameworks and specific approaches or techniques. Depth in relation to other conceptual frameworks or techniques can be integrated post-qualification. Both these arguments clearly have some merit. The latest version of the BACP criteria for the accreditation of training courses has been carefully written to avoid favouring either position. The core curriculum for training embedded in the criteria describes what counsellors and psychotherapists need to understand and be able to do in language that is meaningful both across the range of specific approaches to therapy and from an integrative perspective.

REGULATION OF COUNSELLING AND PSYCHOTHERAPY

Statutory regulation of the profession was on the agenda through most of the term of the last Labour government (until 2010). Members of the public are often surprised to learn that the terms *counsellor* and *psychotherapist* are not protected in any way, so that anyone can legally describe themselves as such regardless of qualifications or experience. The previous government's proposals would have brought regulation of these titles under the auspices of the HPC and set up a national register for counsellors and psychotherapists, intended to ensure standards and safeguard the public. These proposals were controversial in a number of ways and agreement was never reached between the HPC and the various professional bodies. There were disputes about whether there should be one joint register, or separate registers for counsellors and psychotherapists, and if so how the distinction should be made, or indeed if there should also be a separate register for those working with children and young people. Some within the profession also argued vociferously that regulation itself would be limiting of the diversity and creativity currently in existence, both in training and in practice. They also point to the relative lack of consensus or indeed evidence concerning exactly how training contributes to successful outcomes in therapy.

The current government favour an approach of voluntary regulation within the profession, and it is unclear at the time of going to press exactly how this will be developed from the current professional-body schemes such the United Kingdom Register of Counsellors and Psychotherapists (UKRCP). The UKRCP is a voluntary register of counsellors/psychotherapists. A condition of registration is accreditation with either BACP, COSCA (the Scottish professional body), UKAHPP (the UK Association for Humanistic Psychology Practitioners) or FDAP (Federation of Drug and Alcohol Professionals).

RESEARCH AND EVIDENCE-BASED PRACTICE IN COUNSELLING AND PSYCHOTHERAPY

I used to live across the street from a psychology lecturer who frequently taunted me that I was teaching a postgraduate-level course in a discipline that did not have a research base. This was unfair. To generalise somewhat, the psychodynamic approach has a long tradition of research going back to Freud, which is largely based on the single case study methodology; the cognitive–behavioural approach has produced a body of evidence based on the more apparently 'scientific' methodology of the randomised control study; whereas the humanistic approach has tended to favour qualitative research into the client's experience of therapy, in keeping with its values and priorities. There is also a history going back at least forty years of 'outcome studies' in counselling and psychotherapy, which attempt to determine the success or otherwise of therapy in general and of specific approaches. Arriving at a consensus and enabling therapists to speak with confidence about their research base has, however, proved problematic until relatively recently. Eloquent and comprehensive reviews are now available however, for example by Duncan et al. (2010) and Cooper (2008).

Perhaps the most interesting finding to emerge from the research is the so-called 'equivalence of therapies'. Despite frequent attempts to determine which approaches are most successful or indeed which approaches are most successful with specific client issues, the vast majority of the available research indicates that all the different approaches to counselling are roughly equivalent in their effectiveness. However, a deeper examination of the results indicates that not all *therapists* are equal in their effectiveness, and indeed outcomes vary widely between individual practitioners. This would seem to suggest that whatever determines the success or otherwise of therapy, it is not generally the theoretical orientation or approach used. Duncan et al. (2010) draw on the available research to offer a summary of the factors that *do* appear to influence the outcome. They suggest strongly that the most important factor is in fact the client – their resources, preferences, ability to determine a focal problem, see themselves as able to change or bring about change, and the support available to them outside of therapy. The most powerful factor that is, at least to an extent, within the sphere of influence of the therapist is the therapeutic relationship, and specifically the client's perception of the therapeutic relationship. Positive outcomes are most likely to be associated with a relationship in which the client feels understood and accepted by their therapist. The third factor is a sense of confidence in the process of therapy and the therapist, and finally technique or approach is estimated to make only a 15% contribution to the outcome of therapy. In particular Duncan et al. make the case for therapists using techniques and approaches that make sense to the client and are if possible a good 'fit' with their existing ideas about themselves, how people develop, how they change and so on. This contributes powerfully to the argument for therapists to have a range of techniques and approaches available to them and to involve clients actively in deciding how to work together.

A tension therefore exists between the body of evidence available to guide counsellors and psychotherapists in their practice on the one hand, and the approach taken by the 'evidence-based practice' movement and bodies such as NICE on the other, who at least until now have tended to operate from a largely 'medical model' paradigm of attempting to determine the best treatment approach for a particular problem or diagnostic label, and have tended to favour randomised control studies over other forms of evidence. Some indications of a particular fit between therapeutic approach and specific client problems have emerged from this approach – for example CBT for panic disorder – but in general this has not so far proved to be a very productive line of enquiry for counselling and psychotherapy. At least two trends are evident within the profession in response to this. On the one hand there is pressure to 'conform' and begin to generate the kind of evidence that will be recognised and accepted by NICE in order to promote counselling and psychotherapy as a more widespread and officially sanctioned response to a range of problems or conditions. On the other hand there is a movement to lobby NICE to take a wider view of what constitutes evidence-based practice.

CONCLUSION

Counselling and psychotherapy are now practised in a variety of contexts and are accessed by clients seeking help with a wide variety of problems or issues. There is convincing evidence that the most important factor in determining the success of therapy (aside from the client themselves) is the formation of a positive therapeutic relationship characterised by empathy, acceptance and genuineness. Practitioners come from a variety of backgrounds including, but not limited to, psychology. A variety of training routes are available, usually involving a minimum of two years' part-time study, but often longer. Training can be focused on a specific therapeutic approach or theoretical framework (of which there are many in existence) or can be integrative. Building a career as a counsellor/psychotherapist is a challenging endeavour, and many therapists are 'portfolio workers' who divide their time between private practice, sessional or part-time work as a therapist, supervision and/or training and other work related to their particular interests, background or expertise. It is likely that a more robust voluntary regulation scheme for counselling and psychotherapy will be introduced in the near future in the UK.

QUESTIONS FOR REFLECTION AND DISCUSSION

1   How accurately do you think the public perception of counselling and psychotherapy matches the way the profession defines itself?

2   How do you feel about the usefulness or otherwise of a distinction between the terms 'counselling' and 'psychotherapy'?

3   To what extent do you think counsellors and psychotherapists can be 'trained' or educated or is it more about qualities that some people have and others do not?

4   Which approach or approaches to therapy most appeal to you given your current level of knowledge and understanding? (And why?)

5   How do you respond to the arguments for and against statutory regulation of counselling and psychotherapy?

6   How do you respond to the 'equivalence of therapies' finding? What other implications might it have for the training and practice of counsellors and psychotherapists?

SUGGESTIONS FOR FURTHER READING

Bayne, R. and Jinks, G. (2010) *How to Survive Counsellor Training: An A–Z guide.* Basingstoke: Palgrave. Practical information and guidance on preparing for and getting the most from training if you decide to follow that path.

Dryden, W. (2006) *Counselling in a Nutshell.* London: Sage. A concise and very readable overview of the theory and practice of counselling with the working alliance as its central theme.

Duncan, B., Miller, S., Wampold, B. and Hubble, M. (eds) (2010) *The Heart and Soul of Change: Delivering what Works in Therapy.* Washington, DC: APA. A thorough distillation of the available research and its implications for practice, which challenges preconceptions and presents practical and pragmatic guidelines for practice.

Feltham, C. and Horton, I. (2012) *The Sage Handbook of Counselling and Psychotherapy* (3rd edn). London: Sage. An excellent reference text. Clear and authoritative chapters on principles, theory, skills and techniques, client problems and current trends/issues by a wide selection of respected authors.

Rogers, C.R. (2004) *On Becoming a Person.* London: Constable. A classic collection of Rogers' writing from the period when his ideas about therapy were becoming established. Recommended reading as the source text for much of the foundation of contemporary practice.

16

COACHING AND COACHING PSYCHOLOGY

Ho Law and Christian van Nieuwerburgh

This chapter discusses:

- recent developments in coaching and coaching psychology;
- what is coaching psychology?
- the GROW model;
- the universal integrative framework (UIF);
- applications of coaching psychology;
- the way forward and professional issues.

INTRODUCTION

This chapter explores recent developments in coaching and how psychology can be applied to its development and practice. As a central feature, this chapter includes details of what coaching psychologists actually do in practice, the exciting new developments and the day-to-day applications. We shall first describe the historical developments in coaching psychology, some key models of coaching and coaching psychology, and then focus on the application of coaching within the education sector by way of illustration. In the concluding section, we shall discuss some current issues in this branch of applied psychology and its future trends and developments.

Coaching and coaching psychology in the UK

Over the past decade, a new industry has been developing in the UK that is rapidly becoming a mainstream profession. Coaching has become a discipline in its own right as well as a component that can be integrated into all walks of life. When we carried out our research at the Institute of Directors in 2004, the average turnover of the companies that provided coaching was £8 million with £500,000 pre-tax profit in the UK (Law et al., 2007). In 2008 it was estimated to be worth some £150–£250 million (Passmore, 2008). Despite the current financial crisis, the coaching market is predicted to continue to grow.

In the UK, there are thousands of suppliers in coaching, ranging from individual sole traders to large corporations. Training programmes for coaches are available in all parts of the UK, ranging from one-day introductory courses to university-based masters' programmes (for example, at UEL, Oxford Brookes and Sheffield Hallam). The programmes are usually modular in structure. A typical coaching psychology programme consists of the following components (see Figure 16.1):

- introduction to coaching and coaching psychology;
- models of coaching;
- theories of psychology including learning theories and personality types;
- a range of coaching techniques;
- evaluation.

To cater for the diversity of students who are interested in coaching, especially for those students who are in employment, some academic institutions (such as UEL) offer programmes in both full-time and part-time modes, as well as by distance learning. For more information, please see the resources section at the end of the chapter.

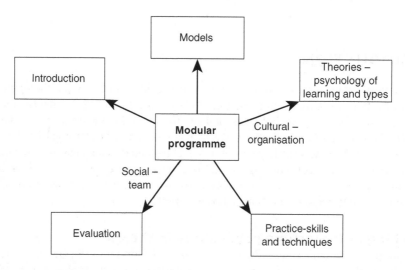

Figure 16.1   A typical modular programme

In practice, coaching programmes and interventions are now implemented in most industries and organisations. These range from external coaches working with senior executives to the development of internal coaching capacity through the training of staff as coaches. Coaching is now also prevalent within the educational sector, with lecturers and teachers involved in peer coaching and mentoring. It seems that coaching in education is an area of increasing interest (as discussed later in this chapter).

These developments have been supported by the BPS. Within its Division for Occupational Psychology, we have witnessed a continuous increase in the number of submissions in coaching practice under the area of 'counselling and personal development' (one of the eight core areas of competence under the area of occupational psychology) for assessment as part of the qualification in occupational psychology. At the same time, it is important to note that this aspect of psychology (coaching) is one that is attracting professionals from a broad range of fields. Leaders and managers from the health, education, commercial and public sectors are moving into the arena of coaching. In addition, some counsellors and psychotherapists are retraining as coaches (Peltier, 2010).

The development of coaching psychology as a profession can be traced back as far as 2002 to a workshop convened by Professor Stephen Palmer at the BPS Annual Conference for the Division of Counselling Psychology. The group initially developed a coaching psychology forum. This provided a discussion platform to develop understanding of coaching psychology. An introductory article for the Division of Occupational Psychology was published to promote the idea of coaching psychology and the forum (Law, 2002). In 2003 it was proposed that a Special Group for Coaching Psychology (SGCP) should be set up within the BPS structure. The BPS SGCP was formed on 15 December 2004 with its inaugural meeting held in London. At the time of writing, the SGCP has over 2300 members. Members are provided 'with an easy and effective means of sharing research as well as practical experiences that relate to the psychology of coaching' (see the resources section).

WHAT IS COACHING PSYCHOLOGY?

'Coaching' is widely understood as a process intended to unlock a person's potential, and thereby 'to *maximize* their own *performance*. It is helping them to *learn* rather than teaching them' (Whitmore, 2002). Coaching has been described as the 'art of facilitating the performance, learning and development of another' (Downey, 1999) and is said to be 'directly concerned with the immediate improvement of performance and development of skills by a form of tutoring or instruction' (Parsloe, 1995).

Even the definitions above raise the question about differences between coaching and a number of related fields, specifically mentoring and counselling. There is no question that all are 'helping conversations' that employ many of the same skills (questioning, listening, being 'present', showing empathy, etc.). It is our view that there are areas of overlap, but also that it may be helpful to discuss what is unique about coaching.

We do not aim to provide a rigid differentiation between coaching, mentoring and counselling here. However, it is our belief that coaching can be distinguished in the following ways:

- coaching is underpinned by psychological and adult learning theories;

- coaching is focused on the attainment of goals (usually set by the coachee);

- coaching is considered to be a conversation between two individuals of equal status.

Law et al. (2007) developed a framework called the universal integrated framework (UIF) that defines coaching as 'underpinned by psychological learning theory in a process that is developmental, brings about change and is culturally mindful'. This definition allows diversity and enables flexibility and fluidity in its practices.

The official definition of 'coaching psychology' adopted by SGCP is:

> ... [the] enhancing [of] well-being and performance in personal life and work domains underpinned by models of coaching grounded in established learning or psychological approaches'. (Palmer and Whybrow, 2007)

COACHING MODELS

Here we define a model as an abstract/simplified description or representation of a complex system or concept to show its essence and how it works. A model can guide practitioners by articulating what to do. It also enables them to provide a rationale to account for their actions. It provides practitioners with a map to help coachees to understand where they are going and how to help them. In recent years, there has been an explosion of coaching models. We believe that it is important for coaches to adhere to a process during coaching. Choice of models should be based on familiarity and the needs of the coachee. In this chapter, we shall describe two models: the GROW model, which is perhaps the most used, and the UIF, which is recognised as a powerful, integrative approach to coaching psychology.

The GROW model

The GROW model was developed by Graham Alexander (2006) based on his coaching experience and popularised by Sir John Whitmore (2002) through his consultancy practice. The model provides coaches with a description of the different stages of the process (see Figure 16.2). It helps coaches and coachees to clarify the expected outcomes (e.g. improved performance in terms of the coachee's goal or specific behaviour change in terms of their action plan in the 'way forward' stage).

The GROW model is a useful tool for structuring a coaching session. It offers a framework for discussing and exploring **g**oals, **r**eality (the current situation), **o**ptions,

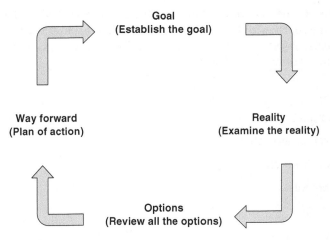

Figure 16.2   The GROW model

and the **w**ay forward/**w**illingness. The natural starting point is the goal. However, this is not always clear until later in the coaching session, so it may need revisiting later. Although it seems a linear structure, it is a reiterative/circular process such that the goal set can be reviewed in future sessions. After discussing the way forward it may be necessary to revisit the options, or realign the goal.

A typical GROW coaching session

One can design a coaching session or even a whole programme according to the GROW model. The first stage is to focus on setting the goals. Next, there is an opportunity to check the reality in terms of the current situation. Possible options are then explored. Finally a way forward is agreed. In some situations, one might find that it is not that easy to identify the goals without exploring the context (**t**opic) or reviewing the current situation (Garvey et al., 2009). Hence, the GROW model may sometimes be referred to as TGROW. In practice, coaches need to be flexible in terms of the ordering of the stages in the process – moving to and fro between each stage as necessary.

Goals

According to GROW, the first stage of coaching is to understand the coachee's goals, aims and/or objectives. Questions include the following.

- What are your hopes and dreams (the bigger picture, long term)?
- What do you hope to achieve (in the short, medium or long term)?
- What do you want to accomplish at the end of this session (immediate term)?
- What are your expectations of coaching (about the process itself)?

In eliciting the coachee's hopes and dreams, the questions asked by the coach would need to help the coachee to clarify and consolidate their aspirations so that SMART or SMARTER goals/objectives can be formulated. SMARTER is an extension from the SMART acronym (Doran, 1981); it stands for:

- **S**pecific

- **M**easurable

- **A**chievable/agreeable

- **R**ealistic/relevant

- **T**ime bound

- **E**valuation

- **R**eview.

Useful questions include the following.

- Specific – what does the 'goal' look like (e.g. in terms of work/life domain)? How will you know when you get there (the journey metaphor)?

- Measurable – how will you measure your success/progress?

- Achievable/agreeable – is it achievable? Would your parents/line manager/ your team agree with this (depending on the context)?

- Realistic – how realistic is this ambition?

- Time bound – when by?

- Evaluation and review – how will you know it is effective? How might you measure the benefits of achieving this? When would you like us to meet again and review this?

According to research (Locke and Latham, 1990), goal-setting is an important factor for success. Goal-setting can make a crucial difference to the coachee in terms of achieving a desirable outcome. The goal needs to be challenging as well as realistic. If it is too difficult, it becomes unachievable; if too easy, if it can be uninteresting. Either case could have a de-motivating effect upon the coachee.

Breaking a large and ambitious vision/mission – a longer-term goal or aim – into a set of inter-related smaller subgoals/objectives/milestones may be desirable. This helps monitor progress and sustain motivation (Lerner and Locke, 1995). The coachee is regarded as the owner of the goals and should take responsibility to achieve them (Gollwitzer et al., 1990), though other stakeholders may be involved along the way.

Reality

The reality stage allows coachees to re-evaluate their current situation and thereby identify the gap between where they are and where they want to be. In coaching, this may involve reviewing their performance, past and present, in terms of what is relevant to their goal, and establishing track records (including 360-degree feedback from others if available). Typical questions may include the following.

- What is the current situation?

- What have you done so far in relation to this? Can you give me some examples?

- What are the barriers?

- What do you mean by that?

- How do you feel about your achievements so far?

Options

This stage consists of two parts. During the early part of the options stage, one should be as creative as possible (with a non-critical, non-judgemental attitude) to generate the maximum number of options. This is intended to open up a whole world of possibilities that the coachees may not have thought of before. There are various tools and techniques to help coachees to generate a list of options, for example Buzan's (2000) mind mapping, Crawford's (1954) attribute listing, de Bono's (1970, 1985) six thinking hats and random words, and Osborn's (1948) brainstorming. Questions include the following.

- What are the options?

- What have you not tried before?

- If you could do anything, what would you do?

- Finally, please give me one more idea.

The second part of the options stage is about evaluation and decision-making. Whereas the early part of this stage was about opening up new possibilities, this part is about narrowing it down to a finite set of options in terms of their feasibility. This enables coachees to decide which options are most realistic and likely to be achieved. Questions include the following.

- Let us look through this list of options one by one ... What are their pros and cons?

- Is this feasible?

- How much would this cost?

- How long would this take?

Way forward

At the final stage of the GROW model, the coaches/mentors and coachees usually agree a way forward and generate an *action plan* that links to the selected options as the output of the session. The coach should also check to see if the coachee is committed to take the plan forward and whether there are any barriers that may prevent them from achieving those actions. Questions may include the following.

- Can you summarise the key points we have agreed in this session?

- What are you going to do?

- What are the possible barriers?

- How would you overcome them?

- Who could help you to overcome those barriers?

- What support/resources do you need?

- Who needs to be involved?

- How will you get there?

- When by?

- When shall we review this?

The universal integrative framework (UIF)

The UIF model provides coaches with a framework for coaching, which is seen as having four dimensions:

1 Personal (self) – this includes one's own self-awareness as well as self-identity.

2 Social – this includes social interaction; and can be applied to the workplace context, e.g. interaction in a team.

3 Cultural – this is not limited to the geographical boundary; and includes the organisational culture in the workplace context.

4 Professional – this includes continued professional development (CPD) as well as wider considerations such as environmental concerns and corporate social responsibility (CSR).

The UIF was developed by Law et al. (2007) based on their consultancy practice in coaching and mentoring. Unlike GROW, it is a non-linear spatial model that links

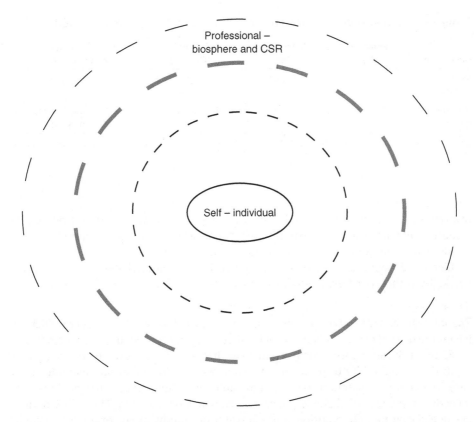

Figure 16.3   Diagram of the universal integrative framework. CSR, corporate social responsibility

Source: Adopted from Law H.C., Ireland, S. and Hussain, Z. (2007) *Psychology of Coaching, Mentoring and Learning.* Chichester: John Wiley.

the four dimensions to learning theories (see Table 16.1 and Figure 16.3). The above dimensions also link to the coach's/mentor's and/or coachee's competence. These are expanded further below (abstracted from Law et al., 2007: Chapter 6).

Dimension I: personal competence
These competencies reflect how we manage ourselves. They consist of two parts:

1 awareness of oneself (self-awareness);

2 management of oneself (self-regulation)/self-management.

Table 16.1   Dimensions and elements of the universal integrative framework

Dimension:	I **Personal (Self)**	II **Social (Other)**	III **Cultural (Culture)**	IV **Professional competence**
Awareness elements:	1 Self-awareness	3 Empathy	5 Enlightenment	7 Reflective practice
Management elements:	2 Self-regulation	4 Social skills	6 Champion	8 Continued professional development

Source: Law H.C., Ireland, S. and Hussain, Z. (2007) *Psychology of Coaching, Mentoring and Learning.* Chichester: John Wiley.

Self-awareness

Awareness of one's own internal states, feelings, emotion, cognition, preferences, resources and intuitions. The extent to which one accepts and values oneself.

Element 1: emotion. Awareness of one's own emotions.

Element 2: cognition. Self-reflection and evaluation – knowledge of one's own values, self-worth, capacities, strengths and weaknesses.

Self-management

The ability to manage and control one's emotions and motivation. The extent to which one invites the trust of others by being principled, reliable and consistent (trustworthiness).

Element 3: motivation. Positive emotion that drives one towards one's goals or aspirations. The ability to perform consistently in a range of situations under pressure. The ability to maintain commitment and take a course of action to achieve one's objective in the face of obstacles, personal challenge or criticism. The ability to manage one's awareness of emotion, and control it productively. For example, resilience measures – whether one is able to pick oneself up and bounce back when things go badly. Realism measures – how one balances optimism with realism.

Element 4: control. Ability to control disruptive emotions and impulses. This explores the extent to which one is emotionally controlled – namely whether one is free to express one's feelings but also in control of whether, how and when one does so.

Element 5: trustworthiness This also means honesty or integrity. It measures whether one invites the trust of others by being principled, reliable and consistent.

Element 6: conscientiousness. Take responsibility for personal improvement and performance.

Element 7: flexibility. Measures whether one is able to adapt one's thinking and behaviour to match changing situations (also adaptable for change).

Element 8: creativity. Innovative; comfortable with new ideas and novel applications.

Dimension II: social competence

These competencies reflect how we manage relationships. Social competence is a learning process as individuals gain insight through social interaction and awareness of others. It consists of the following elements:

- awareness of others (empathy);

- management of others (social skills).

Element 9: understanding (and trust). Ability to see from others' perspectives. Ability to understand the key issues, see the whole picture and draw a clear conclusion when presented with incomplete or ambiguous information. Measures whether one trusts others but also the ability to protect oneself from exploitation.

Element 10: Empowering. Help develop others to satisfy their needs and achieve their aspirations.

Management of others (social skills)

Ability to influence others, collaborate, co-operate with others by identifying a common ground, shared objectives, taking a leadership role, managing team spirit, resolving any conflicts and communicating clearly with a display of interpersonal sensitivity.

Element 11: communication. Listening to others' points of view. Provide clear and convincing messages about one's position and rationale.

Element 12: facilitating conflict resolution. Measures how well one can balance the requirements to be assertive (standing up for what one wants) while staying calm and respecting others. Helps mentees/coachees handle conflict. The coaches and mentors engage with both the emotional and social aspects when confronting conflicts.

Element 13: leadership facilitation. Inspiring; providing guidance to individuals and groups.

Element 14: coaching the team. Creating synergy in team or group coaching to achieve collective objectives.

Element 15: coaching for change. Championing change and modernisation.

Dimension III: cultural competence

The competencies here reflect how we manage organisational change. This dimension includes the organisational environment (from awareness, appreciation and respect of coachee's/mentee's cultures to helping champion organisational and cultural change.) They consist of the following elements:

- awareness of other cultures (enlightenment);

- management of organisational cultures (champion).

Cultural competence measures the extent to which coachees inquire into or respond openly to others' culture, ideas and values; and their willingness to challenge and question their own assumptions as well as others'. Coaches and mentors have the ability to mediate boundaries between cultures, connecting to others and their own culture. In doing so, one can experience oneself as part of a larger, collective consciousness, culturally and spiritually. One recognises that collective awareness and morality can transform the organisation and society as a whole.

Element 16: appreciation. Having appreciation of other cultures and religions.

Element 17: respect. Showing respect for the differences in others' cultures.

Element 18: championing equality and diversity. Achieving high performance through people from different cultures and backgrounds. One contributes one's voice to a collective endeavour.

Dimension IV: professional competence
The final section reviews some coach knowledge and approaches, which have an impact on coaching outcomes. This requires coaches to adopt professional approaches, giving and seeking authentic feedback to and from others.

The priority of the above dimensions and their associated elements may vary according to the type of coachees and their aspirations. For example, coachees may come from the same culture or be working within the same organisation as the coach. One may then be less concerned with the cultural aspects of the interaction, but focus on aspects of their personal development (self) or social interaction (e.g. developing social skills and emotional intelligence and resilience, etc.).

If on the other hand one has coachees working from very different cultures and/or organisations, it may be necessary to pay particular attention to the cultural context that they bring into the coaching space.

The UIF thus offers a highly flexible framework that enables coaches to apply different coaching skills and techniques within different coaching spaces, such as executive coaching (cultural/organisational dimension) and life coaching (self).

A psychometric tool to measure competencies based on the UIF can be used to provide feedback to coachees and identify areas for development. Like any psychometric tool, one needs to be mindful that the results only provide a 'snapshot' of the coachee's condition at the time of responding to the questionnaire. The results may change over time depending on their development. Used sensibly, it can be a powerful tool for guiding the coaching conversation. The tool is now available online, and the reader may contact the authors to access the tool.

APPLICATIONS OF COACHING PSYCHOLOGY

As mentioned previously, there is a growing acceptance and adoption of coaching in a broad range of fields, notably within the corporate sector, but also within the public sector, particularly in health and education. As an example, we will consider how coaching psychology is being used within the educational sector.

Since the beginning of this millennium, there has been a sharp increase in interest from schools and colleges and a clear recognition of the synergy between the goals of education and those of coaching psychology.

Schools and colleges are often highly pressurised and busy workplaces that focus on education and increasing the life chances of learners. Because they can be highly scrutinised and politicised organisations, staff can benefit from coaching support. Educational organisations have recently become more interested in using coaching approaches to support staff, embed professional development and enhance learning opportunities for students. In this section, we will review a number of these applications.

Leaders in education

A growing body of evidence and decades of practice show that coaching can enhance leadership and management in organisations. It has been employed successfully to:

- help leaders to transfer theoretical learning to workplace practice;

- enhance skills and develop new habits;

- develop greater self-awareness;

- enhance motivation;

- strengthen personal confidence and self-regard;

- build resilience and support well-being.

(Passmore, 2010)

Coaching can also have a significant role to play with educational leaders. It already forms a part of the development of school and college leaders. In the UK, coaching training is an integral part of the National Professional Qualification for Headship (NPQH) programme. Furthermore, most newly appointed principals and head teachers benefit from formal and informal coaching arrangements organised by their institutions, professional associations or local authorities (LAs). This, in turn, leads to a greater understanding and awareness of the potential of coaching within educational organisations.

Putting it into practice

Cognitive psychology and cognitive behavioural approaches are often appropriate when working with educational leaders. In the busy and frequently hectic environment of a school or college, leaders value the enforced reflection that coaching conversations can bring. These conversations can also serve to re-energise and motivate educational leaders by reconnecting them with their moral purpose and values.

- What made you want to work in education?

- What is most rewarding about your role?

- What element of your role makes you most proud?

School and college leaders also value the opportunity to have a professional conversation about their vision and strategic plans. The coach can create a safe, non-judgemental context in which the coachee can be explicit about their aspirations for their organisation and the people within it. By contrasting this vision with a thoughtful assessment of 'current reality', educational leaders can start to formulate a clear plan of action for moving towards their vision.

- If you were to draw or verbally describe your vision, what would it look like?

- How will you get others engaged and enthused about this vision?

- What strategy will most increase the chances of your vision becoming a reality?

- What impact will the changes have on students in your classrooms?

Aspiring leaders

In addition to providing valuable support for new and existing head teachers and principals, there are real opportunities to identify and develop future leaders. Coaching can be employed to support aspiring educational leaders to consider their concerns, ambitions and career plans. Often, the confidential, supportive and non-judgemental nature of the coaching relationship is conducive to exploration and 'dreaming' – exploring aspirations and purposes.

Putting it into practice

Once a positive and trusting relationship has been established between coach and coachee, the use of Johari's window (Luft and Ingham, 1955) is particularly effective with aspiring educational leaders. In a five-step process, the coachee is invited first to consider the 'arena' quadrant. The coach asks the coachee to think about how they are currently perceived in their educational organisation. The questioning focuses on how the coachee would describe herself as an educational professional. In keeping with the Johari model, coachees would only include information that they 'know' that their colleagues would agree with. The coach would be supporting the coachee to focus on mostly positive aspects of their professional self. Once that step has been completed, attention can be turned to the 'façade' quadrant. This is also known as the 'hidden area' and includes information that the coachee may know but others might be unaware of. A discussion about this quadrant can uncover what motivates and energises the coachee, as it allows for a discussion of values and beliefs. The third step is to focus on their 'blind spot': information that others 'know' but the coachee is unaware of. This is an interesting concept as, in theory, the coachee does not 'know' what might reside in that box. However, this quadrant contains feedback that the coachee may have had that they do not agree with. This discussion can uncover areas for development, or equally areas of strength that are not being fully exploited. The 'unknown' quadrant is there simply to capture any new information or knowledge that is discovered through the process of coaching. Finally, returning to the 'arena', the coachee can be challenged to talk about how they would like to be perceived, or might need to be perceived in future if they are to achieve their aspirations. By focusing on 'what needs to change' between the current perception and the desired future perception, coachees can formulate a plan of action or strategy that builds on existing strengths. To support their development, coachees should consider which elements from the 'hidden area' they might want to share with others and how to shed more light on the 'blind spot' by soliciting feedback.

The Johari window can be a powerful coaching tool to raise self-awareness and identify potential ways forward (Figure 16.4). It is particularly suited to the educational context because of its exploration of values and moral purpose.

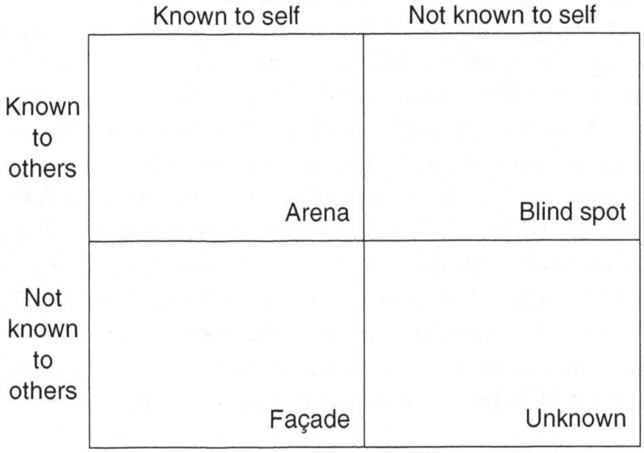

Figure 16.4   Johari window

Source: Luft, J. and Ingham, H. (1955) 'The Johari window, a graphic model of interpersonal awareness' in *Proceedings of the Western Training Laboratory in Group Development*. Los Angeles: UCLA.

Peer-to-peer support

In educational organisations, perhaps more than in others, there is significant opportunity for staff to provide support to one another. One approach to collaborative learning between educational practitioners is 'lesson study', an initiative supported by National Strategies in the UK. It involves a three-step process that can be supported by coaching: a pre-lesson conversation between two educational professionals, observation of the lesson and a post-observation review discussion. The peer observation of a lesson can often be the step that causes anxiety (on both sides). A coaching approach might support the entire process. Instructional coaching is a slightly different yet complementary method that has gained credibility and popularity particularly in the USA. This approach focuses on developing 'instructional coaches' to support other educators to implement agreed 'best practice' in the classroom (Knight, 2007).

Putting it into practice

With peer-to-peer support in educational organisations, it is important to recognise that we are dealing with 'knowledge workers' (Drucker, 1999). The best way of engaging with knowledge workers is to respect their expertise and engage them in the thinking process. The worst way to engage with them is to tell them what to do. For these reasons, a coaching approach between peers that focuses on building trusting relationships between professionals is most likely to lead to better educational practice in schools and colleges.

Embedding professional development

In response to a growing recognition that 'one-off' professional development sessions (e.g. a course or a conference) do little *by themselves* to change practice 'back at the workplace' (Robertson, 2008), schools and colleges are increasingly turning to coaching to build on such events. Through coaching interventions following courses, conferences or seminars, educationalists are able to discuss the application of learning in their organisations and work with others to embed effective practice. Allison and Harbour point out that forward-thinking schools see CPD as 'less about staff training days and training courses and more about a process of ongoing, collaborative professional learning – where professionals support and learn from each other' (2009).

Peer coaching can be used effectively to make the most of learning opportunities. Participants in training activities can be supported to reflect on their learning, plan how to disseminate and integrate new practice into the organisation, and review any implementation.

- What difference will this make to your practice?
- What are the benefits of changing your practice?
- How might this impact on the rest of the organisation?
- How can you get buy-in from your key stakeholders?

Enhancing learning opportunities for students

In their seminal publication *Leading Coaching in Schools*, Creasy and Paterson point out that the use of coaching in education is driven by 'a desire to make a difference to student learning' (2005). They identify five key skills of coaching:

- establishing rapport and trust;
- listening for meaning;
- questioning for understanding;
- prompting action, reflection and learning;
- developing confidence and celebrating success.

Staff from within the educational organisation or external coaches can work with individual students to support them in their studies or with their future plans. When coaching young people in schools and colleges, there is a real opportunity to allow the students to consider their own goals and dreams in a safe, confidential and non-judgemental environment. Often there will be conflicting drivers, sometimes imposed by family members or carers, at other times with direction from their schools. A considerable amount of time can be invested into identifying what motivates students and what they think is worth pursuing in the future. Once this work is done, coaches can focus on what students might do in the present to make their goal more likely in future.

Support for students through coaching can be delivered in a number of ways. Staff can be trained in the appropriate coaching skills and then allocated to individual students. This works well because staff will benefit from a professional development opportunity and students have access to time and attention from key educators in the school or college. It is also possible to train young people to provide coaching to their peers. This has the advantage of building the skills of the young people themselves, enhancing their employability, increasing internal capacity and raising the self-awareness of those trained to be coaches while also providing coaching support to a larger number of students from their peers.

Some of these ideas can also be used in primary schools. Children can be taught peer coaching skills within their primary classroom contexts (Briggs and van Nieuwerburgh, 2010). Schools can develop the coaching-related skills of active listening, asking good questions and giving feedback with children as young as ten years old. These skills can be used in the classroom to provide mutual support and feedback between children.

By developing the coaching skills of staff and students so that they can provide support to one another, the educational organisation builds internal capacity and the newly trained coaches increase their own skills and self-awareness. This can be particularly effective when the student or educator may not perceive the need for coaching for themselves. By learning the process, skills and 'way of being' necessary for coaching, the learners often start to consider how these may relate to their own situations. Furthermore, if they are then given opportunities to have coaching conversations with others, these are often two-way. It may also be the case that coaches are encouraged to set an example and become a role model within the organisation.

Obviously, we have only considered one sector in our discussion of the possible applications of coaching. As we mentioned at the beginning of the chapter, coaching psychology is having an increasing impact across an ever-broadening range of individuals and organisations. Coaching psychology is being embraced in a greater number of countries and cultures, highlighting the growing importance of the approach.

CONCLUSION

This chapter has provided a review of the recent development in coaching psychology as a distinct branch of applied psychology. Coaching psychology is truly coming of age in the twenty-first century (Palmer and Cavenagh, 2012). Future directions in mainstreaming coaching psychology practice in organisations and consultancy include:

- coaching psychology standards and competence;
- coaching and coaching psychology training;
- CPD and supervision;
- evaluation.

We shall discuss each of the above topics in turn.

Coaching psychology standards and competence

The development of standards is part of the professional development of any discipline. The coaching and coaching psychology professions have been engaged in working to develop a set of coaching standards for some years now. These standards need to be based on the core competencies of the discipline, enable one to audit the quality of a model, its processes, procedures and outputs, and also facilitate the evaluation of outcomes.

Sometimes, standards are established by professionals in order to regulate their practice. If the standards are developed too early (before a discipline is mature) it could stifle creativity and hinder development of the discipline. At present, coaching psychology is still on a developmental journey. As a result, the existing standards depend very much on its practice, for instance, through the BPS and HPC accreditation processes, which have established standards of practice. We recommend that coaching practitioners adopt the standard of practice of their own allied professional bodies (such as the BPS, SGCP and ISCP).

Coaching and coaching psychology training

At present, coaching and coaching psychology training provides participants with learning about the established coaching models, and their applications (usually the participants practise among themselves). The epistemology and principles of psychology that underpin these models should be included in this training. Currently, those interested in becoming coaches face a wealth of training opportunities from one-day courses to masters' programmes. Each person will need to carefully consider what will most suit their needs. For a brief introduction to some of the tools and techniques of coaching, a reputable training organisation offering a two-day course may suffice. However, we believe that those intending to take on the role of a coach will want to find a course that delves more deeply into the psychological and adult learning theories that underpin current practice.

CPD and supervision

All registered psychologists who practise psychology in the UK are required to engage in CPD and supervision. As an allied discipline, we recommend that all coaching psychology practitioners and trainers should also engage in ongoing CPD and have peer supervision. This should ensure that practitioners and trainers have adequate resources and support so that they can conduct their practice professionally and ethically.

Evaluation

Law et al. (2007) have provided a thorough evaluation framework that can be applied at different levels, ranging from individuals to large-scale applications in organisations. Evaluation is such an important component for any serious application that coaching psychology practice should embed evaluation as part of its process. We see this as applying not only to coaching psychology practice but also to the whole range of coaching applications.

QUESTIONS FOR REFLECTION AND DISCUSSION

1   In this chapter, the authors linked the UIF coaching model to psychology of learning. Can you identify any other learning theories that might be adapted in coaching applications? Would these learning theories be applicable to education as discussed in the case study?

2   The goal of a coaching conversation is to re-develop the coachees' skills and knowledge by asking them a set of questions. The GROW model provides platforms for participants to step into the near future of their lives. As a coach, you could devise additional questions that encourage coachees to generate new proposals for action. What would these questions look like? What are the characteristics of these questions?

3   In a GROW coaching session, what skills (in addition to questioning) might a coach employ to encourage the coachee to develop new insights and increase their level of motivation?

4   In this chapter, the authors have illustrated how coaching is being used in the educational sector. Which other sectors are already benefiting from coaching in this way?

5   This chapter introduces two coaching models: GROW and UIF. Compare and contrast the two models and make a list of the similarities and differences between the two models.

SUGGESTIONS FOR FURTHER READING

Hawkins, P. and Smith, N. (2007) *Coaching, Mentoring and Organizational Consultancy: Supervision and Development*. Milton Keynes: Open University Press. Read Chapters 5 and 6: Chapter 5 describes coaching within the organisational context and includes the role of cultures; Chapter 6 expands the role of culture further in terms of how to create a coaching culture.

Knight, J. (2007) *Instructional Coaching: A Partnership Approach to Improving Instruction*. Thousand Oaks, CA: Corwin Press. Chapter 3 suggests some key 'ways of being' that are important for a coach. Chapters 4, 5 and 6 – present a way of using coaching to support professional development within schools.

Law, H.C., Ireland, S. and Hussain, Z. (2007) *Psychology of Coaching, Mentoring and Learning*. Chichester: John Wiley & Sons. Read Chapter 6 – it provides a detailed description of UIF.

Law, H.C., Laulusa, L. and Cheng, G. (2009) 'When Far East meets West: seeking cultural synthesis through coaching', in M. Moral and G. Abbott (eds), *The Routledge Companion to International Business Coaching*. Hove: Routledge. pp. 241–255. This chapter describes the application of UIF within the cross-cultural context of the East and the West.

Megginson, D. and Clutterbuck, D. (1995) *Techniques for Coaching and Mentoring*. Oxford: Elsevier Butterworth-Heinemann. Read Chapters 2 and 3. The whole of Chapter 2 focuses on goal-setting. Chapter 3 describes a three-step model for using metaphors to effect change that helps in clarifying the current situation.

Passmore, J. (ed.) (2006) *Excellence in Coaching: The Industry Guide*. London: Kogan Page. Chapter 4 is a good source for learning about how the GROW model works. Also read Chapter 9 (integrative coaching) and look at Figure 9.1. It shows an alternative way to build your own model for improving work performance. Like UIF, it consists of different dimensions – maintaining partnerships to help coachees/mentees increase their self-awareness of unconscious thoughts, linking it to their actions and expected outcomes. Can you identify its elements and link them to the four dimensions within UIF? Are there any missing dimensions that the model needs to further develop?

Training and societies

For further information on studying coaching psychology programmes, please visit the UEL website: http://www.uel.ac.uk/postgraduate/specs/coachingpsychology/

For the distance-learning programme: http://www.uel.ac.uk/programmes/psychology/postgraduate/coachingpsychology-dl.htm

For information on professional membership visit:

the BPS Special Group in Coaching Psychology: http://www.sgcp.org.uk/

the International Society for Coaching Psychology: http://www.isfcp.net/

17

CAREERS GUIDANCE AND PSYCHOLOGY

Jenny Bimrose, Rachel Mulvey and Nelica La Gro

This chapter discusses:

- the work of careers guidance professionals;

- the theoretical frameworks underpinning their current practice;

- training routes into the profession;

- likely future trends.

INTRODUCTION

Careers guidance is a professional pathway open not only to psychology graduates but also to those from other disciplines interested in helping people to navigate and manage their careers. It is a relatively young profession, with the theory underpinning professional practice deriving predominantly from the academic disciplines of psychology and sociology. This chapter considers some of the current issues and challenges for careers guidance. These include the volatile context in which careers guidance is being delivered across the UK and the opportunities for employment opening up, the precise nature of careers guidance services, its origins, and what constitutes best practice. Training pathways are identified, which include postgraduate courses and work-based learning. Along the way, case studies, derived from lived experience, give a flavour of this nascent profession.

THE BIG PICTURE

Each time the social organisation of work changes, so do society's methods for helping individuals make vocational choices (Savickas, 2008). Indeed, methods of helping individuals make successful transitions from compulsory education into and through the labour market have, over time, taken different forms (e.g. advice, coaching, counselling, guidance), occupied various structural locations (e.g. schools, employing organisations) and accumulated a varied nomenclature (e.g. careers guidance, vocational counselling, and careers education, information, advice and guidance). Global economic turbulence has marked yet another set of profound structural labour market changes (Wilson, 2008), posing fundamental challenges to those providing support services for those engaged in labour market transitions globally (Savickas, 2002).

As a result of the changing economic and political landscapes, demand for careers support from a broad spectrum of individuals is on the increase, with the emergence of a plethora of new market players and cross-sector partnerships involving public, private and third sectors. These trends are not unique to careers in the UK, with the Organisation for Economic Co-operation and Development (OECD, 2010) reporting that many governments are increasingly using private and non-profit entities to provide goods and services to citizens. This rising demand for careers support services has occurred in parallel with: increased use of information and communications technologies (ICT) in the delivery of services, which has, in turn, been stimulated by an increasingly ICT-literate generation; high levels of consumer usage online; and new online systems facilitating data exchange between employers, individuals and third parties, such as schools, colleges and universities (Bimrose et al., 2011).

Despite shifting emphases by governments of the day regarding the exact purpose of careers guidance, the policy focus for careers has consistently assumed that if individuals who are in transition (having completed a stage in their education), who are not in employment or who wish to change jobs, are matched with the 'right' jobs, training or education courses as quickly and effectively as possible, then everyone gains. This begs a number of questions. Two important ones are: who defines 'right' in this particular context and what exactly are the forces operating that prevent the matching of individuals to these opportunities without the intervention of careers guidance?

The answer to the first of these questions (Who defines 'right'?) immediately highlights a potential tension between those who practise careers guidance and those who manage and fund services. On the one hand, managers and funders of services demand measurable outcomes from careers guidance, usually in the form of placement into employment, education or training. On the other hand, careers practitioners will typically try to establish what the particular needs of their clients are, then try to support them. For some, placement (into employment, education or training) may not be what they want or need.

The answer to the second question (What prevents clients matching to jobs without the intervention of a practitioner?) highlights a professional practice issue. Do the forces preventing harmonious transition of all individuals from education into employment lie within the individual, or within society? Practitioners subscribing to the first option will assume that all individuals can choose their career path and so prefer to work exclusively with individuals, enhancing self-esteem and empowering them to take the decisions and action required to ensure a positive result – a measurable outcome. Practitioners, however, who believe that individual action is largely constrained by social structures beyond their control (for example, racism and sexism) will be more inclined to work with the systems within which they are making their transitions, in addition to working at the individual level. This is a fundamental issue for careers guidance practice – should its focus rest with the individual client, or on the systems and structures in which clients, and indeed practitioners, are located, or indeed both?

Wherever and however careers guidance is delivered, it offers a wealth of opportunity for practitioners who can find employment in a range of organisations, increasingly across public, private and third-sector careers organisations, colleges of further education and universities, and community-based and voluntary organisations. People completing their training in careers guidance in recent years have secured employment in a wide variety of employment contexts. In addition, many initiatives delivering lifelong learning or economic regeneration embed careers guidance within their programmes. Whether called a careers adviser or a careers consultant, a careers coach or an outreach worker, it should be possible to locate a space in which to practise careers guidance congruent with your own value system.

THE NATURE OF CAREERS GUIDANCE

For many years, a clear-cut definition of careers guidance has remained elusive. It has been argued that 'career' has undergone something of a transformation, with a distinction made between career choice as a point-in-time 'event' (Osipow and Fitzgerald, 1996: 50) and career choice as a developmental 'process' over a longer period of time (p. 54). Career as 'the evolving sequence of a person's work experiences over time' has also been proposed (Arthur et al., 1989: 8), whereas Young and Collin (2000) identify a range of meanings. These include career as an abstract concept (referring to the 'individual's movement through time and space'); as a construct used in academic, professional and lay discourse; as a construct used in organisational and social rhetoric (to motivate and persuade employees); as a construct embracing attitudes and behaviours associated with work-related experiences over a lifespan; and finally, as a construct involving self-identity, hopes, dreams, fears and frustrations (p. 3). 'Overall, career can be seen as an overarching construct that gives meaning to the individual's life' (p. 5).

A breakthrough was reached towards the end of the twentieth century, with the publication of an extensive, international review of national policy on careers guidance, undertaken by the OECD (2004) in close co-operation with the European Commission. This report offered a comprehensive definition of careers guidance, its intention, its scope and its delivery mechanisms; careers guidance:

> covers services intended to assist individuals, of any age and at any point throughout their lives, to make educational, training and occupational choices and to manage their careers. These may include services in school, in universities and colleges, in training institutions, in public employment services, in companies, in the voluntary/community sector and in the private sector. The

services may be on an individual or group basis; they may be face-to-face or at a distance (including helplines and web-based services). They include careers information (in print, ICT-based and other forms), assessment and self-assessment tools, counselling interviews, careers education and careers management programmes, taster programmes, work search programmes and transition services. (OECD, 2004: 19)

PROFESSIONAL ASSOCIATIONS FOR CAREERS

The OECD definition of careers guidance has gained currency, and has been used by policymakers in countries who are in the process of setting up formalised careers guidance services. Closer to home, it was formally adopted by the largest professional association for careers guidance within the UK, the Institute for Career Guidance (ICG), which may set a precedent for universal adoption. Because of this ongoing debate, a number of terms that variously combine 'guidance', 'counselling' and 'careers' are currently used to imply subtle but important distinctions in practice: guidance, careers guidance, vocational guidance, vocational counselling, adult guidance, educational guidance, careers counselling, and careers education and guidance (Bimrose, 1996: 54).

An examination of practice in the area reflects this confusing picture. The Careers Profession Task Force (CPTF), which reported on the careers guidance workforce, considered evidence from no fewer than five professional associations in the UK (CPTF, 2012). In order of largest membership numbers they were: the ICG, the Association of Graduate Careers Advisory Services (AGCAS), the Association for Careers Education and Guidance (ACEG), the National Association for Educational Guidance for Adults (NAEGA) and the Association of Career Professionals International (ACPI), which represents those working in the private sector (CPTF, 2010). Worldwide, the International Association of Educational and Vocational Guidance (IAEVG) represents approximately 21,000 careers professionals, mainly through national associations. Its members come from fifty-three countries and from all continents. The CPTF welcomed action taken by relevant professional associations to establish one overarching group, to be named the Career Development Institute, responsible for developing common professional standards to apply to all members. The government also welcomed the progress made by the CPA, particularly the development of a 'licence to practise', building on the ICG's Register of Practitioners.

WHAT DO CAREERS PRACTITIONERS DO?

Careers guidance is a relatively new occupational area, which is emerging as a knowledge base in its own right and establishing its own identity as a profession. Just as there is a plethora of names for practitioners, and a wealth of contexts within which to practise, so there is variation within what constitutes typical practice. What, then, could careers guidance practitioners find themselves doing, and what do they actually do?

Box 17.1   Generic careers practitioners

As a generic careers practitioner you would:

- help clients to understand themselves and move on in careers decision-making through individual interviewing and some group activity;

- help clients make sense of opportunities in education, employment or training, evaluate their options and implement a plan of action;

- if necessary, use referral and advocacy to meet particular client needs;

- use software and databases as part of your toolkit with clients; and

- liaise with employers, training providers and other organisations.

Box 17.2   Careers practitioners in further and higher education

As a careers practitioner in further or higher education you would:

- offer services that help students to develop careers management skills;

- work with individual students either through drop-in sessions or booked interviews to devise and implement career plans;

- run career development programmes or workshops;

- devise innovative approaches to job search strategies;

- work with academic tutors on career development through curriculum design; and

- manage careers resources, including ICT or web based.

Box 17.3   Careers practitioners working with adults

As a careers practitioner working with adults you would:

- help individual clients navigate the labour market by making informed choices about work and employment;

- administer psychometric testing where called for;

(Continued)

> *(Continued)*
>
> - support adults currently in employment who want a career change or development;
>
> - devise and deliver group-based programmes for career decisions; and
>
> - work with community groups (e.g. refugees).

DOES CURRENT THEORY SERVE CURRENT PRACTICE?

This is an important time for the development of careers guidance: the policy spotlight is on current practice, and the profession have to clarify who they are and what they do. Emergent issues question the adequacy of traditional theory to sustain developing, dynamic practice. Savickas (1995) traces current problems with theory to the fundamental issue of differing philosophical origins. He identifies inherent tensions that arise from the academic traditions of different theories: 'sharp lines have been drawn on which philosophy of science to choose' (p. 15). Arguing for theoretical convergence, he concludes that:

> vocational psychology could benefit simultaneously from refinements forged within the distinct career theories, from advances produced by convergence among career macrotheories and from break-throughs induced by divergence in work-role microtheory. (p. 29)

As a result of comparing theories, Osipow and Fitzgerald (1996: 323) conclude that they differ not only because of the different philosophical orientations of authors, but also because they are trying to achieve different objectives. They distinguish: those that focus on explanations of the choice process; those that focus on career development over time; and those that focus more on providing practical techniques. A common weakness of these theories is their tendency to claim universality for their concepts (Osipow and Fitzgerald, 1996), a claim that seems not to be justified in practice.

This, in turn, has given rise to two distinct trends in the development of theory – trends that are sometimes overlapping. One is towards developing theories that attempt to meet the needs of specific client groups, like minority women or ethnic groups. Traditional theories were developed in relatively homogeneous Western capitalist contexts that were strongly individualised, masculine, secular and action- and future- focused (Bimrose, 2001). They tend to assume choice and autonomy for the individual, whereas some critics question this as a reasonable assumption for some client groups within their social and cultural contexts. For example, serious weaknesses in applying theory to girls and women have been identified (Bimrose, 2008) and a number of theoretical approaches have been developed over the past few decades specifically for women that are more holistic in their conceptualisation (e.g. Cook et al., 2002).

Other theories have been promoted as having particular relevance to women, in addition to other client groups, because they stress the complex and dynamic nature of individual career development (August, 2011). A particular example is systems theory. Specifically, the systems theory framework (STF) of career development (McMahon and Patton, 1995; Patton and McMahon, 1999, 2006) depicts the myriad intrapersonal, social and environmental–societal influences on career development. It also considers the random influence of chance, locating career development within the context of time by considering the inter-relationship of past and present experiences with individuals' hopes and plans for the future. The STF highlights the microsystem of the individual, with the recursive influences of a broad range of interconnected intrapersonal influences (e.g. gender, age) as well as the social and environmental–societal influences (e.g. family, socio-economic circumstances, globalisation) that derive from the macrosystem in which individuals live.

The second trend within the development of career theory is a move towards a post-modern approach (Collin and Watts, 1996; Savickas, 1993). Savickas (1993) discusses this move away from 'logical positivism, objectivist science, and industrialism' towards 'a multiple perspective discourse' (p. 205), and summarises key differences between the modern and post-modern era (p. 209). Careers counselling, he suggests, has produced six notable innovations to mark its entry within the post-modern era (Savickas, 1993). These are as follows.

- First, a rejection of the notion that careers practitioners are experts: 'instead of portraying themselves as masters of truth, counselors are creating a space where those involved can speak and act for themselves' (p. 211).

- Second, the replacement of the concept of 'fit' with 'enablement', and the affirmation of diversity.

- Third, recognition of the importance of context and culture, together with the broadening of focus beyond a preoccupation with work-role; together, these signal a move towards life-design counselling and grand narratives (p. 212).

- Fourth, there is a questioning of the legitimacy of separating the career from the personal, with a move towards the greater integration of these two domains.

- Fifth, the realisation that career theory has provided objective guidance techniques that practitioners have increasingly had to combine with subjective techniques derived from counselling theory for their practice. Embryonic career theories are thus being developed that focus more on meaning, invention and construction, and move towards 'co-construction or social construction of meaning' (p. 213).

- Finally, a shift away from objectifying clients by measurement to a preference for autobiography and 'meaning-making'.

Savickas (1993) suggests that changes in careers counselling re-define the practitioner as a co-author and editor of career narratives. Instead of diagnosing abilities and achievements, assessing potential and matching clients to the most suitable education, training or employment opportunities, practitioners would authorise careers by narrating coherent stories; invest career with meaning by identifying themes and tensions in the story line; and help clients learn the skills necessary for the next episode in the story (Savickas, 1993). So, an exploration of significant events, turning points or positive role models in a client's life history confirms for the clients that these events or people may, legitimately, be important and influential to their future personal development. Indeed, by sifting through life history, patterns might very well emerge. For example, a client might identify two or three significant people who have had a positive influence on them during a particular event or period in their lives. The careers practitioner would then tease out patterns or similarities among these people with their client and discuss possible meanings to identify lessons to be learnt, thus indicating pointers or preferences for their future career development.

CAREERS GUIDANCE FOR THE TWENTY-FIRST CENTURY: HOW POLICY IS SHAPING PRACTICE IN THE UK

Three separate, but overlapping, major policy agendas continue to have careers at their centre.

- First is the up-skilling agenda that seeks to address key skill gaps in the workforce, so that the UK can compete globally and play a leading role in economic growth (e.g. Department for Business, Innovation and Skills, 2010a; UK Commission for Employment and Skills, 2010).

- Second is the lifelong learning agenda, which aims to facilitate the development of a knowledge society through individuals' engagement in learning and training (e.g. Department for Children, Schools and Families (DCSF), 2009).

- Third is the social equity agenda, which focuses on fair, inclusive and just processes and practices in the delivery of public services (e.g. DCSF, 2007; The Cabinet Office, 2009).

To meet these policy agendas, careers services across the UK have been reviewed. Strategies and government policies across the UK have all emphasised the importance of careers guidance to economic growth and development (for Wales: Edwards et al., 2010; for Scotland: The Scottish Government, 2011; and for Northern Ireland: Department of Education & Department for Employment and Learning, 2009).

In England, the past fifteen years have seen three distinct waves of radical restructuring to careers guidance services. This started with the privatisation of careers services, in which private providers bid for contracts to deliver services through a competitive tendering process. Within a few years, under New Labour's social inclusion agenda, these careers services, though still contracted out to providers, were subsumed into integrated youth support services under the Connexions remit. This required a dramatic shift in emphasis from universal to targeted services. So instead of every user enjoying equal access to the services on offer, more services (and resources) were directed at specific user groups; in Connexions, the focus was on young people not in education, employment or training, also known as the NEET group (Mulvey, 2006).

The latest restructuring saw integrated youth support services come back under LA control. This resulted in the reduction in the services offered (and therefore massive reduction in the number of careers guidance professionals employed) because of the intense pressure on reducing LA spending as a consequence of reduced budget allocation. However, an all-age careers service, launched in England in 2012, replaced the previously separate services for young people and adults (Department for Business, Innovation and Skills, 2010b) and brought England in line with the all-age provision in Wales, Scotland and Northern Ireland. It also forced the introduction of a free market into the provision of careers that is not the case elsewhere in the UK.

As a consequence of these policy changes, there are a number of key issues facing careers practitioners (Box 17.4)

Box 17.4   Issues and trends: the practitioner's view

A continuous flow of policy initiatives has resulted in a continuous process of change that can at times seem relentless:

- Careers guidance is firmly on the policy agenda in the context of economic regeneration and lifelong learning.

- Challenges to established ways of working in careers guidance can be perceived as threatening.

- New opportunities are emerging for both practitioners and their clients, across the public, private and voluntary sectors.

- Digital technologies and social media will play an ever-increasingly important role in the delivery of careers services.

- Labour market information is regarded increasingly by policymakers across the UK as pivotal to high-quality careers guidance, with pressure to integrate more centrally to service provision.

TRAINING FOR THE PROFESSION

Government policy has paid attention both to the organisation of careers guidance delivery and appropriate training for careers practitioners, particularly with regard to those working with young people. Policymakers for careers guidance uncritically accepted the ideology underpinning narrow forms of work-based assessment in the early 1990s. National Vocational Qualifications (NVQs) for guidance (Levels 3 and 4) were introduced in the mid-1990s with no account taken of published critiques that discussed problems with (NVQ) competence-based assessment in practice in other occupational areas (for example, Hodkinson and Issit, 1995; Hyland, 1994; Wolf, 1995). The development and implementation of a new 'Qualification in Careers Guidance' (QCG) for practitioners, with renewed emphasis on work-based learning and competency, was implemented nationally from the academic year 2001/2002. There are, therefore, currently two distinct routes into the profession: either education-based or work-based. The education-based route involves either a one-year full-time or two-year part-time course in higher education. The workplace route sees practitioners working towards occupational competence over a period of at least eighteen months, and typically two years. In adult careers services, including Jobcentre Plus, there has been far greater emphasis on the work-based (NVQ) qualifying route.

Anomalously, those successfully completing a postgraduate QCG were then required to complete some parts of the NVQ4 in Guidance in their workplace, before being deemed occupationally competent for the purposes of contract compliance. The Skills Commission (2008) took evidence on both training routes in terms of how well they equipped advisers to practise across the spectrum – from adult to young people, school to workplace, public to private service – and concluded that neither route was without its flaws. A key recommendation made (The Skills Commission, 2008) was that a taskforce be convened to scrutinise the workforce and identify those actions necessary to secure a high standard of professional practice for effective careers education and guidance. This was the impetus for the Careers Profession Task Force (CPTF). The CPTF (2010) made clear recommendations that both work-based and higher-education routes should continue to be offered, that all practitioners should have a specialist careers qualification, which should be at Level 6 (which equates to a final-year honours degree) and that this should be achieved by 2017, subsequently with achievement of a postgraduate qualification.

BECOMING QUALIFIED: INDIVIDUAL JOURNEYS TO PROFESSIONAL PRACTICE

At the time of writing, training centres are being closed or suspended in higher education institutions as a result of austerity measures resulting from public spending cuts. Successful study in full- or part-time mode leads to the award of a postgraduate Diploma in Career Guidance (Qualification in Career Guidance – QCG). Details of course centres can be obtained from the website of the professional association.

The QCG programmes have a history of being highly successful in terms of employability. Diplomates work in the statutory (youth) sector, adult guidance agencies, careers services in further and higher education, and the private and voluntary sectors. The course offers the opportunity to engage in reflective professional learning and to combine academic with practical work. In line with recommendations from the CPTF (2010), there is an increased emphasis on how professionals in training can be helped to exploit developments in information technology within careers guidance work, recognise the importance of labour market information and intelligence, and place increased emphasis on the importance of science, technology, engineering and maths (STEM) subjects in their practice.

A number of course centres increasingly offer a range of associated qualifications (e.g. Postgraduate Certificate in Careers Education, postgraduate programmes in careers coaching). Progression from the initial professional qualification QCG typically takes the form of a master's degree in careers guidance. In most universities this comprises a part-time research-based programme.

Work-based routes for practitioners who are employed within the field of guidance involve assessment on the job towards vocational qualifications within the Qualifications and Credit Framework (QCF) such as the Level 4 Diploma in Advice and Guidance or Level 6 Diploma in Careers Guidance and Development.

The following case studies are compiled from actual experiences of people who have undertaken professional training , but do not relate to a specific individual. They offer illustrations of the types of trajectories that lead to professional careers guidance practice.

Box 17.5   Saima

Having completed a degree in business studies, Saima found employment in an LA housing department, working directly with members of the public. She most enjoyed the aspects of the work in which she felt she was developing positive relations with people and 'making a difference'. After several years, however, Saima felt her role was limited and the scope of her work predictable. She undertook the QCG and, once qualified, secured employment in a local school as a learning mentor, working to boost achievement and raise aspirations.

Box 17.6   Andy

Some years after leaving school, Andy started a part-time degree course in modern languages. Unsure what he wanted to do once he graduated, he took a job in a national bookstore chain. Once he and his partner started a family, Andy went part time to combine employment and childcare. He also became involved in a local community group, working with refugees, which allowed him to develop effective interpersonal and communication skills. Realising that this was an area of work he found fulfilling, he wanted to undertake formal training and came on the QCG course. On completion, he went to work for a local careers company, working with young people in inner city schools.

> ### Box 17.7   Wendy
>
> Wendy left school at sixteen and went to her local further education college where she gained a Distinction in GNVQ Level 3 Business Studies. She found work in a local employment agency, and enjoyed helping local people get local jobs. From there she moved to the economic development team of her local council, and undertook a Higher National Diploma (HND) in Public Management. She found herself managing a local project to regenerate a neglected housing estate. As part of her own training needs she is undertaking the Level 4 Diploma in Advice and Guidance, developing competence in the workplace, and gathering evidence for her portfolio.

Of course, where there are students, there are also teachers. The recent changes in training routes have made demands on those delivering professional training to adapt to a rapidly moving external environment. Issues that currently exercise trainers are detailed in Box 17.8.

> ### Box 17.8   Training: the trainer's view
>
> - Safeguard standards and embrace change.
>
> - Develop blended approaches to initial training.
>
> - Embed careers guidance in wider provision.
>
> - Straddle professional and academic agendas.
>
> - Maintain a professional presence within the spectrum of practice.
>
> - Contribute to the knowledge base underpinning practice.

CONCLUSION

Despite public spending cuts, careers guidance remains a developing professional area. It offers varied employment opportunities in a range of contexts. Indeed, as the practice of careers guidance has become more established, policy requirements in the UK have increased its range of clients and tasks. The new professional contexts and roles for guidance practitioners are being accompanied by the development of new theories for practice that signal a rejection of scientific, positivist approaches to careers and their replacement with paradigms embracing more holistic, fluid models of human behaviour. The process of working out (and working through) the implications of new approaches for practice is underway. A key challenge for this community of practice is likely to be reconciling new approaches and thinking to policy directives embedded in traditional theory.

QUESTIONS FOR REFLECTION AND DISCUSSION

1   In terms of policy, is careers guidance part of the welfare provision, there to look after people, or is it part of a national economic strategy to get everyone (who can be) engaged in work or training?

2   Thinking about your own career path up to this point, would you see psychology (individualistic) or sociological (structural) factors playing the greater part?

3   When considering your future career planning (either immediate or long term), would a rational-positivist or a post-modern approach be more helpful to you?

4   Where do you think real learning as a professional takes place – in the classroom or in practice?

SUGGESTIONS FOR FURTHER READING

Athanasou, J.A. and Esbroeck, R.V. (eds) (2008) *International Handbook of Career Guidance*. Dordrecht: Springer. A comprehensive and wide-ranging text that brings together thirty-two chapters on various aspects of international theory and practice.

Hodkinson, P., Sparkes, A.C. and Hodkinson, H. (1996) *Triumphs and Tears: Young People, Markets and the Transition from School to Work*. London: David Fulton Publishers. This is a good text for getting the sociological perspective on careers guidance, and a close understanding of what careers mean for the individuals involved.

Swanson, J.L. and Fouad, N.A. (2010) *Career Theory & Practice: Learning through case studies*. (2nd edn). Thousand Oaks, CA: Sage Publication. Offers different perspectives that selected theories provide for working with clients and their career concerns.

Savickas, M.L. (1995) 'Current theoretical issues in vocational psychology: convergence, divergence, and schism', in Walsh, W.B. and Osipow, S.H. (eds) *Handbook of Vocational Psychology: Theory, Research and Practice* (2nd edn). Mahwah, NJ: Lawrence Erlbaum Associates. pp. 1–34. While the Savickas chapter in particular is good for the postmodern perspective, the *Handbook* overall gives a good insight into the issues currently engaging the careers guidance community of practice. A subsequent edition, Walsh, W.B. and Savickas, M.L. (eds) (2005) *Handbook of Vocational Psychology: Theory, Research and Practice* (3rd edn), offers further discussion of theory and practice.

18

THE PROFESSIONAL ACADEMIC

John Radford[1]

This chapter discusses:

- the nature of professions;

- how far academics can or should be professional;

- the changing nature of higher education, and pressures on the system;

- the United Kingdom 'binary experiment' and lessons that were lost;

- the academic job, and preparation for it;

- an ideal of professionalism as 'responsible autonomy', for institutions, academics and students.

SUMMARY

Many branches of Psychology are recognised as professional, but academics are in an anomalous position for various reasons, including a divided allegiance to a discipline and an institution. The criteria for what constitutes a profession are summarised. Academics only partially meet them. They are professional in the sense of being paid, and to a large extent in the way they approach their work and their students (considered to be clients). New academics in the UK are now required to take a qualification in teaching, but the nature of this is currently under debate. At the same time their disciplinary qualifications, normally a first degree and increasingly a PhD, can be criticized. The nature of academic work is rapidly changing with economic and technological developments. It is suggested nevertheless that professionalism, considered as *responsible autonomy*, is an ideal at which to aim.

---

[1]Some paragraphs of this appeared first in *PsyPag Quarterly*, Issue 77, December 2010.

INTRODUCTION

If you are a real scholar you are thrust out in the cold. Unless you are a money-maker, I say, you will be considered a fool, a pauper. The lucrative arts, such as law and medicine, are now in vogue, and only those things are pursued which have a cash value (John of Salisbury, died 1180).

All professions are conspiracies against the laity. (Character Sir Patrick Cullen in the play *The Doctor's Dilemma,* by George Bernard Shaw, 1911).

The system is not working together. It is changing so fast, developing contradictory patterns. And there is no overall planning for it. We are striving to monitor it, but we have no power to change things. Monitoring shows up absurdities; all we can do is drink coffee and complain. (Anonymous professor, quoted in Leisyte et al., 2009)

The various branches of Psychology discussed in this volume are generally recognised as professional ones. Academics are in a somewhat anomalous position. For a long period the British Psychological Society (BPS) managed its business through two boards, for professional and scientific affairs respectively. I always thought this carried the unfortunate, if unintended, implication that professionals could not be scientific, and scientists – who largely overlap with academics – could not be professional. The word 'academic' itself has overtones of 'abstract, unpractical, cold, merely logical' (*Concise Oxford English Dictionary*). When the Society wanted to create a (professional) division for such persons, 'academic' was rejected in favour of 'teachers and researchers'. Two decades ago Barnett and Middlehurst (1993) wrote, 'academics are changing from being a status group to a proletariat without ever having been a profession'. Smyth (1995) suggested they had been reduced to 'workers in the knowledge factories'. More recently I have been inclined to say they are, rather, slaves in the graduate mines.

Nevertheless, I argue that professionalism, rightly considered, is an ideal to which we should aspire.

THE ACADEMIC 'PROFESSION'

Professionalism

There is no legal definition of what constitutes a profession. But there are several generally recognised characteristics (Eraut, 1994; Radford, 1997, 2003b; Slater et al., 2008; Warren Piper, 1992). I think they should apply, with some variations, to the academic, scientific, applied, professional and any other activities of psychologists (to say nothing of other disciplines).

- First, formal and intellectual training, based on a shared body of knowledge, both practical and theoretical. This means much more than a set of skills, important though these are. There must be a grasp of the range of knowledge underlying the practice, and of its fundamental principles.

- Second, a commitment to the best interests of the client, and acceptance of codes of conduct, enforceable when necessary. One expects a physician or lawyer to do what is best for the client, not what they prefer or find convenient. They should do so although the client may not be able to tell the difference. In other words, the professional must be trustworthy. In the case of academics, the client is the student. There is an obligation to teach what students need (not the same as what they want, though that is a legitimate concern), rather than what interests you (though that is also a valid concern).

- Third, exclusion of the unqualified. A piece of paper does not guarantee good practice, but it should mean that a standard has been reached, and it is often something that can be withdrawn if that is not maintained. In education, it is absurd to insist that no one can teach on a course without a formal qualification in that particular area. There have been distinguished professors with no academic qualifications at all. Any discipline can benefit from outsiders. But one does not want complete charlatans teaching.

- Fourth, accountability for what is achieved, rather than for specific actions. What you need from your GP, or your clinical psychologist, is to get better, without assessing the particular treatment. In education the results are, or should be, long term as well as short. Students need to pass exams, itself a medium-term rather than immediate result. The real test is the rest of their lives, though evidence is hard to come by. It makes little sense to try to assess teaching by whether enough handouts are given or forms filled in, though these are (perhaps) necessary tools. Indeed it is counter-productive.

- Fifth, responsible, autonomous work without direct supervision. Once again, the professional must be trusted, this time by those in authority.

- Sixth, autonomy and self-regulation of the profession itself. There must be a robust system, not only to direct the profession's affairs, but also to monitor the behaviour of its members, in line with the accepted codes of conduct. This should include a significant input from outside the profession itself, to ensure objectivity.

There are dangers in professionalism, and Sir Patrick Cullen's charge is indeed one of them. A profession may become arrogant, secretive and defensive. When something goes wrong it closes ranks to protect its members. That is why the sixth point above is vital. Another major danger is stagnation. Professional training and practice may become hidebound, and reject anything new. Physicians at first refused to accept anaesthetics or antiseptics, and there are many other examples. These dangers must be actively guarded against. But professionalism can and should also, indeed mainly, provide protection for the 'laity', that is, the clients or public. And it is far better if this is done willingly and with full commitment by individual members, rather than reluctantly under compulsion from outside. Regulations and systems are necessary, but they are not sufficient. The failure of Members of Parliament to grasp this was a major factor in the recent furore over their expenses.

Academics as professionals

It is obvious that academics only partially meet these criteria. The vast majority are 'professional' in that they are paid at least something (unless emeritus). They work long and conscientiously without direct supervision or sticking rigidly to rules or hours, although such behaviour is ever more eroded by numbers of students combined with continual bureaucratic demands. They still frequently put their clients' interests ahead of their own, willingly giving up extra time to keen, or weak, students. On the other hand academics are hardly organized at all as such and, consequently, lack self-regulation. They cannot exclude those unqualified – indeed many would strongly object to such an idea – and they are in general inappropriately trained, though this is, to an extent, changing. It has long been argued that it is odd that those who are, in a sense, gatekeepers to nearly all professions should not themselves constitute a profession (Elton, 1989; Perkin, 1987; Radford, 1994). Perkin pointed to some of the reasons, which still obtain. Their loyalties are often divided between discipline, institution and occupation (one might add, sometimes in terms of trade union membership). They have often failed to guarantee the worth of what they are doing and to make the public aware of it. In the past they relied too much on an assumption of 'effortless superiority' and (up to about forty years ago) on a comfortable security in a pleasant and reasonably rewarding occupation. Such was the situation described in Halsey and Trow's classic *The British Academics* (1971) and which still, perhaps, colours public perceptions. Universities' claims of excellence are not always based on good evidence (Wangenge-Ouma and Langa, 2010). In general the autonomy of professions, including the academic, is under attack and diminishing (Slater et al., 2008). The starting salaries of lecturers are not much above the national average wage, while professors are far below medical GPs, let alone consultants to whom they might be considered comparable in training and expertise.

THE TIMES THEY ARE A-CHANGING

Higher education

The times always were 'a-changing', but recently, it seems, more rapidly than ever. All advanced societies have had some system of higher education, concerned largely to produce leaders, civil, military, scientific, religious or other. Western universities originated as training schools for law, medicine and theology, upon a foundation of general education. I have sketched the story elsewhere (Radford et al., 1997; Radford 2003a). As they proliferated, universities diverged in various ways. England possessed only two until the nineteenth century and they followed an unusual pattern (Scotland was rather different). The professional aim was largely lost, and Oxford and Cambridge became by the eighteenth century a preparation for Church of England clergy and a sort of finishing school for sons of the gentry. After this came the ideal of what S.T. Coleridge called the 'clerisy', a classically educated, enlightened, Christian, non-specialised elite fitted to lead the nation. In 1935 the University Grants Committee could still ask, 'When the young graduate puts on the gown and hood of his [sic] degree, of what inward and spiritual graces are these the outward and visible signs?' (Shinn, 1986). In the interim the aim had shifted from the moral to the intellectual, 'to cultivate the mind and form the intelligence', as Mark Pattison, Rector of Lincoln College, Oxford, put it in 1867. It was not training for a specific occupation, a view reiterated in 2002 by the former Chief Inspector of Schools, Chris Woodhead. The intellectual activity *par excellence* came to be research, though this became dominant in the UK only in the twentieth century. With the phenomenal growth of science and technology, new knowledge was at a premium, and universities, now including the new civic institutions, were major suppliers of it. Concomitantly, the prevailing mode of first degrees came to be the single-subject pattern, three years full time away from home. Another influential view of what universities should be was exemplified in the ideals of Wilhelm von Humboldt and the University of Berlin after the Napoleonic Wars (Michelsen, 2010). He conceived of a body of scholars and students, free to learn and free to teach, and of all knowledge as united under the aegis of 'philosophy'. It was in a sense a reversal of the mediaeval pattern, with general education now taking precedence over professional (Nybom, 2003). A few UK universities are currently exploring such a wider approach; for example the Dumfries Campus of the University of Glasgow has included in its undergraduate curriculum since 1999 'core courses' in critical thinking, textual analysis, communication, ethics, politics, history and sociology of science and rhetoric (letter, *Times Higher Education*, 26 February 2011). The Humboldt university would not, however, prepare students for mundane occupations. For that, another sort of institution was needed.

The binary experiment

Such a binary system is still the norm in many European countries, where it seems to provide 'different but equal' opportunities (Hoyningen-Huene, 1992; Kivinen and Nurmi, 2010). Here, it was partially experimented with between 1970 and 1992, when polytechnics were created, mainly from former colleges of technology, to provide degree-level education that would be more practical than the university version, and incidentally cheaper, since they were not to do research, and less independent as they came under local government. Like most national education policies, it was political rather than educational. And like other policies, it did not work. The polytechnics on the whole provided a good education, and developed a good new way of assuring quality under the Council for National Academic Awards (CNAA), based essentially on the method of peer review. But you can't stop academics doing research merely by failing to fund it, and there was a strong tradition of research and development with local industry. At the same time science and technology, in which many polytechnics had been strong, largely fell away. Student interest diminished, British industry with its local demand for training was declining, and the Robbins Report in 1963 specifically called for more science in the universities. The CNAA became more influential than intended; the 'public' institutions became larger in total than the universities, as well as more like them in the courses they offered and the experience and qualifications of academic staff. They themselves pressed for the more prestigious status. They were created universities by statute. The opportunity was taken to dismantle the more democratic internal governance on which the CNAA had insisted, and to replace peer review, and the relative independence of universities, with a central inspectorial system. We are left with a nominally unitary, but really hierarchical, system. The subsequent two decades have seen a sort of trench warfare between successive governmental agencies and the universities, in which academics, of course, are the foot-soldiers. It is too complex to unravel here, and no end is clearly in sight (see Silver, 2007). The main obvious outcome is a great increase in bureaucracy.

The changing context

Meanwhile, all sorts of other influences are shaping what academics have to do. The implications of the Bologna Declaration on European harmonization of higher education (Schriewer, 2009) have yet to become apparent in the UK. Meanwhile, courses everywhere have become modular, so that, in theory, a degree is made up of free-standing units. In principle, the main advantage of these is that students could construct a flexible course, full or part time, with choices to suit their inclinations and career plans. In practice, many qualifications allow little real choice, and the adoption of university-wide programmes means that it is extremely difficult to change any part of them, or adapt modes of teaching to new demands (see e.g. Schmidt et al., 2010). Students do not or cannot switch readily between full and part time, but at the same time decreased funding means they often have to work anyway while technically full time. At the moment of writing (February 2011) the effects of a new radical change in student funding have yet to be worked out. Another innovation is the semester system now bizarrely superimposed on the three-term pattern, itself apparently derived from two Christian festivals plus a bigger break to bring in the harvest. The latter was once known as the long vacation, but for academics it is now replaced by a much more modest 'annual leave'. Universities are under constant pressure to be more economically relevant (Lambert, 2003; Sandelin, 2010) or 'entrepreneurial' (Etzkowitz, 2010; Rae and Matlay, 2010). John of Salisbury would be unsurprised. Greatly increased numbers of students, with more varied capabilities and demands, have the obvious results of bigger workloads and less satisfaction in the teaching process. Some claim it is simply no longer possible to monitor and maintain standards (e.g. Alderman, 2009). Many academics feel they are not only perpetually overworked, but also are not doing the job they could and should do.

WHAT DO ACADEMICS DO?

Academic tasks

What then is that job? There have been various studies of how academics spend their time, usually in terms of a small number of categories such as 'teaching', 'research' and 'other'. I have suggested before (Radford, 2003b) that these conceal a host of different activities. 'Teaching', for example, may be lecturing, to small classes or several hundred, one-to-one tutorials, seminars and small group work, supervision of labora-tory classes, fieldwork or projects, workshops and so on. A short reflection shows that academics may need to carry out, to varying degrees and at varying times, any of the following.

- *Teaching* in multiple modes, with concomitant preparation and marking, both enormously time-consuming.

- *Research* in the refereed journal sense.

- *Submissions* and reports in relation to research.

- *Student assessment*, including formal examinations, course work, qualitative assessment, etc.

- *Scholarship* and study.

- *External examining.*

- *Professional practice* in an applied field.

- *Consultancy*.

- *General writing*, course materials, text books, mass media, etc.

- *Membership* of professional or learned bodies, with varied duties and functions.

- *Counselling* and individual student guidance and advice.

- *Course development*, including curriculum and syllabus design.

- *Internal validation* processes.

- *Student recruitment* and selection.

- *Administration*, from record-keeping to co-ordinating the work of colleagues or assistants, timetable construction, ensuring supplies of equipment or source material, etc.

- *External relations* with the general public, parents, schools and colleges, employers and professional bodies.

- *Internal politics* and negotiations, including committee work as member, chair or secretary.

- *Clerical work* including word processing, filing, PowerPoints, etc.

- *Meeting demands of external accreditation bodies* and perhaps taking part else-where as an assessor.

This is just to illustrate the sheer range of activities. In terms of time allocation, many can be grouped together as teaching, research or administration. The widely heard complaint is that the last of these takes up too much time. At least one colleague has told me that it is her largest single activity. Tight (2009) reviewed the ten major surveys of academic workload that were carried out between 1961 and 2004. They show that during the 1960s weekly hours increased from about forty to something over fifty, but not greatly after that (up to 2004, note). Such surveys need some caution if self-reported, as academics do not generally work set hours but, in professional fashion, carry on until the job is done. Also, it is not always easy to distinguish the activities; for example, is preparing a PowerPoint teaching or administration? Academics feel the load is increasing, but this, Tight thinks, is due to the greater demands of administration at the cost, particularly, of research. This, he says, 'reflects the decreasing trust in academics on the part of their key funder, the state; yet, paradoxically, the increasing amount of time spent on it threatens the quality of the teaching and research it is meant to protect.' Personally I tend to a more cynical view. Administration, by and of academics, increases partly because it is an instrument of control, which is an aim, explicit or implicit, of central government, as has long been clear (Jenkins, 1995; Salter and Tapper, 1994). Partly too, due to Parkinson's Law (1958), which expressed in a light-hearted way what is a real effect. The basic law is 'work increases so as to fill the time available for its completion'; by extension, administration increases regardless of what is being administered. For example, it is always easier to add regulations and procedures than to remove them. Once an ethics committee, health and safety provisions, or validation processes are introduced, it is almost impossible to remove or reduce them.

Research

Apart from sheer workload, and the administrative burden, the main arguments have been about the relationship of teaching and research. Students, and the general public, expect both of universities (Radford and Holdstock, 1996, 1997). Jenkins and colleagues (2003), reviewing the evidence, show not unexpectedly that many academics hold strongly to a functional link of teaching and research. But this is not easy to demonstrate. There is a good deal of evidence, but Jenkins et al. conclude it shows a much more complex link than simple causality. Whether research benefits teaching, or vice versa, depends on particular balances of time and interests. Elsen et al. (2009) suggest it essentially depends on the involvement of students. Leisyte and colleagues (2009), from documentary evidence plus interviews with forty-eight Dutch and English academics, concluded that 'teaching and research are increasingly falling apart as two distinct entities'. There is certainly a clear tendency to concentrate research funding in a few institutions. At the same time research continues to be important for prestige and promotion, and indeed for personal satisfaction. Parker (2008) found that for appointments as senior and principal lecturer, universities had largely adopted parity of teaching and research. But for reader and professor most require research excellence exclusively, and do not allow similar applications based on teaching. Post-1992 universities are most likely to recognise teaching and research equally.

Research also plays a very large part in the various rankings of institutions that have become so influential. It has long been apparent that these rankings are inconsistent and unreliable (Berry, 1999; Stolz et al., 2010). It is perhaps somewhat reassuring that Gunn and Hills (2008) suggest that rankings initially had a large effect on recruitment, but that this rapidly fell off, although the post-1992 universities are far more variable than the older ones. They point out that students may apply to places they think they will get into, rather than on the basis of high ranking. And, of course, applications do not say anything about the quality of students, or their suitability for particular courses. The fact is that recruitment and selection of students are a very haphazard process. Psychologists know a lot about this but it is seldom applied, even by them. My own subjective feeling is that if a department or similar unit is to offer first degree teaching, it is important that there is a significant degree of professional activity: research, scholarship, consultancy, practice, writing. This does not mean all members of staff, but the department as a whole. Students may be actively involved in some of these activities, but should at least be aware of them, and feel they are in an outfit that cuts the mustard, to put it colloquially.

EDUCATION FOR ACADEMICS

I have always advocated that academics should have practical experience outside academia. But dealing only with formal preparation, this obviously has two parts, the discipline and the profession. Until recently, at least in the UK, the second part has been unconsidered.

Discipline

The first part normally consists of a first degree (occasionally more than one), and frequently a PhD: currently about 63% in pre-1992 universities, 29% in the later ones, in both cases increasing (*Times Higher Education*, 17 February 2011). It may be surprising to learn that the first PhDs in this country (actually DPhil Oxon) were only awarded in 1917. There were mediaeval doctors of philosophy, but the modern PhD derives ultimately from the Humboldtian concept of the university, although it is a far cry from the 'unity of knowledge' ideal, and is now generally an extreme specialization (Radford, 2001). This has been criticized for some time, e.g. Noble (1994). In the USA more than 40,000 PhDs are awarded annually, by more than 400 institutions, though half are from 50 universities (Nerad, 2004). Major US surveys present several widespread criticisms. The education is too narrow; graduates lack key professional skills (e.g. collaborative, managerial, organizational); they are ill-prepared to teach; they are ill-informed about employment outside academia. Nerad suggests also that there is too long a gap between completion and employment. Undoubtedly at least some of these points apply in the UK also, particularly in respect of preparation for an academic career. The PhD student resembles the expert who knows more and more about less and less, and may have only a first degree to fall back on when it comes to teaching a range of courses. Modular courses may have failed to provide a wide overview of the discipline. He or she may have done some teaching, but generally with little support or instruction. There are considerable differences between doctorates from different universities. During 2011, the Quality Assurance Agency was consulting on a draft document designed to achieve comparability of all UK doctorates, but this appeared not to address the issues above.

Profession

Here we come to the professional side. Following a recommendation of the Dearing Report (National Committee of Enquiry into Higher Education, 1997), every higher education institution in the UK is required to have in place some form of professional development for all new teaching staff. It is now typically a Postgraduate Certificate in Education, currently accredited by the Higher Education Authority (HEA) (Gosling, 2009). This is registered as both a company limited by guarantee and a charity, and is owned by Universities UK and Guild HE, which are representative bodies for universities, comprising their executive heads (generally vice-chancellors or principals). The criteria adopted by the HEA – the UK Professional Standards Framework – are concerned solely with teaching and student learning. However, these are currently (February 2011) under review, and may well be considerably widened, to include for example public information, career enhancement, professional standards, etc. The HEA also seeks to encourage professional development by established staff, who can be eligible for Fellowship of the Academy. I have argued (Radford et al., 1997), as have many others, that if education is to be termed 'higher' it must be far more than teaching and learning, even if combined with research. Dearing, indeed, in line with the criteria for a profession at the start of this chapter, stated:

> the essence of professionalism is a thorough and up-to-date grasp of the fundamental knowledge base of the occupation; sufficient understanding of the theoretical principles to be able to adapt to novel circumstances and to incorporate research findings into practice; and appropriate practical skills and professional values.

This should, of course, apply both to the academic's discipline and to education itself. I would go further. In terms of the criteria for professions suggested above, the HEA provisions apply most exactly to the third, exclusion of the unqualified. Continuity of higher education policy has not been noticeable in the past sixty years, but if the present arrangements persist, all academics in the UK will eventually have a teaching qualification. Whether this also satisfies my first criterion, which is essentially that of Dearing, depends on the exact nature of that qualification. The possible shortcomings of the discipline training – arbitrarily selective modular degrees, narrow PhDs – remain. The other four criteria are not being systematically addressed. In particular, academia is not developing the kind of independent but monitored self-regulation that I would regard as desirable. Perhaps it never will. Individually, many, probably most, academics function as professionals towards their students. But they lack the knowledge to take an overview of policy, and the power to direct it. The daily pressures are such that they appear often to be in a looking-glass world where they are running as hard as they can to stay in the same place. As I put it in the first edition of this book, the younger ones in particular lack the confidence and the skill to resist the more grossly absurd demands put upon them, and the knowledge to show why these are unacceptable and that there are better ways. They need to be able to defend the rationale of their professional practice. Further, there is a risk of being swept along helplessly by a tide of changes in society and in education itself, of which the massive increase in demand for higher education is just the most obvious. In the UK and elsewhere this is accompanied by inability or unwillingness of the state to foot the bill, despite its becoming the dominant force in policy (see Shattuck, 2008). In this country, we are only beginning to see alternatives in the shape of private and for-profit institutions, the latter in particular radically altering the nature of academic work (Lechuga, 2006).

PURPOSES OF HIGHER EDUCATION

And there are yet wider questions that concern the whole purpose of higher education, questions that go back to Confucius and Lao-Tse and to classical Greece (Beck, 1964; Chaplin, 1978; Tweed and Lehman, 2002), for example the interests of the individual or society, of training or wider education and so on. Far-reaching decisions are made about education based on unchallenged assumptions or political expediency. It is surely the role of academics, if anyone, to take a broader view. Nearly all the vast literature devoted to the purpose of higher education stresses values and qualities beyond formal training and qualifications, important as these are. What such values and qualities are, and how they may be achieved, is too complex to debate here (see Radford et al., 1997). But academics surely should be aware of these issues, and be prepared and able to lead the debate. With few exceptions this does not happen at present. As Pascarella (2001) put it, 'The academy has the unfortunate tendency to apply scientific standards of evidence to every field of study except itself.' I have suggested before (Radford, 1994, 1997, 2008) that psychologists should be leaders in such debates, inasmuch as our discipline is fundamental to education, more so than any other. Training for education must draw on many disciplines such as Philosophy, Anthropology, History, etc., but Psychology is specifically concerned with basic processes such as mental and behavioural development, learning and thinking, social relations and social skills, assessment and measurement, communication and so on. We can claim established knowledge and methodology that provide a sound basis for practice; certainly a far better one than is often found. I have also suggested the possibility of innovations such as, for example, a professional doctorate in higher education, comparable with those in other branches of Psychology, although it might well apply in other disciplines also. Such a doctorate would combine theory, method and practice with a significant but not dominant element of research. It would be appropriate for academics (and administrators) in a system that must necessarily be largely but not wholly concerned with teaching (see Radford, 2011).

CONCLUSION

Two decades ago Altbach (1991) wrote: 'Without a well-qualified, committed and adequately compensated professoriate, no academic institution can be fully successful.' In 2003 I commented: 'Whether it will be possible, at this late stage, to evolve a true breed of professional academics is dubious' (p. 128). It now seems more so than ever. A stream of publications detail the problems facing higher education worldwide, and the need for, or inevitability of, changes (more or less radical), e.g. d'Ambrosio and Ehrenberg (2007); Eckel and Kezar (2003); Gordon and Whitchurch (2010); iPED Research Network (2009); Welch (2005) and, more as a speculative fantasy, Radford (2012). The tone of many is 'not particularly optimistic' (Stromquist, 2007). Brown (2005, 2008), among others, has sought reasons, and remedies, for the current deficiencies of the present UK system, with responsibility falling both on government and on the higher education sector itself. In the second paper he urges that there should be a reduced role for government, with more pragmatic and less ideological policies, while education needs more effective representative bodies, and should as a whole become more questioning and professional.

Responsible autonomy

But one might say, who will bell the cat? Personally, I summarise my concept of professionalism as *responsible autonomy* (Radford, 2010; see also Huisman, 2007): the ability to make more informed decisions and take more effective action, while having regard to the interests of others. That is what ideally, in my view, should characterise institutions of higher education, those who work in them, and those they produce. The obstacles are certainly great; yet I think it is still possible for individuals to do a little more than drink coffee and complain.

QUESTIONS FOR REFLECTION AND DISCUSSION

1 Academic psychologists: parasites, priests, proletariat or professionals? (see Radford, 1997.)

2 Why are academic salaries so low?

3 What would be the ideal preparation for an academic career, in your view?

4 Have we anything to learn, from a professional point of view, from academia in other countries?

5 What, if any, practical steps can academics take to improve their status?

SUGGESTIONS FOR FURTHER READING

Gordon, G. and Whitchurch, C. (eds) (2010) *Academic and Professional Identities in Higher Education: The Challenge of a Diversifying Workforce*. New York: Routledge.

Papers on academic training and careers, different national contexts, professionalism, 'borderless education', etc.

A special issue of the journal *Higher Education Policy*, 2007, 20 (3). Special issue on autonomy. Topics include the problem of increasing dependency on outside agencies, academic freedom in Europe and USA, and quality assurance.

A special issue of the journal *Higher Education Policy*, 2007, 20 (4). Special issue on sustaining diversity: differentiating higher education systems in a knowledge society. Topics include massification and diversity, funding, academic training, student mobility, organization and governance of universities.

A special issue of the journal *International Journal for Academic Development*, 2010, 15 (1). Issue on diversity in academic development. Papers on different European higher education contexts, engaging students, curriculum revision, peer review, supervision of studies, etc.

iPED Research Network (2009) *Academic Futures: Inquiries into Higher Education and Pedagogy*. Newcastle upon Tyne: Cambridge Scholars Publishing. (iPED is Inquiring Pedagogies). Topics include research communication, intellectual development of students, a sustainable academic future, competitive funding, academics as entrepreneurs, network collaborative learning, problem- vs. project-based learning.

Silver, H. (2007) *Tradition and Higher Education*. Winchester: Winchester University Press. Discussion of changing views of what universities can and should be, over the last half-century.

PART THREE

New Directions

19

NEW DIRECTIONS IN APPLIED PSYCHOLOGY: A ROUNDTABLE

Edited by Rowan Bayne

For the roundtable, I invited expert psychologists to write about five hundred words in answer to the question: 'Which new direction(s) would you like to see in your branch of applied psychology?' I negotiated longer pieces with several of the contributors. Replies to the question are organised in three sections:

1   Areas of applied psychology that have potential for careers and that are either not discussed or only touched on in earlier chapters.

2   Supplements to some of the areas discussed in earlier chapters.

3   General.

The roundtable and the book end on two contrasting notes, one bleak (but suggesting a way forward), the other upbeat. Colin Feltham argues that 'psychology has not lived up to its early promise' and suggests two reasons: psychology's 'neurotic attachment to a scientific identity' and 'little sense of priority or urgency'. In marked contrast, Nicky Hayes celebrates the increasing dynamism of modern applied psychology and hopes for a place for routine consultation with specialist or generic applied psychologists in any project that involves people.

SECTION 1: SOME FURTHER AREAS OF APPLIED PSYCHOLOGY

THE HUMANITARIAN AND THIRD SECTORS

Sarah Davidson

More than ever, in times of financial crises the humanitarian and third sectors, which include charities and humanitarian organisations, are increasingly relied upon to deliver services locally, nationally and globally. As humanitarian and third sectors have recognised the significance of psychosocial support, psychologists have contributed to guidance, strategy and practice (e.g. Davidson, 2010a, 2010b; Wessells, 2006). Critical within these has been the identification of minimum standards to prevent and respond to crises (e.g. Hobfall et al., 2007; Inter-Agency Standing Committee (IASC), 2007; The Sphere Project, 2011) and the management of stress and trauma (see e.g. Antares, 2008; McKay, 2005).

Psychosocial support has usefully been defined as: 'the dynamic relationship that exists between psychological and social effects, each continually interacting with and influencing the other' (Save the Children, 2005: 1). Drawing from a vast body of theory and research, including community psychology, attachment theory, organisational and positive psychology and systems theory, this emerging area of applied psychology has tried to address the linkages between the individual, community and socio-political arenas. Leaning (2008), for example, has explored several key elements of human security among individuals and their community, including: the importance of 'place'; the system of social networks that enable familiar, secure and repeated interactions; and the need for hope. She explores conditions in Mogadishu and Afghanistan in which the destruction of 'place' and 'social networks' are intimately linked to a personal and collective sense of dislocation and alienation.

Psychologists in this area need to be familiar with elements that facilitate trust and therapeutic relationships, as well as what constitutes an outcome, output and good evaluation. Awareness of contexts is especially fundamental, as is working at various levels of analysis, focusing on prevention and the sharing of psychological skills and principles with non-professionals (e.g. Orford, 2008). Cultural awareness and sensitivity is key (IASC, 2007) as is self-awareness and having strong consultation skills.

In terms of training, programmes can be found on a range of subjects, such as in developing management skills in voluntary organisations and NGOs (e.g. CASS Business School, organisations London); in interpersonal skills for the voluntary sector (e.g. Lampeter, University of Wales); peace building (e.g. Peace Operations Training Institute, USA); and security (e.g. Cranfield University, UK). A fairly recent development is the MSc in International Humanitarian Psychosocial Consultation offered by distance learning at UEL. On this programme, students from countries including Afghanistan, Haiti,

Malawi and Vietnam are able to study and exchange learning and different perspectives through discussion boards and virtual seminars. Modules are offered on: international contexts, humanitarian contexts, psychosocial consultation, well-being and resilience, and research. Networking is all the more important when one is working with diverse groups, without an obvious team or group of peers. Psychologists or psychosocial professionals working in the humanitarian and third sectors are often lone advisors, so the need to connect with others in similar positions can be critical.

Historically those working as psychosocial professionals for humanitarian organisations have included those with both clinical qualifications and international experience:

- Pat Bracken qualified as a psychiatrist before working in Uganda for the Medical Foundation for the Care of Victims of Torture in the late 1980s. He has described how this experience was important in teaching him about the crucial role played by social and cultural contexts in terms of how people's emotional reactions are shaped and their attempts to understand them. Finding traditional psychiatric approaches unhelpful, particularly in their individualistic focus, he worked instead at a community level. He went on to conduct consultancy work for Save the Children in Liberia, Sierra Leone and Nepal (Fannon, 2008).

- Another UK psychiatrist who found Western-centric psychiatry inappropriate and detrimental when applied in international humanitarian contexts is Derek Summerfield. A consultant to Oxfam, Summerfield has argued for the need to be critical of diagnostic labels such as PTSD and the mass globalisation of individualistic interventions at the cost of adequate assessments and consideration of cultural differences (Summerfield, 1999).

- Mike Wessells is a US psychologist who has worked extensively with humanitarian organisations across Africa and in South-East Asia. He has advocated the importance of self-reflection and critical thinking in humanitarian psychosocial approaches to ensure the core principle of 'do no harm' (Wessells, 2008). He has also co-chaired the Task Force on Mental Health and Psychosocial Support in Emergency Settings, which developed the first inter-agency, consensus guidelines for the field of mental health and psychosocial support in humanitarian crises (IASC, 2007).

- Lisa McKay qualified as a forensic psychologist before gaining international humanitarian experience and then working at the Headington Institute in California, USA. The Headington Institute, like the Antares Foundation, the Mandala Foundation and the Centre for Humanitarian Psychology, focuses specifically on issues of stress and resilience as they relate to international humanitarian workers. Each of these organisations also provides a range of useful online materials to support delegates. As well as writing of her own experiences, McKay has noted the significance of spirituality for the resilience of those working in the humanitarian sector and has written an online training module on the subject (McKay, 2010).

- My own experience is as a clinical psychologist who has worked in the UK's NHS as well as with a number of humanitarian and third sector organisations. As both the psychosocial advisor to the British Red Cross and a trainer of clinical psychologists and humanitarian delegates, I believe the importance of understanding different contexts and their implications for people's needs and access to resources is imperative. By not recognising the specific requirements associated with the context of age, of the young or old for example, it is known that children and older people's needs go unmet (e.g. HelpAge, 2010, and Humanitarian Emergency Response Review (HERR), 2011). Also important is the need to stand back and notice and check on the assumptions underpinning our actions. This is particularly needed when these actions are in a place or with a group of people about whom we are less familiar, or even with those we believe we are familiar with, but have not checked that this is the case. By not checking with those with whom we are working, we risk causing harm through our assumptions, by being misguided or blinkered, such as offering individual therapy rather than engaging a family, community or organisation; or by offering assistance through an inappropriate channel, such as a mixed-gender group. Self-reflection is also required, together with the need to remember our own needs and not have them met only through our work with others.

Although having an applied psychological qualification has been important in terms of carrying credibility, there are many who work directly with individuals and communities who undertake a wide range of roles and who are well placed to enable, support and empower. Increasingly, professionals from a range of disciplines will be expected to conduct more psychosocial activities, promoting the resilience of individuals and communities through ensuring better access to key resources, undertaking consultation to promote a better fit between what is wanted and from whom it is delivered, and eliciting and understanding the impacts and outcomes of different services and programmes.

The HERR (2011) conducted of the UK's Department of International Development would seem to support this direction. The Review noted that a combination of climate change, urbanisation, continuing conflicts, scarcity of resources and increasing pressure on commodities such as oil and food will result in more global humanitarian crises in the future. As a consequence, the Review concluded that more people will be required to respond; people who will need to put resilience at the top of the priority list, working innovatively in partnerships with others, consulting effectively to promote meaningful engagement and accountability to and for all (HERR, 2011).

Psychosocial competencies that promote the effective engagement of and collaboration with individuals, couples, families, groups and communities will be essential. So too will the ability to look beyond pathologising and stigmatising labels (e.g. PTSD) to the opportunities, resources and alternative narratives available. Maintaining a critical awareness of the disparities that inhibit access to rights, such as safety and dignity, will also be required; particularly when it is known that natural disasters and their subsequent impact on average kill more women than men, or kill women at an earlier age (Neumayer and Plümper, 2007), and that women and girls living in the makeshift camps in Haiti, a year on, were at greater risk of rape and sexual violence (Amnesty International, 2011).

Applying psychosocial competencies will be the province of all who work within the humanitarian and third sectors, which is why it will be important for there to be accessible courses supporting the development and maintenance of relevant competencies. Networks of professionals and partnerships between agencies will be required in order to meet the increasing demands, develop and monitor standards and provide peer support. An example of such partnerships can be found between InterHealth, RedR UK, the Kenyan Red Cross and Amani Counselling Centre, who together deliver workshops in Nairobi in order to promote the awareness of security and listening skills to enhance the resilience of those delivering humanitarian assistance.

At the same time, such partnerships must place each stakeholder on an equal footing, avoiding some of the more colonial attitudes and power imbalances traditionally seen in the relationships between richer donors, who have exported aid and dominant ideologies, to poorer beneficiaries. Here too psychosocial skills and research offer a way of both considering and talking about power, and of introducing methods to increase its visibility and challenge the taking-up and maintenance of unhelpful power positions. Lessons can be learnt from the processes of reconciliation, to the benefit of community empowerment and resilience (Lederach, 2001).

Psychologists are not, will not and cannot be alone in meeting the demand for psychosocial activity within the humanitarian and third sectors. However, with their understanding of developmental factors and the importance of context, with their research skills and critical thinking, and with their applied skills in engagement, consultation, problem-solving and self-reflection, they should be able to respond constructively and usefully to the increasing humanitarian demands that lie ahead.

GREEN LIVING

Nicky Hayes

As Moscovici (Moscovici and Faucheux, 1972) showed, minority influences, if consistently maintained, can gradually change the social representations held by society as a whole. For example, environmental awareness as a motivator of everyday behaviours was very much a minority view in the 1970s and 1980s, but gathered momentum gradually until by the end of the 2000s it had become an accepted social representation.

Beliefs about waste management, for example, became transformed. The general shortage of consumer goods in the post-Second World War era meant that people tended to live frugally, with little waste, and that consumer goods were built to last. But the growth of consumer capitalism in the 1960s produced planned obsolescence, in which consumer goods were designed to wear out and be replaced with new ones in a relatively short period of time. The result was an ever-increasing number of consumer goods and packaging, and an ever-increasing amount of waste.

In the 1970s, this was seen as largely unproblematic; by 2010 reducing waste was perceived as a fundamental social responsibility. Psychologically, this change was not achieved through large public programmes, but through smaller manageable goals, none of which was particularly arduous in itself. Recycling began simply with depositories for glass bottles and newspapers, and gradually extended to other substances; LA waste collections were introduced in most places; and a growing dissatisfaction with excessive packaging was responded to by commercial businesses adopting more responsible packaging strategies. Psychologically, each step contributed to people's sense of self-efficacy and challenged the earlier perceived helplessness.

Many psychological studies conducted during the 1970s and 1980s showed how people were concerned about environmental problems, but felt helpless to do anything about it personally. A powerful illustration of the importance of self-efficacy beliefs happened in the 1970s, as consumer pressures removed chlorofluorocarbons (CFCs) from supermarket shelves almost instantly, when it was shown that these were seriously damaging the ozone layer. The widespread nature of this action showed that it was not a matter of public unwillingness that was holding back affirmative environmental action, but a general sense of learnt helplessness. Once it was clear that an unequivocally effective action could be taken, people were prepared to take it, and did.

For the most part, however, it needed something more to convert the general social representations; and this occurred through the process of figuration: a summary metaphor used as an everyday illustration of the issues. This was the idea of the 'carbon footprint', now an everyday idea, but if you had talked about a carbon footprint to someone in the early 1990s, they would have looked at you blankly, and probably asked what on earth you were talking about.

The 'carbon footprint' summarised energy use in day-to-day living, bringing together many different manageable goals. It reduced learnt helplessness by showing how small or less obvious actions, such as a more economical use of electricity or the use of public transport, could be a positive contribution, and it challenged the earlier and puritanical idea that only living a pure and pollution-free lifestyle would be acceptable.

Small-scale behavioural changes have repeatedly been shown to be far more effective than large public programmes, whether that be in water management schemes, the use of public transport or the management of everyday waste. What we saw in those two decades was a major change in social representations, brought about by the enhancement of personal self-efficacy beliefs through the use of manageable goals to challenge learnt helplessness.

Suggestions for further reading

Bandura, A. (1989) 'Perceived self-efficacy in the exercise of personal agency', *The Psychologist*, 2: 411–24.

Moscovici, S. (1984) 'The phenomenon of social representations', in R.M. Farr and S. Moscovici (eds), *Social Representations*. Cambridge: Cambridge University Press. pp. 3–70.

Moscovici, S. and Faucheux, C. (1972) 'Social influence, conformity bias and the study of active minorities', in L. Berkowitz (ed.), *Advances in Experimental Social Psychology, Volume 6*. New York: Academic Press. pp. 149–202.

Seligman, M.E.P. (1975) *Helplessness: On Depression, Development and Death.* San Francisco, CA: Freeman.

Seligman, M.E.P. (1991) *Learned Optimism: How to Change Your Mind and Your Life.* New York: Knopf.

Wagner, W. and Hayes, N. (2005) *Everyday Discourse and Common Sense.* Basingstoke: Palgrave Macmillan.

COMMUNITY PSYCHOLOGY

Carolyn Kagan

Community psychology is a relative newcomer to the applied psychology field and has a focus on social change and social justice (Kagan et al., 2011). As a field it can be understood in three ways (Kagan et al., 2011: 471). First, as a psychological paradigm distinct from other applied fields: a form of critical psychological praxis with a particular ontology, epistemology, methodology, ethics and politics. Second, as a perspective that can inform and be integrated with other forms of applied psychology (as in community counselling psychology, community organisational psychology, community environmental psychology, community clinical psychology and so on). Third, it can be seen as a practice that can sometimes lie disguised in other community practices, such as community development, community organising, community health promotion and community work. In order to stimulate and support community psychology, we will need to:

- be flexible about the nature of community psychology but retain a reflective and critical stance on both it and other forms of psychology praxis;
- recognise that theory and practice, and research and action, are inseparable;
- retain a focus on social marginalisation and social change, and work with and celebrate diversity in all its forms with a focus on reducing inequality;
- collaborate with those who might be at the receiving end of practice from the start;
- identify the value base underpinning work for social justice and social change and be clear about how to ensure these values are not compromised in practice;
- think and work interprofessionally and interdisciplinarily, and prepare practitioners through interprofessional and non-professional learning opportunities;
- recognise that expertise by experience is as valuable as professional expertise and that popular (lay) and scientific (expert) knowledge should be combined;
- be prepared to acknowledge the contribution other people have made to the work – change is rarely achieved by community psychologists who at best can facilitate change;
- adopt a systemic approach that sees individual behaviour and experience as embedded in numerous social institutions and a wider social, historical and cultural context;

- not be precious about method and adopt a pluralistic approach that is determined by the issue at stake, the practical possibilities and the potential for the impact of any findings;

- seek to identify the implications of praxis at local, regional and global levels and find ways to maximise the impact of work undertaken through the development of partnerships and international links;

- be prepared to stand up and speak for what is right and to promote practice-based evidence;

- recognise that communities are made of people with experience and knowledge, but that connections between communities can be supported in order to achieve wider-scale impetus for change and social justice;

- understand the interconnectedness of things and find new ways to promote community resilience in the face of global financial, environmental, economic, population and food crises;

- be prepared to be open to new learning, to the taking-up of new challenges and to expose the impact that social policies and practices have on the most marginalised groups;

- share the joy of living.

For example, if we are going to think and work interprofessionally and interdisciplinarily and prepare practitioners through interprofessional and non-professional learning opportunities, we may need to change how we think about the preciousness of psychology training. We may need to open up both undergraduate and postgraduate training to shared learning with students from other disciplines, greater exposure to non-psychology trained staff, and work experiences where they are supervised by people with diverse professional backgrounds. This sounds relatively simple, but taken seriously would radically change student learning within accredited psychology undergraduate and postgraduate programmes.

APPLYING PSYCHOLOGY TO THE LAYOUT OF PRINTED TEXT

James Hartley

Consider the layout of this text and the page that you are reading now from a typographical point of view. The text is set in *portrait* style, i.e. taller than it is wide. Such an arrangement is fairly common. But texts can be set in *landscape* style too – where the text is wider than it is tall. Texts set in print (or on screen) can be considered from a vertical and a horizontal point of view. Normally this is not problematic for textbooks, but it can be so with other kinds of text – such as medical leaflets, concert programmes and the like. Psychologists (and type-designers) often vary the layouts of text to see which versions are more readable, but psychologists are more likely to test the differences between versions with samples of appropriate users or readers. Psychologists like to have evidence to support any decisions that they make.

Now let us examine this piece of text:

> For adults and children over 12 take 1 or 2 tablets with food 2 or 3 times a day. Do not take more than 6 tablets in 24 hours. Leave at least 4 hours between doses. Do not give this medicine to children under 12. Do not take this medicine during pregnancy. It may delay labour or make it last longer.

And then consider when happens to the readability of the text when the clauses and sentences are separated from each other:

> For adults and children over 12
> take 1 or 2 tablets with food 2 or 3 times a day.
> Do not take more than 6 tablets in 24 hours.
> Leave at least 4 hours between doses.
> Do not give this medicine to children under 12.
> Do not take this medicine during pregnancy.
> It may delay labour or make it last longer.

Next, let's see what happens when indentation is used to clarify the content:

> For adults and children over 12
>   take 1 or 2 tablets with food 2 or 3 times a day.
> Do not take more than 6 tablets in 24 hours.
> Leave at least 4 hours between doses.
> Do not give this medicine to children under 12.
> Do not take this medicine during pregnancy.
>   It may delay labour
>   or make it last longer.

Finally, consider the same piece of original text spaced by computer using psychological rules for the spacing of text to make things clearer (courtesy Randall Walker).

> For adults and children
>   over 12,
>   take 1 or 2 tablets
>   with food,
>   2 or 3
>   times a day.
>
> Do not take
>   more than 6 tablets
>   in 24 hours.
>
> Leave at least 4 hours
>   between doses.

Do not give
   this medicine
      to children under 12.

Do not take this medicine
   during pregnancy.
      It may delay labour,
         or make it last longer.

Well what do you think? Could you use this computer-based text as the basis for producing a final version of this text? Would it be helpful if we used computer programs to space text for us first, rather than doing it all ourselves? Would some versions be better than others? How would we find out?

Activities for reflection and discussion

Working with a friend (or in small groups) examine any medical information leaflet provided with an off-the-shelf medical treatment. Consider how it might be improved in terms of its page size, page orientation, typesizes and weights, the spatial arrangement of the text, the clarity of the headings, the sequence of the information presented, the clarity of any graphics, and its readability. Does the leaflet seem fine to you or not? Why has it been printed in this way? What might you do to improve it?

Suggestions for further reading

Abraham, C. and Kools, M. (eds) (2012) *Writing Health Communication*. London: Sage.
Hartley, J. (2000) 'Could this be easier to read? Tools for evaluating text', in J. Hartley and A. Branthwaite (eds), *The Applied Psychologist* (2nd edn). Buckingham: Open University Press. pp. 113–125.

Useful journals

Information Design Journal; *Journal of the American Society for Information Science & Technology*; *Visible Language*.

PERSONALITY THEORY

Rowan Bayne

The most prominently studied and widely accepted personality theory since the 1980s is five-factor or 'Big Five' theory, whereas the most widely used applied personality theory in the same period is psychological type theory in its Myers-Briggs Type Indicator (MBTI) sense. Remarkably, the two theories are closely related in some respects; in particular the main associated questionnaires correlate highly, with the clear implication that the evidence for the validity of one of these theories generally supports both. Critics of MBTI theory often fail to appreciate this fact.

   I would like to see MBTI theory more accepted by mainstream psychology. A different name might help – preference theory rather than 'psychological type'. Although the term 'type' has some strengths (Bayne, 2005) it is too tainted by association with charlatans and sounds too rigid. Moreover, the validity of type dynamics, though this concept is stimulating and central for many writers about type, is not well supported (e.g. Reynierse, 2009).

Two ways in which MBTI and Big Five theory differ are the concept of preference and the tone of their personality descriptions. Preference can be defined as 'feeling most natural and comfortable with a particular way of behaving and experiencing', and MBTI theory suggests that eight preferences are the most useful. Box 19.1 indicates their meanings. People who prefer E (Extraversion) for example and given normal development generally behave in E ways but some of the time behave introvertedly.

Box 19.1   Brief descriptions of the preferences in MBTI theory

E	More outgoing and active ...... More reflective and reserved	**I**
S	More practical and interested in facts and details	
	More interested in possibilities and an overview	**N**
T	More logical and reasoned	
	More agreeable and appreciative	**F**
J	More planning and coming to conclusions	
	More easy-going and flexible	**P**

EI is Extraversion versus Introversion. SN is Sensing versus Intuition

TF is Thinking versus Feeling. JP is Judging versus Perceiving.

Table 19.1 illustrates the differences in tone between four of the preferences and four of the Big Five factors. The broadly parallel Big Five terms are in brackets in the first column.

Three examples of MBTI theory in action from a variety of areas of applied psychology follow. The first is for those who give feedback to themselves or others, the second for those who wish to exercise more, and the third for those involved in any kind of selection, e.g. for teams, jobs, training and possibly romance.

First, Smith (1993) compared the comments on an essay of six lecturers with a preference for Thinking and six with a preference for Feeling. All the lecturers were experienced teachers and all had preferences for Intuition and Introversion. They generally agreed on a fairly low mark for the essay and on the essay's strengths and weaknesses. However, and even though their department had agreed guidelines on giving feedback on essays, lecturers who preferred Feeling praised the essay twice as much and wrote twice as many suggestions for improvement.

Smith (1993) interpreted these differences and qualitative data from interviews with the lecturers in terms of contrasting philosophies of teaching – people who prefer Thinking tend to focus on what is wrong and how to improve it whereas those who prefer Feeling tend to focus on strengths and to show more concern about

Table 19.1   Comparing four of the preferences and four of the five factors: some examples

Personality characteristic	Example of preference theory description	Example of Big Five theory description
Introversion (Low Extraversion)	Depth	Inhibited
Sensing (Low Openness)	Observant	Unimaginative
Thinking (Low Agreeableness)	Analytical	Unsympathetic
Perceiving (Low Conscientiousness)	Adaptable	Weak-willed

students' emotional reactions to their comments. Further research (and as far as I know, Smith's study has not been replicated or extended) could investigate the impact of the two styles of feedback on students with preferences for Thinking and Feeling.

Second, Brue (2008) found relationships between the combinations of the preferences and choice of enjoyable forms of exercise. She uses a colour system based on MBTI theory, and there is a brief – eight minute – quiz to indicate which colour represents you at www.the8colors.com. The results indicate which forms of exercise and environment for exercise are most and least likely to suit you; e.g. people who prefer INTJ and INFJ are whites in her system and tend to enjoy exercising alone in a calm, familiar and pleasing setting and letting their minds drift – exercise as a 'moving meditation', whereas ESTPs and ESFPs (reds) tend to want lots of stimulation, variety and quick responses – exercise as absorbing action. As these examples suggest, the key variables may be motives such as a need for routine or to be alone, with the actual activity a way of fulfilling them and the health benefits a side effect.

Third, a low but positive correlation has been consistently found between high scorers on the personality characteristic of Conscientiousness (the broad parallel to preference for Judging) and job performance. This has been interpreted in strong terms. For example, Mount and Barrick (1998) wrote, 'There are now two dispositional predictors in our field whose validity generalises: general mental ability and Conscientiousness. Thus, no matter what job you are selecting for, if you want employees who turn out to be good performers, you should hire those who work smarter and harder' (p. 856).

The MBTI interpretation is radically different. For example, it suggests that organisations following this advice will miss the strengths of those who prefer Perceiving, e.g. their flexibility, and the strengths of those who prefer Sensing and Perceiving, e.g. their calmness and practical intelligence in a crisis. Robertson et al. (2000) approached this more even-handed conception from the opposite direction when they commented that 'some of the characteristics associated with high Conscientiousness may also serve to undermine certain aspects of managerial performance' (p. 173). However, the dominant view in psychology is still the Mount and Barrick one (e.g. Kuncel et al., 2010).

SECTION 2: SUPPLEMENTS TO AREAS REVIEWED IN THE MAIN CHAPTERS

CLINICAL PSYCHOLOGY

Susan Llewelyn

On most important questions there are, of course, always many perspectives: the same is true for how optimistic we can feel about the future of clinical psychology, and what future directions it should ideally take. The recent growth, uptake and influence of ideas from clinical psychology across society as a whole has meant that many more people have had access to clinical psychology services over the last decade or so than in the past, but it has also meant that demand has grown so fast that supply of qualified practitioners has not been able to keep pace with expressed need. One of the consequences of this has been the controversial growth of alternative forms of psychological interventions, alongside clinical psychology, of which the most obvious in the UK has been the increasing access to psychological therapies (IAPT) programme (Layard, 2006). The intention of IAPT has been the delivery of state-funded mental health services, often with a preventative slant, to populations who previously did not have such access, at an affordable rate, by using manualised evidence-based psychological treatments, by people with specifically focused and relatively brief trainings, sometimes (but by no means always) supervised by clinical psychologists. Evidence suggests that this programme has been broadly successful (Richards and Suckling, 2010) although others have pointed to its limitations, particularly in the use of brief targeted interventions when clinical problems may be complex and long standing.

It is here perhaps that the future of clinical psychology is assured: there will always be a need for an approach (or profession) that can drawn on a variety of theoretical insights and models to understand and resolve more difficult clinical problems. It seems very unlikely that there will be any fewer or simpler mental health or psychological challenges in the future as society becomes ever more complex and fluid, where many taken-for-granted assumption about personal relationships can no longer be taken for granted. So initiatives like IAPT must be welcomed, but their limitations acknowledged, and the clear importance and relevance of clinical psychology as a robust discipline based on the science of psychology must be underscored. One consequence of this may be paradoxical: the numbers of clinical psychologists in training and practice may decrease somewhat, as cheaper alternatives built on psychological ideas are developed, but the importance of the advancement of the discipline may actually grow, through the growth of good practice and theory.

Hence, what is really important for the future of the discipline is the maintenance of professional standards and the development of confident and competent practitioners who can act as leaders, teachers and supervisors in the provision of innovative and psychologically informed services for patients. There are two very welcome developments in clinical psychology that auger well for the profession – first the increased willingness to take on a clearer leadership role (Llewelyn and Cuthbertson, 2009), and second the high level of innovation in research, thinking and practice in a whole range of areas particularly outside the traditional mental health context, such as learning disability, physical health rehabilitation and the looked-after-children sector (see for example work in these areas by Samuel, 2009; Kennedy, 2008; and Golding, 2008 respectively). Overall, I believe that there are grounds for optimism, but also that as a professional group, clinical psychologists need to be much more than psychological practitioners; most crucially we need to think, develop, initiate, lead and diversify.

EDUCATIONAL PSYCHOLOGY

Irvine Gersch

The profession of educational psychology is changing considerably, and although we have been hearing this fact for the past 25 years, I believe that we are now seeing a major change in the role educational psychologists (EPs) are expected to undertake. In my view, the changing career patterns and the working environments in which EPs are now finding themselves are likely to persist and intensify during the next decade. These changes relate to:

1   training

2   the role

3   employment pathways.

Training

In the past five years we have seen a dramatic change in the training of EPs, with the move from a one-year full-time MSc training requirement to a three-year full-time doctoral qualification to practise. This has, in my view, enhanced the research skills and expertise of graduates, and served to ensure that graduates are confident, reflective and up to date.

Many programmes, including that within UEL, have extended the title from 'educational psychology' to 'educational and child psychology', and hopefully, devoted time to recent research on child development. I feel sure that, in the future, this will also include greater use of the growing evidence emanating from the fields of child development, parenting, neuroscience and children's spiritual development (e.g. Gersch et al., 2008).

The traditional focus within EP training on 'assessment' has been replaced by a focus on *assessment **and** intervention*, reflecting the changes within the role of the EP as well as trainee interest. Indeed, many trainees have expressed the view that, for the future, they will need greater training on specific interventions.

In a small-scale study more than ten years ago, some trainees predicted that the skills and qualities that will continue to matter for the future will include personal and human qualities, adaptability and flexibility, keeping their knowledge up to date, being independent and looking after themselves and their career, and emotional intelligence (Kelly and Gersch, 2000).

However, it is likely that, even within three years, training courses will have limited time available to cover such a wide curriculum as is now required by the width of the role for which trainees are preparing, and which employers and others expect. After their initial training has been completed, many EPs may need to go on to undertake further, specific training courses in specialist, therapeutic or intervention areas, once they have started work as an EP.

The role

The EP role has been reviewed nationally in recent years (e.g. Department for Education and Employment (DfEE) 2000a, 2000b; Farrell et al., 2006); and now in 2011, as part of the green paper review of special educational needs (DfE, 2011), training is to be reviewed yet again. Thus far, the evidence indicates that users of the service want a great deal from EPs. Clearly, EPs provide consultation, assessment, intervention, training, project work, systems work, advice to the LA on policy and parent support, to name but a few of the key areas of work. All of these are valued (DfEE, 2000b) and many groups want faster and greater access to EPs, e.g. schools, parents, nurseries and social workers. Time and staff are limited, and educational psychology services have to make hard decisions about priorities. Such hard decisions are unlikely to get easier during the next five years, given the economic constraints within which LAs and other employers are working.

Educational psychologists have changed their regulatory body from the BPS, which was voluntary, to the HPC, which is now statutory. There remain many benefits for EPs to retain membership of their main union, the Association of Educational Psychologists (AEP), as well as the BPS, which provides professional support, up-to-date literature, courses, guidance and much more.

I think legal challenges will increase in the future; more complaints are likely to be made to the HPC, and other bodies, in line with increased public information and a litigious public attitude and orientation. Consequently, secure professional and legal insurance cover, membership of the AEP (which also includes legal support), and easy access to a professional help line are all very important, for those who are self-employed, as well as those working for LAs and other employers, and certainly for those with mixed patterns of employment.

Employment pathways

In the context of economic and political changes (economic austerity and cuts), localism (whereby the aim is for local communities to have more say over their services) and loss of staff, the number of those who are self-employed seems to be an increasing trend. Such individuals and groups already appear to be highly professional, well organised, with attractive websites and good marketing, offering transparent and attractive services to parents, schools and others.

At the risk of making predictions that end up coming back to haunt me, and in spite of the warning given by the physicist Niels Bohr that 'prediction is extremely difficult ... especially about the future', or following the example of getting things totally wrong, like Lord Kelvin, who as President of the Royal Society said in 1893, 'X-rays will prove to be a hoax' (cited in Nown, 1985: 6 and 67), I do want to make a few predictions about the profession of educational psychology.

My own prediction for the future is that EPs will tend to have portfolio careers, a career mix (e.g. Handy, 1984), perhaps involving a range of work including some for LAs, on a part-time basis, private or self-employed casework, work for charities, and/ or for other agencies, providing services and direct work to schools or groups of schools. This will involve a mix of employers and self-employment, as well as services and activities provided. There will be greater choice than ever in future career paths. This will be both exciting and, at the same time, anxiety laden. New thinking about insurance and professional indemnity, legal protection, pricing, costing, business planning as well as high-quality supervision and meticulous, ethical professional practice in all these different domains will be needed.

In surviving these changes, my personal view is that EPs should offer relevant and helpful services (Gersch, 2004, 2009); they need to be professional, flexible, legally protected, and all EPs should monitor global and national changes very carefully. They need to be up to date with the fast-developing literature on child development, educational research, neuroscience, the national and international news, and, wherever they work, they will need to ensure that they receive high-quality supervision, mentorship and ongoing CPD in new techniques.

For the brave new world, the old adage 'fortune favours the brave' may well apply to EPs in more ways than we think possible at this time.

OCCUPATIONAL AND ORGANISATIONAL PSYCHOLOGY

Clive Fletcher

As an applied field, occupational psychology faces considerable challenges at the time of writing, with the continuing fall-out of the economic crisis leading to cuts in universities as well as in the consultancy budgets of many large organisations – thus rendering both academics and practitioners vulnerable. The increased government-funding emphasis on supporting the applied aspects of academic teaching and research may exacerbate an issue I raised in the first edition of this book, namely the drift of occupational psychology from psychology departments into business schools. Concern over the ramifications of that trend underlies two of the three main developments I would like to see in the future direction of the field.

The first is a greater awareness of ethical perspectives. To take but one example, it is somewhat worrying that the influential International Task Force on Assessment Centers 2009 Guidelines should say virtually nothing about the well-being of candidates, despite their purporting to cover ethical considerations and the evidence suggesting that some individuals may be vulnerable in the assessment centre setting (Fletcher, 2011). There is a danger that in becoming more aligned with business schools, psychologists may increasingly take the perspective of the organisation rather than that of the individual. The time given to studying ethical issues and perspectives on MSc courses in occupational psychology should probably be greater. In addition, more space given to articles with ethical themes (e.g. Kwiatkowski and Duncan, 2006) in our journals is desirable.

The second development I would wish to see is a much enhanced knowledge of theory and research in personality, not only being provided in undergraduate psychology degrees and MSc programmes, but also underpinning assessment practice in the occupational field. Most students are content to read potted accounts of different theories, and seldom read the sources (e.g. Allport, Eysenck, Cattell, Kelly) themselves. Practitioners mostly seem to take their ideas on personality from whatever questionnaire measures they are familiar with and the 'Big Five', which leaves them with a rather limited and somewhat mechanistic perspective; how many users of the MBTI or the Sixteen Personality Factor Questionnaire (16PF) have read any of Jung's or Cattell's work respectively? This, in turn, detracts from the richness they can bring to understanding and describing the role of personality in an individual's behaviour at work.

Indeed, the danger is that they become little different from HR practitioners who have a Level B test user certificate and attended several courses relating to specific personality inventories.

Finally, it would be to the benefit of both academics and practitioners if their interests were brought closer together. A classic example of the current divide between them is that one of the main offerings of practitioners is carrying out individual psychological assessments – usually a process whereby a candidate for a job is given a battery of tests and a lengthy interview to assess their suitability. Despite the frequency with which this is done, there is virtually no research on it. To improve our evidence-based practice, and to increase the dialogue between practitioners and academics, we need to make our occupational psychology research more relevant to current issues and methods in the applied arena.

OCCUPATIONAL PSYCHOLOGY

Chris Lewis

The future of occupational psychology does not look as bright as it should. It continues to fall further into the realm of producing 'technicians' rather than 'technologists'. It has been highjacked by the belief that it is a discipline where knowledge of business is more important than knowledge of psychology. This is evidenced by the growth in size of the Association of Business Psychologists and the common plea, by newly qualified occupational psychologists, that master's programmes should provide them with a broader training in business matters.

It is true that training should be broader than the rather stifling eight content areas indicated by the BPS – but the breadth is not about business skills. Business knowledge is outside the fundamental discipline of occupational psychology, as are other knowledge areas that a practising occupational psychologist might need to have in order to operate in particular contexts. For example, structural engineering, foreign languages and neuropsychology are just three others that come to mind. Outside knowledge is crucial, but is a matter for responsible professional practice and what CPD is required.

So, what should this increased breadth look like? It should build on the uniqueness that occupational psychologists have to offer as experts on the world of work. They are trained psychologists with an understanding of methodological issues. The breadth of training should be about facilitating the exploration of these knowledge areas still further. Those in training have to be helped to understand what occupational psychology does not know and how this might be rectified. Without this, for example, the occupational psychologist using psychometric tests in selection becomes indistinguishable from the HR professional trained on one or two five-day courses on the topic.

There are so many consuming issues that the occupational psychologists (and psychologists in general) need to address. They must at least be making progress, as psychologists, in understanding the implications that not resolving these issues has on professional practice.

By way of illustration here are a few that might be considered.

- All psychological variables have no objective zero point; they are arbitrary, and therefore have no meaning beyond the individual. Attaching a scale to a psychological variable does not resolve this (Kline, 1998).

- Predictive validity of a test does not allow any prediction to be made about an individual who has taken the test. Predictive validity is demonstrated by using sizable samples to remove error variance. For the individual, that error variance may still exist (Blanton and Jaccard, 2006).

- Although it is easy to understand the mathematical description of probability, it is impossible to internalise the implications of it. Interpreting probability is a qualitative activity that involves emotion (Taleb, 2007).

- The interaction between emotion, personality and cognition in predicting work performance is not measurable. Attempting to measure the interaction between scales that have been used to assess these is pointless as what they are measuring cannot be generalised across individuals (LeDoux, 1998).

- The content of effective leadership is very much more than the scales, used by occupational psychologists, can ever identify. Seeking predictive traits is too narrow an approach (Rooke and Torbert, 2005).

These are tough questions to address, but failure to do so might mean that occupational psychologists, and other professional groups who they are training or coaching, are doing things that are just wrong.

Solutions to some of these fundamental problems are being explored through such things as focusing on 'outcome content validity', 'heuristic modelling' and the relevance of concepts such as 'bounded rationality', and even daring to look at 'energy' and non-religious notions of 'spirituality', but the search must continue.

In the market place, therefore, the 'unique selling point' of the occupational psychologist should be that they explore ways to overcome the troublesome psychological and methodological obstacles and take the discipline further for the benefit of other professional groups. Without this, occupational psychology will become submerged in a generic category labelled 'professionals involved in the people part of work'.

INVESTIGATIVE INTERVIEWING

Ray Bull

A new direction in forensic psychology now being taken up in some countries around the world is concerned with the interviewing of suspects, victims and witnesses. This initiative seeks to enhance how much information such people provide (e.g. to the police), the reliability of this information and the likelihood that truthfulness/deception can be detected (see Bull et al., 2009 for an overview). In many countries the 'old' style of 'interrogating' is still practised (and trained). However, psychological research has demonstrated that coercive/oppressive styles of interrogation can produce false confessions. A 'new direction' here would also be to build a body of research and theory on 'reactance' (e.g. guilty suspects deciding not to provide much/any relevant information because of the way they are questioned – which may well happen more frequently than false confessions). One reason why coercive interrogation is still practised is the common belief that guilty people will not normally confess. However, research by psychologists is revealing that, for example, of a large sample of sex offenders now in prison (many of whom had not confessed) only half said that they had entered the police interview having already decided whether to deny or confess. In fact, less than 20% had planned to deny (and around 30% had planned to confess). The other 50% entered the police interview not yet having decided whether to deny or confess (Kebbell et al., 2006).

In the UK the police in collaboration with psychologists have developed and refined the 'PEACE' approach, which emphasises interviewing to gather information rather than a confession. Recently some other countries have considered this development to be worthy of national adoption there (e.g. New Zealand and Norway), which has been based on peer-reviewed research (e.g. Walsh and Bull, 2010).

For decades research on the detecting of deception found that people were very poor at determining whether someone (e.g. seen in a video-clip) is lying or not. However, in these many dozens, if not hundreds, of studies the 'judges' focused on what was *visually* available. An emerging theme is that the detection of deception is more likely to occur if the persons being evaluated (for truth/lies) provide sufficient *verbal* information. Thus, interviewing people using the 'PEACE' procedure is more likely to provide such information than is an accusatory or oppressive approach.

For a considerable period of time, psychologists (and others) have claimed to have developed methods of 'linking' unsolved and solved crimes committed by the same person. This can involve ways of linking (1) an unsolved crime to a solved crime, or (2) two (or more) unsolved crimes. Some of these claims have lacked an empirical foundation. The success of such methods depends considerably on the quality of the information available, some of which comes from victim/witness interviews, which need to be conducted to a high standard. More recently research of greater quality is being conducted on this topic (e.g. Tonkin et al., 2011).

FORENSIC PSYCHOLOGY IN THE PRISON AND PROBATION SERVICES

Ruth E. Mann

Forensic psychology is concerned with all aspects of criminal behaviour, but this article focuses specifically on the work of psychologists in the prison and probation services. Forensic psychology in the UK has boomed as a profession over the past twenty years. In the 1980s, forensic psychologists mainly engaged in individual work with prisoners, particularly assisting them cope with the experience of imprisonment, with some additional time spent on parole and lifer reports. In the past twenty years, research findings that certain psychological interventions with offenders can reduce reoffending have prompted considerable government investment in such approaches in correctional settings. Simultaneously, research knowledge of the psychological correlates of reoffending has developed, and enabled validated structured procedures for assessing risk by identifying the presence of these 'risk factors'.

With evidence-based assessments and interventions having quickly become the mainstay of forensic psychologists' work, we face a number of challenges. Two examples are described below.

1   The increased emphasis on structured schemes for risk assessment, and the power that psychologists are perceived to wield in this process, have damaged the relationship between psychologists and offenders (Crewe, 2009; Maruna, 2011). Where prisoners used to see psychologists as part of their support system, now they view psychologists with distrust and fear. Some psychologists have resolved this dissonance by deciding that their 'client' is the public and not the individual in front of them. As Crewe (2009) pointed out, it is noteworthy that a former chief psychologist for the National Offender Management Service listed, *in the following order*, the stakeholders for psychological services in prisons as being: 'the public, victims of crime, prisons and probation staff, and offenders' (Towl, 2003: 6). Prisoners have used terms like 'pure fear' to describe their experience of being the subject of risk assessment (Attrill and Liell, 2007). Structured risk assessment performs much better than clinical judgement but is limited by its failure to acknowledge the role of biological, situational and social factors in crime, and by biases such as the fundamental

attribution error causing assessors to prefer internal stable explanations of crime (Maruna and Mann, 2006). So, one issue that forensic psychologists need to tackle is how to repair our reputation with the people who actually most need psychological services.

2   There is uncertainty among both psychologists and offenders about the purpose of psychological interventions delivered across prison and probation settings. Should psychological interventions aim purely to reduce reoffending and protect communities? Or should they aim to improve the participants' quality of life and well-being? Generally this conundrum has been resolved by arguing that the aims are one and the same – decreasing an individual's risk of reoffending is equivalent to increasing the quality of his life. But some have argued that interventions intended to reduce reoffending are better described as punishment than rehabilitation (e.g. Ward, 2010). Forensic psychologists cannot ignore or downplay these criticisms. Like all psychologists, we must continually reflect upon our behaviours and assumptions, and listen to the voices of those with whom we work, in order to ensure that our practice is not unconsciously subverted by the pervasive societal belief that those who commit crime do not deserve the same respect as more 'upstanding' members of society.

Forensic psychologists work with clients who are frequently stigmatised and socially excluded. Consequently, these clients are often difficult to engage and suspicious of professional help, especially when it is offered within a system that otherwise is designed to punish and restrict freedom. The context in which many forensic psychologists work therefore produces many challenges; but the personal and social value when positive outcomes are achieved can also provide great reward.

THE USE OF VIRTUAL REALITY-BASED ENVIRONMENTAL ENRICHMENT FOR PATIENTS RECOVERING FROM BRAIN INJURY

Paul R. Penn and F. David Rose

De Wit et al. (2005) reviewed the amount of time spent by stroke patients in formal therapy across four rehabilitation centres within Europe, and concluded: 'Patients spent a large amount of the day in their rooms, inactive, and without any interaction' (p. 1983). This is broadly in line with earlier European research (e.g. De Weerdt et al., 2000; Lincoln et al., 1997; Newall et al. 1997).

The paucity of environmental interaction that can be experienced by patients in the days and weeks following a brain injury is a real concern from a fundamental neuroscience perspective. An extensive body of animal-based laboratory research dating back to the early 1960s has consistently shown that the quality of an environment that an animal is exposed to post-experimentally induced brain injury has profound effects on its recovery. Stated very crudely, researchers make the distinction between enriched environments and impoverished environments. An enriched environment is actually a composite of a number of elements, e.g. opportunities for increased exercise, sensory stimulation, learning/training and social interaction. An impoverished environment is one that is lacking in all of the above respects.

Nithianantharajah and Hannan (2006) reviewed research on enrichment, plasticity and disorders of the nervous system. This research has pointed to their effectiveness in ameliorating the impairments associated with a diverse range of different types of central nervous system damage, for example: spinal cord contusion; brain damage of genetic or developmental origin; traumatic brain injury; degenerative disease and damage of pharmacological or teratogenic origin (Will et al., 2004). The same body of research has also consistently pointed to the deleterious effects of impoverished environments on the recovery from brain damage.

The animal-based literature provides clear impetus for examining the effect of environmental enrichment in human populations. Unfortunately, constraints on NHS budgets, staff availability, resources, in addition to limitations imposed by health and safety concerns make it very difficult to modify the physical environment of a hospital ward, or physically transport a patient to a less impoverished environment.

Just over a decade ago, Rose et al. (1998) suggested that if one cannot provide an enriched real-world environment for a patient, then it should be possible to provide them with an enriched virtual environment via the use of virtual reality. Virtual reality is defined as: 'An advanced form of human-computer interface that allows the user to interact with and become immersed in a computer-generated environment in a naturalistic fashion' (Schultheis and Rizzo, 2001: 299). Over the past twenty years virtual reality has found numerous domains of application within neuropsychological assessment and rehabilitation (e.g. see Penn et al., 2009; Rizzo et al., 2004; Rose et al., 2005 for reviews). However, the authors are not aware of any research that has investigated its use in enriching recovery environments post-brain injury, yet, intuitively, this would seem to be its most obvious application.

There are a number of significant conceptual and methodological issues to address in implementing the use of virtual enriched environments for human populations, not least of which is identifying the parameters that differentiate an enriched environment from a standard rehabilitation environment. However, researchers at UEL believe that the argument for rigorous empirical investigation into virtual environmental enrichment is too compelling to ignore.

STRENGTHS

P. Alex Linley

Capp's (Centre for Applied Positive Psychology) work in strengths applications has led the way with innovations in research and practice in this space. In this short article, my intention is to do two things. First, to overview some of the ways in which strengths are being applied across the employee life cycle. Second, from this basis, I will make recommendations for how I would like to see the field develop in the next decade.

When people use their strengths, they achieve a host of positive psychological benefits, including greater happiness and well-being, more resilience, increased self-confidence and self-esteem, and less stress. They are also more engaged at work and perform better, being more likely to achieve their goals. With all of these positives coming from a single intervention – using one's strengths – it is not surprising that organisations have woken up to the potential for applying strengths across the employee life cycle.

For example, Ernst & Young, the Big Four professional-services firm use strengths as an attractor proposition for their target graduate population, and then recruit and select their successful applicants on the basis of their strengths. Standard Chartered Bank use strengths at the heart of their performance management processes to help people deliver on their organisational goals through using their strengths. Numerous organisations, including Avery Dennison, HSBC, Birmingham Children's Hospital and Aviva, use strengths approaches in the development of their teams. Other organisations, including Thomson Reuters, are using strengths approaches in relation to how they assess their future talent.

All of these approaches represent a shift from the traditional competency mindset that 'you can develop anyone to do anything'. In contrast, strengths approaches focus more on building on the best of what people bring, while managing any weaknesses that may get in the way. This provides a fundamentally different perspective for how organisations work, and how the people within those organisations experience their work. It is this that provides the basis for my hope and recommendations for the future.

First, it is inevitable that the speed of practice will always outpace the speed of research. As a result, practitioners cannot wait for the research basis to inform their 'best practice'. Instead, I propose the concept of 'best judgement', allowing practitioners to innovate and deliver on their views of what is most likely to deliver the results the organisation needs.

Second, this 'best judgement' approach to what can become 'research in practice' can then be used to inform more traditional academic research agendas. Rather than the direction of information flow being that research must always inform practice, we can instead see how practice and experience can help to shape interesting and worthwhile questions for research.

Third, the shift towards strengths rather than competencies suggests that we will be able to cast our nets wider and increase the diversity of the people we employ, and the positions in which we employ them. By appreciating that different strengths can achieve the same outcomes, we can make the most of the powerful demographic trends that are propelling more female talent and more Asian talent into the workplace.

Finally, this positive shift in approaches to work heralds significant potential to change the working experience of thousands and thousands of people around the world. We can create work as the place where people come together to give of the best of themselves and make their greatest contributions. This may seem like a utopian vision, but when we start to realise the best of people, it is amazing what we can achieve – as positive psychology and its applications have consistently shown.

SECTION 3: GENERAL PERSPECTIVES

PSYCHOLOGICAL ETHICS: THE GOOD, THE DEFENSIVE AND THE UTILITARIAN

Richard Kwiatkowski

Psychologists are ethical. They, in large part, define their professional values and consequent behaviour through their ethical code, which clearly emphasises respect, competence, responsibility and integrity. Through socialisation via a long process of education and apprenticeship they have embedded this way of being into who they are, not unquestioningly, but in full cognisance of the importance of context, thought and action.

Having emphasised that, I will put forward two contentious themes. First that registration by the HPC may, over time, actually change the relationship between psychologists and their clients in the direction of a defensive stance, and unwittingly lead to loss within the profession; and second, that the rise of utilitarian ethics can insidiously compromise psychology's traditional ethical perspective. I shall conclude that psychology is a force for good because of its ethical nature, but that there are interesting dangers ahead.

The rise of defensive psychology

The vast majority of psychologists are ethical; but of course it is vitally important that any rogue psychologists are brought to book. After the category of 'Chartered Psychologist' was created, the BPS set up and maintained a voluntary code of ethics, and disciplined members who had behaved badly.

In 2009 the HPC took over this function but as the *statutory* regulator of applied psychology. In each case the primary aim was to protect the public. However, the style is very different. With the old, more person-centred BPS regulatory affairs department, psychologists could phone and speak informally about issues troubling them. Hundreds of calls were received each year from psychologists and members of the public asking for advice about ethically complex situations – these might involve a possible breach of confidentiality, concern about the drinking habits of a colleague, alarm about late return of essays, a dispute over a psychometric instrument or even allegations of serious abuse. The regulatory-affairs department staff would facilitate decision-making in a non-directive way, through raising issues and drawing the attention of the enquirer to the code of ethics, or to legal or moral obligations (e.g. child safety, honesty, research ethics guidelines, legal obligations, etc.). If mediation and discussion were possible this would be suggested or even facilitated (for instance between two psychologists complaining about each other).

The HPC is a very different organisation. It is a body set up by Act of Parliament; it has legal power; it is a regulator; it has one master (or 'key stakeholder'): the law; and it necessarily acts in strict adherence to the letter of the law. Nothing can really be off the record. (This would be seen as unfair to the registrant and the complainant – and the Council for Healthcare Regulatory Excellence might have a rather negative view on informal conversations.) All conversations are recorded, and anything disclosed can be used in pursuance of a complaint. The *raison d'être* of the HPC is protection of the public, so it must take a precautionary approach: every complaint is considered very seriously; there is no informal mediation process; evidence is taken; and, if there are grounds for a case to proceed, a legal case is presented.

Let us return to the (not so hypothetical) case of two psychologists bickering and making allegations against each other. There is now no one to say, 'Don't be silly, sit down and talk'. Both sets of complaints, however flimsy, will start the legal process moving. This has consequences our squabbling psychologists may not have antici-pated, for example, if there seems to be a potential case to answer, the allegations will go onto the HPC website until the hearing can take place, which may take several months. Once on the internet these allegations will potentially be available for ever, even if 'no case to answer' is eventually found. If there seems to be a case to answer, the investigation and hearing process itself might take a couple of years and cost each psychologist tens of hundreds if not tens of thousands of pounds (e.g. in legal fees), as well as potentially causing huge reputational damage and almost inevitably enor-mous personal stress. They may be approached by the press, or photographed in the street. The allegations may be the subject of journalistic speculation, commentary and blogs. (All of these have already happened in some cases that were eventually dismissed.)

It may be argued that this is unlikely – a mischievous allegation from another psy-chologist, tit-for-tat rebuttals and yet ... and yet the reputations of two psychologists damaged perhaps for ever. Who will seriously employ them? Perhaps an employer will have felt obliged to suspend them while the case proceeds. Is there no smoke without fire? The knowledge that this sort of process may happen will spread into the profession, and behaviour may subtly change, and unfortunately, 'defensive psychol-ogy' may well then be the result.

As in 'defensive medicine', the first priority will thus be to avoid litigation, to have a clear audit trail, to have pristine paperwork, to always act so as to prevent a com-plaint. This may mean that certain clients are viewed with suspicion (or even avoided); and what becomes reality is the paper or electronic record, not the act itself. At worst, this may have a negative impact on the person-to-person relationship that is so criti-cal in many branches of applied psychology, stifling that openness and transparency that is a hallmark of good psychological practice. Further, as has already happened to an extent in occupational psychology, some psychologists may decide that this sort of regulator is not for them, and opt out. Calling yourself a 'consultant' may actually allow more freedom and creativity than calling oneself a 'psychologist'. This would be a loss for psychology as well as for individual clients.

Is a utilitarian perspective harming psychology?

Turning to my second theme, there is a tension between the deontological nature of the traditional British psychologist's approach to ethics and the utilitarianism that is becoming increasingly common. To paraphrase and summarise at the risk of distorting the approaches through oversimplification, the deontological approach suggests that each action of itself needs to be 'good', and that we should perform such good acts because we would wish those sorts of act to be done to us, and we understand that society will function better if people, for example, tell the truth, stick to their agreements and do not kill anyone.

The BPS Code of Ethics is framed in this tradition:

> ... Immanuel Kant gave expression to this in his Categorical Imperative: 'Act on such maxims as you could will to become universal law'. Our capacity to act on rational moral principles bestows on us the dignity of free moral agents and this leads to a further formulation of the Categorical Imperative: 'Treat humanity in your own person and that of others always as an end and never only as a means'. This position forms the basis of the code. (BPS, 2006: 4–5)

In contrast, the utilitarian perspective, again to paraphrase, suggests that the goodness of an act is best understood by examining its consequences – in simple terms, is the sum of happiness increased by that act? It therefore follows that the utility of an act often increases as more people are made happy. 'The greatest good for the greatest number' is a phrase associated with this position. In an increasingly interdependent world, with organisations and other conglomerates increasingly determining what is seen as 'good', a utilitarian perspective is often the framework of choice.

The essentially personal interactional relationship between a psychologist and the people they are working with depends on trust and is often at its best when it moves beyond the transactional and technical into the creative and transformational. The danger of a utilitarian – and even market-forces – perspective is that professions are reduced to technical 'servants of power' as so eloquently argued by Baritz back in 1960. Psychologists simply become technicians, and because their interactions with people become technical acts then those acts inevitably become shaped in the name of efficiency and utility. Economic considerations intertwine with utilitarian considerations – organisations are essentially utilitarian (Preuss, 1998) – and the notion of profit and loss increasingly informs the relationship of psychologist and client. Thus, ten easy cases of mild anxiety (six sessions each) are a more cost-effective use of a psychologist's time than two complex cases of borderline psychosis (open-ended commitment). Cognitive–behavioural therapy is argued to be more 'cost-effective' than person-centred counselling. This rise of utilitarianism, particularly within the Western or 'developed' world may serve to insidiously undermine the nature of the relationship between the psychologist and the client. Insofar that the context within which we operate is often unexamined and simply taken for granted this process may well already be taking place. The pressure will be to serve 'power' because by serving power we will keep our jobs in this 'time of austerity' or if working independently, attract more clients. Cognitive dissonance would indicate that we will, in our heads, readily minimise any differences between the positions of our masters and our own.

There may seem to be a tension between this utilitarian push and the role of the HPC, but actually they are complementary. The caution engendered by defensive psychology feeds beautifully into being a technician and serving the organisation, for that is where safety lies. And where, then, is individual ethical responsibility?

A gloomy conclusion?

Despite these dangers, I am actually optimistic. I believe that it is no coincidence that the first of the National Occupational Standards for psychology is 'ethics'. Psychologists are ethical. Our codes of ethics will be used by other professions in the future, as now, as models for their own ethical thinking. Research councils, funders and government will continue to consult psychologists about best practice. Given our liberal, humanistic and ethical tradition, psychology is a force for good (Kwiatkowski et al., 2006). However, there are real ethical dangers of which we should be aware; these have to be seen in order to be addressed, and I hope this look at potential dangers has acted as a sort of inoculation against 'mindlessness' as the ethical domain inevitably changes. So, finally, and here is the rub – we can be aware, and through the awareness of these subtle threats to our ethical stance, resist.

REFLECTIONS ON THE PLACE AND USEFULNESS OF PSYCHOLOGY

Colin Feltham

As a non-psychologist counsellor and theorist I draw on psychology somewhat but usually in order to validate something I already experience or observe, or on occasions when there is a serious challenge to my own views that I want to confront. Unfortunately, I am among those who believe that psychology has not lived up to its early promise and shows little sign of bringing any major or revolutionary findings to bear on clinical or social problems.

It is true that psychology has shifted fruitfully from a behavioural to a cognitive focus in recent decades; it has embraced the topics of happiness, mindfulness, forgiveness and compassion; it has produced further interesting theory in the evolutionary and neuroscience domains; and of course it has churned out copious experimental evidence for or against one claim and another. There is a certain amount of stimulation and rigour in all this. My reservations, however, lie in two main areas.

First, like sociology, political science and economics, psychology has yielded no major, surprising and world-changing discovery. Compared with cosmology, physics, evolutionary science, genetics and neurology then, psychology looks decidedly feeble. Oddly enough, it may be within its neglected older, speculative contributions in Freudian and Jungian psychology that much more progress could be made. Also, evolutionary psychology still holds great promise for explaining the most stubborn of dysfunctional human behaviours. In both these areas psychology, fails to make much progress, due, I suspect, to its neurotic attachment to a scientific identity.

Second, psychology, like other disciplines, has little sense of priority or urgency. Climate science and the sustainable technology inspired by its findings is a useful comparison here. Globally significant matters of life and death are at stake and solutions are urgently needed. This is not the case for psychology: it has no clear agenda or products. Feasibly, a meaningful ecopsychology, eco-psychoeducation and ecopsychotherapy might emerge to help steer us towards greater environmental sensitivity and (probably) less damaging consumerist behaviours. I see no real sign of this happening, again I suspect due to the neurotic attachment problem.

If there is a solution or more fruitful direction I think it lies first in a turn back to philosophical psychology, something akin to theoretical physics. By mapping out the most significant problems of human behaviour we might begin to establish a meaningful agenda. I hope I have gone a little way in this direction in my *What's Wrong With Us? The Anthropathology Thesis* (Feltham, 2007). I would commend Nick Maxwell's *From Knowledge to Wisdom: A Revolution for Science and the Humanities* (2007) and Lee McIntyre's *Dark Ages: The Case for a Science of Human Behavior* (2006) for work in similar exhortative and agenda-setting directions.

In the purely psychotherapeutic domain one sees an awful lot of recycled hope and theory, and little that is really new. Too much energy is devoted to cognitive–behavioural and psychopharmacological research in relation to radical therapies attempting to understand socioeconomic, environmental, somatic and affective links. Psychology by its very nature shies away from these.

PSYCHOLOGY TODAY

Nicky Hayes

In my view, the most significant new issue or direction in applied psychology today is the way that psychology has opened out, developing and welcoming new areas of expertise and application.

Applied psychology has never been as dynamic as it is right now. In recent years, many new areas of psychology have been opened up, and many older but less well-recognised areas have strengthened and grown in popularity. This has happened for several reasons. One of them is the effect of the huge expansion of teaching of psychology at general education levels during the past two decades, which has produced a significantly greater general awareness of what psychology has to offer on the part of other professionals, managers, and the public as a whole, creating a climate that is far more receptive to contributions and innovation from psychologists than was the case in previous decades.

Another is the way that psychologists themselves have changed. We have become far more confident about interacting with the media and putting ourselves in the public view; and also more confident generally about the value of our discipline and its relevance to both everyday and special problems. This in turn has stimulated an increased respect for the psychologist as a professional, and a readiness on the part of the media and other professionals to consult psychologists on a wider range of issues, and that in turn has led to the recognition and institutionalisation of several new areas of professional practice. Health psychology is one of the clearest examples of this, but applied psychologists in many other fields are making their presence felt, and sharing their professional innovations with other psychologists – a process that directly facilitates the emergence of new areas of applied psychology.

The third reason for the dynamism of modern applied psychology has to do with the way that psychology itself has changed over the past two decades. Psychological methodology has broadened out: two decades ago, laboratory research in psychology was venerated whereas field-based research was generally regarded as inferior; but in the modern context both types of research are seen as equally valid contributors to psychological knowledge. Similarly, the balance between quantitative and qualitative approaches to data collection has become more even, in that both are now acknowledged as playing an important role in psychological research. These changes have resulted in a discipline that is much more at home with the complexities and diversity of the modern world, and much better equipped to address real-world challenges and questions.

Other challenges still remain, not least of which is our need to capitalise on new approaches and methodologies, and on the insights obtained from applied research, in the form of integrative theory building of value to a wide range of psychologists. But the breadth and diversity of applied psychology, and the number of applied psychologists who are exploring new issues and opening up new areas, are indicators of a healthy dynamism right across the spectrum of applied psychology.

What new directions would you like there to be?

I would like to see psychology involved in even more aspects of everyday living: in design, in architecture, in public communication, in transport and planning, in our everyday understandings of human relationships and ideas and – perhaps most of all – in the understandings of decision makers.

It is right and proper that specialised fields of applied psychology should grow up and be maintained by the psychological profession. But there is also a need for a more general type of applied psychology – for the flexibility to apply psychology as and where it appears to have relevance. This can range from something as trivial as the locations of street crossings, to something as wide-ranging as the decisions of politicians.

Several of my own experiences of applied psychology have been in fairly unexpected areas. My first experience of consultancy in industry, for example, was solicited by IBM research laboratories, and concerned a problem wherein trainees were underachieving on their day-release courses at local colleges. The result was a programme of workshops, consultations, and individual exam counselling, drawing on well-established psychological knowedge. This was a relatively new way of approaching the problem at that time; but it ultimately contributed to the development of the BPS Diploma in the Applied Psychology of Teaching and Learning in the mid-1980s.

In 2000, I attended a series of seminars at the International Congress of Psychology in Stockholm, in which Miles Hewstone and other social psychologists were demonstrating the relevance of modern social psychological insights for political diplomacy and conflict resolution. The diplomats also involved in these sessions were extremely interested, and saw considerable potential in this area.

Another example, in which I am still involved, concerns the understanding of interactive science exhibits and how they engage people. An increased psychological understanding of the social and motivational aspects of these exhibits has shown itself to be of direct use to those commissioning exhibits, to those evaluating them and in some cases to the designers themselves.

These are illustrations, but they show how broad-ranging applied psychology can be. Sometimes, as in my first example, initiatives may link with others and eventually grow into a new area of applied psychology. But many other examples remain as stand-alone instances of applied psychology, as far as professional structure is concerned. But they also become integrated into the knowledge base and experience of other professional groups, and that, in my view, is also a positive thing.

I would like to see generic applied psychologists consulted routinely, whenever a project has relevance for people and does not fall into an established area of applied psychology. I am not claiming that we know everything there is to know – but I am claiming that we have insights which are useful. In my experience psychologists can work positively with just about any other professional group, and to our mutual benefit. If psychological knowledge can help those engaged in decision-making, planning or design to avoid some of the glaringly obvious stupidities that are so common in modern day-to-day living – and I firmly believe it can – then we will have made a positive contribution to society.

REFERENCES

Adams, J. and Neville, S. (2009) 'Men who have sex with men account for nonuse of condoms', *Qualitative Health Research*, 19 (12): 1669–77.

Agnew, S., Carson, J. and Dankert, A. (1995) 'The research productivity of clinical psychologists and psychiatrists: a comparative study', *Clinical Psychology Forum*, 86: 2–5.

Alderman, G. (2009) 'Defining and measuring academic standards: a British perspective', *Higher Education Management and Policy*, 21: 9–22.

Alexander, G. (2006) 'GROW coaching', in J. Passmore (ed.), *Excellence in Coaching: The Industry Guide*. London: Kogan Page. pp. 61–72.

Altbach, P.G. (1991) 'The academic profession', in P.G. Altbach (ed.), *International Higher Education: An Encyclopaedia*. New York: Garland Publishing.

Alvesson, M. (1992) 'Leadership as social integrative action: a study of a computer consultancy company', *Organization Studies*, 13 (2): 185–209.

Amnesty International (2011) *Aftershocks: Women Speak Out Against Sexual Violence in Haiti's Camps*. London: Amnesty International. Retrieved 18 July 2011 from: www.amnesty.org/en/library/asset/AMR36/001/2011/en/57237fad-f97b-45ce-8fdb-68cb457a304c/amr360012011en.pdf

Anderson, N.B. (2006) 'Psychology in the public eye, Part 2', *APA Monitor on Psychology*, 37 (3): 8.

Antares (2008) *Managing Stress in Humanitarian Work: A Systems Approach to Risk Reduction*. Amsterdam: Antares Foundation. Retrieved 29 May 2012 from: http://www.antaresfoundation.org/download/risk_reduction_booklet.pdf

Argyris, C. (1989) *Reasoning, Learning and Action – Individual and Organizational*. San Francisco, CA: Jossey Bass.

Arthur, M.B., Hall, D.T. and Lawrence, B.S. (1989) *Handbook of Career Theory*. Cambridge: Cambridge University Press.

Atkinson, R.C. and Shiffrin, R.M. (1968) 'Human memory: a proposed system and its control processes', in K.W. Spence and J.T. Spence (eds), *The Psychology of Learning and Motivation*. New York: Academic Press.

Attrill, G. and Liell, G. (2007) 'Offenders' views on risk assessment', in N. Padfield (ed.), *Who to Release? Parole, Fairness, and Criminal Justice*. Cullompton: Willan. pp. 191–201.

August, R.A. (2011) 'Women's later life career development: looking through the lens of the kaleidoscope career model', *Journal of Career Development*, 38 (3): 208–36.

Baddeley, A.D. and Hitch, G. (1974) 'Working memory', in G. Bower (ed.), *The Psychology of Learning and Motivation, Volume 8.* New York: Academic Press.

Bagozzi, R., Gurhan-Canli, Z. and Priester, J.R. (2002) *The Social Psychology of Consumer Behaviour (Applying Social Psychology).* Milton Keynes: Open University Press.

Bailey, C. (2010) 'What is the point of psychology? A mixed methods exploration of the public image of psychology', presented at the *PSYPAG Annual Conference*, Sheffield, 21–23 July 2010 . Retrieved 29 May 2012 from: http://www.psypag.co.uk/psypag-conference/conference-abstracts-2010/

Balkundi, P. and Kilduff, M. (2005) 'The ties that lead: a social network approach to leadership', *The Leadership Quarterly*, 16 (6): 941–61.

Bandura, A. (1977) 'Self-efficacy: toward a unifying theory of behavioural change', *Psychological Review*, 84: 191–215.

Banister, P., Burman, E., Parker, I., Taylor, M. and Tindall, C. (1994) *Qualitative Methods in Psychology: A Research Guide.* Buckingham: Open University Press.

Banks, S.M., Salovey, P., Greener, S., Rothman, A.J., Moyer, A., Beauvais, J. and Epel, E. (1995) 'The effects of message framing on mammography utilization', *Health Psychology*, 14: 178–84.

Baritz, L. (1960) *The Servants of Power: A History of the Use of Social Science in American Industry* (Science edn). New York: John Wiley and Sons, Inc.

Barkham, M. and Mellor-Clark, J. (2003) 'Bridging evidence-based practice and practice-based evidence: developing and rigorous and relevant knowledge for the psychological therapies', *Clinical Psychology and Psychotherapy*, 10: 319–27.

Barkham, M., Shapiro, D.A. and Firth-Cozens, J. (1989) 'Personal questionnaire changes in prescriptive vs exploratory psychotherapy', *British Journal of Clinical Psychology*, 28: 97–107.

Barnett, R. and Middlehurst, R. (1993) 'The lost profession', *Higher Education in Europe*, 18: 110–28.

Baron, H. (2011) *Selection of Clinical Psychologist Trainees: Job Analysis to develop selection tools. Final Report.* Commissioned by the Selection Working Group of the GTiCP.

Bateman, N. (2000) *Advocacy Skills for Health and Social Care Professionals.* London: Jessica Kingsley.

Bayne, R. (2005) *Ideas and Evidence: Critical Reflections on MBTI Theory and Practice.* Gainsville, FL: CAPT.

Bayne, R. and Jinks, G. (2010) *How to Survive Counsellor Training: An A–Z Guide.* Basingstoke: Palgrave.

Bayne, R., Jinks, G., Collard, P. and Horton, I. (2008) *The Counsellor's Handbook* (3rd edn). Cheltenham: Nelson Thornes.

Beaver, R. (2003) *Educational Psychology Casework.* London: Jessica Kingsley.

Beck, F.A.G. (1964) *Greek Education 450–350 BC.* London: Macmillan.

Bekerian, D.A. and Levey, A.B. (2005) *Applied Psychology: Putting Theory into Practice.* Oxford: Oxford University Press.

Belsky, J. and Pluess, M. (2009) 'Beyond diathesis-stress: differential susceptibility to environmental influences', *Psychological Bulletin*, 135 (6): 885–90.

Beresford, B. (1995) *Expert Opinions: A National Survey of Parents Caring for a Severely Disabled Child*. Community Care into Practice Series. Bristol: The Policy Press.

Berry, C. (1999) 'University league tables: artefacts and inconsistencies in individual rankings', *Higher Education Review*, 31: 3–10.

Biddle, S. and Mutrie, N. (2008) *Psychology of Physical Activity: Determinants, Well-Being and Interventions* (2nd edn). New York: Routledge.

Bimrose, J. (1996) *Counselling and Guidance for Higher Education*. Cheltenham and Strasbourg: UCAS and the Council of Europe.

Bimrose, J. (2001) 'Girls and women: challenges for careers guidance practice', *British Journal of Guidance and Counselling*, 29 (1): 79–94.

Bimrose, J. (2008) 'Guidance with Women', in J.A. Athanasou and R.V. Esbroeck (eds), *International Handbook of Career Guidance* (1st edn). Dordrecht: Springer. pp. 375–404.

Bimrose, J., Hughes, D. and Barnes, S.-A. (2011) *Integrating New Technologies into Careers Practice: Extending the Knowledge Base*. London: UK Commission for Employment and Skills. Retrieved 30 May 2012 from: www.ukces.org.uk/upload/pdf/Integrating%20New%20Technololgies%20into%20careers%20practice.pdf

Birnbaum, M.H. (2004) 'Human research and data collection via the internet', *Annual Review of Psychology*, 55: 803–32.

Biswas-Diener, R. (2011) 'Applied positive psychology: progress and challenges', *The European Health Psychologist*, 13: 24–6.

Blanton, H. and Jaccard, J. (2006) 'Arbitrary metrics in psychology', *American Psychologist*, 61 (1): 27–41.

Bogart, L. (ed.) (1966) *Psychology in Media Strategy*. Chicago, IL: American Marketing Association. p. 3.

Boniwell, I. (2006) *Positive Psychology in a Nutshell*. London: PWBC.

Boniwell, I. (2008) *Positive Psychology in a Nutshell* (2nd edn). London: PWBC.

Boniwell, I. and Osin, E. (in preparation) 'Validation of a well-being curriculum for Y7 and Y10 school students in the Haberdashers' Aske's Federation'.

Boring, E.G. (1967) *A History of Experimental Psychology*. New York: Appleton-Century-Crofts.

Bowlby, J. (1944) 'Forty-four juvenile thieves: their characteristics and home life', *International Journal of Psychoanalysis*, 25: 19–53.

Bowlby, J. (1951) *Maternal Care and Mental Health*. Geneva: World Health Organization.

Boyle, C. and Lauchlan, F. (2009) 'Applied psychology and the case for individual case-work: some reflections on the role of the educational psychologist', *Educational Psychology in Practice*, 25 (1): 71–84.

Boyle, M. (1990) *Schizophrenia: A Scientific Delusion?* London: Routledge.

Boyle, M. (1999) 'Diagnosis', in C. Newnes, C. Dunn and G. Holmes (eds), *This is Madness: A Critical Look at Psychiatry and the Future of Mental Health Services*. Ross-on-Wye: PCCS Books.

Boyle, M., Baker, M., Bennett, E. and Charman, A. (1993) 'The selection of ethnic minority and majority applicants for clinical psychology training courses', *Clinical Psychology Forum*, 56: 9–13.

BPS (British Psychological Society) (no date). *Types of Psychologists*. Leicester: British Psychological Society. Retrieved 7 June 2012 from: www.bps.org.uk/careers-education-training/how-become-psychologist/types-psychologists/types-psychologists

BPS (British Psychological Society) (1998) *National Occupational Standards in Applied Psychology (Generic)*. Leicester: BPS.

BPS (British Psychological Society)/Committee on Training in Clinical Psychology (2001) *Criteria for the Accreditation of Post-graduate Training Programmes in Clinical Psychology*. Leicester: BPS.

BPS (British Psychological Society) (2002) *The Directory of Chartered Psychologists and The Directory of Expert Witnesses*. Leiceister: BPS.

BPS (British Psychological Society) (2005) *Professional Practice Guidelines*. Leicester: BPS. Retrieved 30 May 2012 from: http://dcop.bps.org.uk/document-download-area/document-download$.cfm?file_uuid=10932D72-306E-1C7F-B65E-875F7455971D&ext=pdf

BPS (British Psychological Society) (2006) *The Code of Ethics and Conduct*. Leicester: BPS.

BPS (British Psychological Society) (2007) *Report of the Working Party on Conducting Research on the Internet: Guidelines for Ethical Practice in Psychological Research Online* (REP62/06.2007). Leicester: BPS.

BPS (British Psychological Society) (2010)

BPS (British Psychological Society) (2011). *Qualifications in forensic psychology (Stage 2) Candidate Handbook*. BPS Qualifications Office, Leicester. The information can also be downloaded from www.bps.org.uk/qualifications

(British Psychological Society) BPS (2012)

British Psychological Society (BPS), Care Services Improvement Partnership (CSIP) and National Institute for Mental Health in England (2007) *Good Practice Guide on the Contribution of Applied Psychologists to Improving Access for Psychological Therapies*. Leicester: BPS.

BPS (British Psychological Society)/Division of Clinical Psychology (DCP) (2000) *Recent Advances in Understanding Mental Illness and Psychotic Experiences*. Leicester: BPS.

BPS (British Psychological Society)/Division of Clinical Psychology (DCP) (2010a) *Core Purpose and Philosophy of the Profession*. Leicester: BPS.

BPS (British Psychological Society)/Division of Clinical Psychology (DCP) (2010b) *Clinical Psychology Leadership Development Framework*. Leicester: BPS.

Bracken, P. and Thomas, P. (2000) 'Putting ethics before effectiveness', *Open Mind*, 102: 22.

Bradley, C. (2001) 'Importance of differentiating health status from quality of life', *The Lancet*, 357 (9249): 7–8.

Brammer, L., Alcorn, J., Birk, J., Gazda, G., Hurst, J., Lafromboise, T., Newman, R., Osipow, S., Packard, T., Romero, D. and Scott, N. (1988) 'Organizational and political issues in counselling psychology: recommendations for change', *The Counseling Psychologist*, 16: 407–22.

Braun, V. and Clarke, V. (2006) 'Using thematic analysis in psychology', *Qualitative Research in Psychology*, 3: 77–81.

Briggs, M. and van Nieuwerburgh, C. (2010) 'The development of peer coaching skills in primary school children in years 5 and 6', *Procedia – Social and Behavioral Sciences*, 9 (239): 1415–22.

Broadbent, D.E. (1973) *In Defence of Empirical Psychology*. London: Methuen.

Bromley, D. (1986) *The Case Study Method in Psychology and Related Disciplines*. Chichester: John Wiley.

Bronfenbrenner, U. (1979) *The Ecology of Human Development: Experiments by Nature and Design*. Cambridge, MA: Harvard University Press.

Brown, J. (1998) 'Helping the police with their inquiries', *The Psychologist*, 11 (11): 539–42.

Brown, P. (ed.) (1973) *Radical Psychology*. London: Tavistock Publications.

Brown, R. (2005) 'Education, education, education – but will government policies produce an excellent higher education system?', *Higher Education Review*, 38: 3–31.

Brown, R. (2008) 'How do we get more effective policies for higher education? Reflections of a policy maker', *Higher Education Review*, 41: 3–20.

Brown Travis, C. and Compton, J.D. (2001) 'Feminism and health in the decade of behavior', *Psychology of Women Quarterly*, 25 (4): 312–23.

Brue, S. (2008) *The 8 Colors of Fitness*. Delroy Beach, FL: Oakledge Press.

Bryman, A. (2004) 'Qualitative research on leadership: a critical but appreciative review', *The Leadership Quarterly*, 15 (6): 729–69.

Buckworth, J. and Dishman, R.K. (2002) *Exercise Psychology*. Champaign, IL: Human Kinetics.

Bull, R., Valentine, T. and Williamson, T. (eds) (2009) *Handbook of Psychology of Investigative Interviewing*. Chichester: Wiley-Blackwell.

Burt, C. (1925) *The Young Delinquent*. London: University of London Press.

Buzan, T. (2000) *The Mind Map Book*. London: Penguin.

Cabinet Office, The (2009) *Unleashing Aspirations: The Final Report of the Panel on Fair Access to the Professions*. London: Panel on Fair Access to the Professions. Retrieved 30 May 2012 from: http://webarchive.nationalarchives.gov.uk/and http://www.cabinetoffice.gov.uk/media/227102/fair-access.pdf

Cahill, J., Barkham, M. and Stiles, W.B. (2010) 'Systematic review of practice based research on psychological therapies in routine clinic settings', *British Journal of Clinical Psychology*, 49: 421–53.

Camerer, C.F. (2000) 'Prospect theory in the wild: evidence from the field', in D. Kahneman and A. Tversky (eds), *Choices, Values and Frames*. Cambridge: Cambridge University Press.

Campbell, C. and Murray, M. (2004) 'Community health psychology: promoting analysis and action for social change', *Journal of Health Psychology*, 9 (2): 187–95.

Campbell, D. and Stanley, J. (1963) 'Experimental and quasi-experimental designs for research in teaching', in N. Gage (ed.), *Handbook of Research on Teaching*. Chicago, IL: Rand McNally.

Careers Profession Task Force (2012) *Composite Progress Report to Ministers*, March 2012. Retrieved from: http://www.aceg.org.uk/wp-content/uploads/CPTFFinal-report-publishedMay-2012.pdf

Carr, A. (1990) 'Doctoral degrees in clinical psychology', *Clinical Psychology Forum*, 25: 35–7.

Carroll, M. and Walton, M. (1997) *Handbook of Counselling in Organisations*. London: Sage.

Carson, D. (1995) 'Law's premises, methods and values', in R. Bull and D. Carson (eds), *Handbook of Psychology in Legal Contexts*. London: Wiley. pp. 29–40.

Chamberlain, K., Camic, P. and Yardley, L. (2003) 'Qualitative analysis of experience: grounded theory and case studies', in D.F. Marks and L. Yardley (eds), *Research Methods for Clinical and Health Psychology*. London: Sage.

Chaplin, M. (1978) 'Philosophies of higher education, historical and contemporary', in A.S. Knowles (ed.), *The International Encyclopaedia of Higher Education*. London: Jossey-Bass.

Chase, V.M., Hertwig, R. and Gigerenzer, G. (1998) 'Visions of rationality', *Trends in Cognitive Sciences*, 2: 206–14.

Cheshire, K. (2000) 'Clinical training in the 1990s: trainees' perspectives', *Clinical Psychology Forum*, 145: 37–41.

Child, D. (2007) *Psychology and the Teacher* (8th edn). London: Continuum.

Chomsky, N. (1957) *Syntactic Structures*. The Hague: Mouton.

Chomsky, N. (1959) 'Review of Skinner's "Verbal behaviour"', *Language*, 35: 26–58.

Clegg, J. (1998) *Critical Issues in Clinical Practice*. London: Sage.

Clifford, B.R. (1995) 'Psychology's premises, methods and values', in R. Bull and D. Carson (eds), *Handbook of Psychology in Legal Contexts*. London: Wiley. pp 13–27.

Clifford, B.R. (1997) 'Hugo Munsterberg: American Psychology's enigma', in A. Chapman, N. Sheehy and W. Conroy (eds), *Biographical Dictionary of Psychology*. London: Routledge. pp. 412–13.

Clifford, B.R. (2002) 'Methodology: law's adaption to and adoption of psychology's methods and findings', in D. Carson and R. Bull (eds), *Handbook of Psychology in Legal Contexts* (2nd edn). London: Wiley.

Clifford, B.R. (2008) 'Role of the expert witness', in G.H. Davies, C. Hollin and R. Bull (eds), *Forensic Psychology*. Chichester: John Wiley & Sons. pp. 235–61.

Clifford, B.R. (2010) 'Expert testimony', in G.J. Towel and D.A. Crighton (eds), *Forensic Psychology*. London: BPS and Blackwell Publishing. pp. 47–61.

Clifford, B.R. (2012) 'Role of the expert witness', in G.H. Davies and T. Beech (eds), *Forensic Psychology* (2nd edn). Chichester: John Wiley & Sons. pp. 287–303.

Collin, A. and Watts, A.G. (1996) 'The death and transfiguration of career – and career guidance?', *British Journal of Guidance and Counselling*, 24 (3): 385–98.

Cook, E.P., Heppner, M.J. and O'Brien, K.M. (2002) 'Career development of women of colour and white women: assumptions, conceptualization, and interventions from an ecological perspective', *The Career Development Quarterly*, 50 (4): 291–305.

Coolican, H. (1998) 'Research methods', in M.W. Eysenck (ed.), *Psychology: An Integrated Approach*. New York: Longman.

Coolican, H., Cassidy, A., Cherchar, A., Harrower, J., Penny, G., Sharp, R., Walley, M. and Westbury, A. (1996) *Applied Psychology*. London: Hodder and Stoughton.

Cooper, C.L. (2003) 'Work-life balance', in R. Bayne and I. Horton (eds), *Applied Psychology*. London: Sage. pp. 203–5.

Cooper, M. (2008) *Essential Research Findings in Counselling and Psychotherapy: The Facts are Friendly*. London: Sage.

Cornish, F. and Gillespie, A. (2009) 'A pragmatist approach to the problem of knowledge in health psychology', *Journal of Health Psychology*, 14: 800–9.

Coulter, A. and Collins, A. (2011) *Making Shared Decision-Making a Reality: No Decision about Me without Me*. London: The King's Fund.

CPTF (Careers Profession Task Force) (2010) *Towards a Strong Careers Profession: An Independent Report to the Department for Education*. Runcorn: DfE. Retrieved 29 May 2012 from: http://www.education.gov.uk/publications/standard/publicationdetail/page1/DFE-00550-2010_

Crawford, R. (1954) *Techniques of Creative Thinking*. New York: Hawthorn Books.

Creasy, J. and Paterson, F. (2005) *Leading Coaching in Schools*. Nottingham: National College for School Leadership.

Crewe, B. (2009) *The Prisoner Society: Power, Adaptation and Social Life in an English Prison*. Clarendon Studies in Criminology. Oxford: Oxford University Press.

Cushway, D. (1992) 'Stress in clinical psychology trainees', *British Journal of Clinical Psychology*, 31: 169–79.

D'Ambrosio, M.B. and Ehrenberg, R.G. (eds) (2007) *Transformational Change in Higher Education: Positioning Colleges and Universities for Future Success*. Cheltenham: Edward Elgar.

Danzinger, K. (1985) 'The methodological imperative in psychology', *Philosophical Science*, 15: 1–13.

Dart, J. and Davies, R. (2003) 'A dialogical, story-based evaluation tool: the most significant change technique', *American Journal of Evaluation*, 24: 137–55.

Davey, M.P., Davey, A., Tubbs, C., Savla, J. and Anderson, S. (2012) 'Second order change and evidence based practice', *Journal of Family Therapy*, 34 (1): 72–90.

Davidoff, J. and Warrington, E.K. (1999) 'The bare bones of object recognition: implications from a case of object recognition impairment', *Neuropsychologia*, 37 (3): 279–92.

Davidson, S. (2010a) 'The development of the British Red Cross' psychosocial framework: CALMER', *Journal of Social Work Practice*, 24: 29–42.

Davidson, S. (2010b) 'Psychosocial support in a global movement', *The Psychologist*, 23 (4): 304–7.

de Bono, E. (1970) *Lateral Thinking, Creativity Step by Step*. New York: Harper & Row.

de Bono, E. (1985) *Six Thinking Hats*. London: Penguin.

De Weerdt, W., Selz, B., Nuyens, G., Staes, F., Swinnen, D. and Van de Winckel, A. (2000) 'Time use of stroke patients in an intensive rehabilitation unit: a comparison between a Belgian and a Swiss setting', *Disability Rehabilitation*, 22: 181–6.

De Wit, L., Putman, K., Dejaeger, E., Baert, I., Berman, P., Bogaerts, K., Brinkmann, N., Connell, L., Feys, H., Jenni, W., Kaske, C., Lesaffre, E., Leys, M., Lincoln, N., Louckx, F., Schuback, B., Schupp, W., Smith, B. and De Weerdt, W. (2005) 'Use of time by stroke patients: a comparison of four European rehabilitation centers', *Stroke*, 36: 1997–83.

Department for Business, Innovation and Skills (2010a) *Skills for Sustainable Growth: Strategy Document*. London: BIS.

Department for Business, Innovation and Skills (2010b) *New All-Age Careers Service: John Hayes*. London: BIS. Retrieved 30 May 2012 from: http://www.bis.gov.uk/news/speeches/john-hayes-icg-conference

Department for Children, Schools and Families (DCSF) (2007) *The Children's Plan: Building Brighter Futures*. Norwich: HMSO. Retrieved 30 May 2012 from: http://www.educationengland.org.uk/documents/pdfs/2007-children's-plan.pdf

Department for Children, Schools and Families (DCSF) (2009) *Raising Expectations: Supporting all Young People to Participate until 18*. Nottingham: DCSF.

Department for Education (DfE) (2001) *The Code of Practice*. London: DfE.

Department for Education (DfE) (2011) *Support and Aspiration: A New Approach to Special Educational Needs and Disability. A Consultation (The Green Paper)*. London: TSO/Department for Education. Retrieve 27 June 2011 from: https://www.education.gov.uk/publications/standard/publicationDetail/Page1/CM8027

Department of Education and Department for Employment and Learning (2009) *Preparing for Success: Careers Education, Information, Advice and Guidance*. London: Department for Employment and Learning. Retrieved 30 May 2012 from: http://www.deni.gov.uk/index/80-curriculum-and-assessment/116-careers-strategy.htm

Department for Education and Employment (DfEE) (2000a) *Educational Psychology Services (England): Current Role, Good Practice and Future Directions – Report of the Working Group*. London: DfEE Publications.

Department for Education and Employment (DfEE) (2000b) *Educational Psychology Services (England): Current Role, Good Practice and Future Directions – The Research Report*. London: DfEE Publications.

Department of Health (1999) *National Service Framework for Mental Health*. London: Department of Health.

Department of Health (2001) *Treatment Choice in Psychological Therapies and Counselling*. London: HMSO.

Department of Health (2004) *The NHS Knowledge and Skills Framework (NHS KSF) and the Development Review Process*. London: Department of Health.

Department of Health (2010) *White Paper: Equity and Excellence – Liberating the NHS*. London: Department of Health.

Dessent, T. (1992) 'Educational psychologists and "The case for individual casework"', in S. Wolfendale, T. Bryans, M. Fox, A. Labram and A. Sigston (eds), *The Profession and Practice of Educational Psychology: Future Directions*. London: Cassell.

Dichter, E. (1949) 'A psychological view of advertising effectiveness', *Journal of Marketing*, 14 (1): 61–7.

Diener, D., Lucas, R., Schimmack, U. and Helliwell, J. (2009) *Well-Being for Public Policy*. Oxford: Oxford University Press.

Division of Counselling Psychology (2001) 'Chartered Counselling Psychologists' training and areas of competence: statement from the Division of Counselling Psychology', *Counselling Psychology Review*, 16 (4): 41–3.

Dixon, K. (1973) *Sociological Theory: Pretence and Possibility*. London: Routledge and Kegan Paul.

Donaldson, S., Csikszentmihalyi, C. and Nakamura, J. (2011) *Applied Positive Psychology: Improving Everyday Life, Health, Schools, Work and Society*. New York: Routledge.

Doran, G.T. (1981) 'There's a S.M.A.R.T. way to write management's goals and objectives', *Management Review*, 70 (11): 35–6.

Doyle, C. (2003) 'Occupational and organisational psychology', in R. Bayne and I. Horton (eds) *Applied Psychology: Current Issues and New Directions*. London: Sage.

Drucker, P. (1999) *Management Challenges of the 21st Century*. New York: Harper.

Duffy, M. (1990) 'Counselling psychology USA: patterns of continuity and change', *Counselling Psychology Review*, 5 (3): 9–18.

Duncan, B., Miller, S., Wampold, B. and Hubble, M. (eds) (2010) *The Heart and Soul of Change: Delivering what Works in Therapy*. Washington, DC: American Psychological Association.

Dunsmuir, S., Brown, E., Iyadurai, S. and Monsen, J. (2009) 'Evidence-based practice and evaluation: from insight to impact', *Educational Psychology in Practice*, 25: 53–70.

Eckel, P.D. and Kezar, A. (2003) *Taking the Reins: Institutional Transformation in Higher Education*. Westport, CT: American Council on Education, and Praeger.

Edwards, H., Sanders, D. and Hughes, D. (2010) *Future Ambitions: Careers Services in Wales*. Cardiff: Welsh Assembly Government.

Egan, G. (2010) *The Skilled Helper* (9th edn). Monterey: Brooks Cole.

Ellenberger, H. (1994) *The Discovery of the Unconscious: The History and Evolution of Dynamic Psychiatry*. London: Fontana Press.

Elliott, R. (1994) 'Addictive consumption: function and fragmentation in postmodernity', *Journal of Consumer Policy*, 17 (2): 159–79.

Elliott, R. (2012) 'Qualitative methods for studying psychotherapy change processes', in D. Harper and A.R. Thompson (eds), *Qualitative Research Methods in Mental Health and Psychotherapy: An Introduction for Students and Practitioners*. Chichester: Wiley.

Elsen, M., Wisser-Wijnveen, G.J., van der Rijst, R.M. and van Ariel, J.H. (2009) 'How to strengthen the connection between research and teaching in university education', *Higher Education Quarterly*, 63: 64–85.

Elton, L. (1989) *Teaching in Higher Education: Appraisal and Training*. London: Kogan Page.

Engel, G. (1977) 'The need for a new medical model: a challenge for biomedicine', *Science*, 196: 129–36.

Engel, J.F., Blackwell, R.D. and Miniard, P.W. (2002) *Consumer Behaviour* (9th revised edn). Fort Worth: Thomson Learning.

Eraut, M. (1994) *Developing Professional Knowledge and Competence*. London: Falmer.

Etzkowitz, H. (2010) 'Entrepreneurial universities for the UK: a "Stanford University" at Bamburgh Castle?', *Higher Education*, 24: 251–6.

Eysenck, H.J. (1964) *Crime and Personality*. London: Paladin.

Fadul, J.A. and Canles, R.Q. (2009) *Chess Therapy*. Morriville, NC: Lulu Press Inc.

Fagan, T.K. and VandenBos, G.R. (1993) *Exploring Applied Psychology: Origins and Critical Analysis*. Washington, DC: American Psychological Association.

Falzon, L., Davidson, K.W. and Bruns, D. (2010) 'Evidence searching for evidence-based psychology practice', *Professional Psychology: Research and Practice*, 41: 550–7.

Fannon, D. (2008) 'Pat Bracken', *The Psychiatrist*, 32: 240.

Farrell, P., Woods, K., Lewis, S., Rooney, S., Squires, G. and O'Conner, M. (2006) *Review of Function and Contribution of Educational Psychologists in Light of the 'Every Child Matters: Change for Children' Agenda*. Nottingham: DfES.

Faulkner, A. (2012) 'Participation and service user involvement', in D. Harper and A.R. Thompson (eds), *Qualitative Research Methods in Mental Health and Psychotherapy: An Introduction for Students and Practitioners*. Chichester: Wiley.

Faulkner, A. and Thomas, P. (2002) 'User-led research and evidence-based medicine', *British Journal of Psychiatry*, 180: 1–3.

Feltham, C. (2007) *What's Wrong With Us? The Anthropathology Thesis*. Oxford: Wiley.

Feltham, C. and Horton, I. (eds) (2012) *The Sage Handbook of Counselling and Psychotherapy* (3rd edn). London: Sage.

Finn, S.E. (1996) *Manual for Using the MMPI-2 as a Therapeutic Intervention*. Minneapolis, MN: University of Minnesota Press.

Fletcher, C. (2011) 'The impact of ACs and DCs on candidates', in N. Povah and G. Thornton (eds), *Assessment and Development Centres: Strategies for Global Talent Management*. London: Gower.

Ford, J. (2010) 'Studying leadership critically: a psychosocial lens on leadership identities', *Leadership*, 6 (1): 47–65.

Fox, D. (no date) *Critical Psychology*. Brighton, MA: dennisfox.net. Retrieved 7 June 2012 from: www.dennisfox.net/critpsy/

Fox, D., Prilleltensky, I. and Austin, S. (eds) (2009) *Critical Psychology: An Introduction*. London: Sage.

Fox, M. (2009) 'Working with systems and thinking systemically – disentangling the crossed wires', *Educational Psychology in Practice*, 25 (3): 247–58.

Fox, S. (1984) *The Mirror Makers: A History of American Advertising and Its Creators*. New York: William Morrow.

Foxall, G. (1997) *Marketing Psychology: The Paradigm in the Wings*. London: Macmillan.

Foxall, G. (2000) 'Radical behaviourist interpretation: generating and evaluating an account of consumer behaviour', *The Behaviour Analyst*, 21: 145–78.

Frankland, A. and Walsh, Y. (2010) *Counselling Psychology*. Leicester: BPS. Retrieved from 27 August 2011 from: http://dcop.bps.org.uk/dcop/home/values/values_home.cfm

Frederickson, N. (2002) 'Evidence-based practice and educational psychology', *Educational and Child Psychology*, 19: 96–111.

Freire, P. (1970) *Pedagogy of the Oppressed*. London: The Continuum Publishing Company.

Furnham, A. (1992) 'Prospective psychology students' knowledge of psychology', *Psychological Reports*, 70: 375–82.

Furnham, A. (2005) *The Psychology of Behaviour at Work: The Individual in the Organization*. Hove: Psychology Press.

Gale, A. (2002) 'A stranglehold on the development of psychology?', *The Psychologist*, 15: 356–9.

Gallwey, T. (1974) *The Inner Game of Tennis*. New York: Viking.

Garvey, R., Stokes, P. and Megginson, D. (2009) *Coaching and Mentoring: Theory and Practice*. London: Sage.

George, E., Iveson, C. and Ratner, H. (1999) *Problem to Solution: Brief Therapy with Individuals and Families* (2nd edn). London: BT Press.

Gersch, I.S. (2004) 'Educational psychology: in an age of uncertainty', *The Psychologist*, 17 (3): 142–5.

Gersch, I.S. (2009) 'A positive future for educational psychology – if the profession gets it right', *Educational Psychology in Practice*, 25 (1): 9–19.

Gersch, I.S., Dowling, F., Panagiotaki, G. and Potton, A. (2008) 'Children's views of spiritual and metaphysical concepts: a new dimension to educational psychology practice', *Educational Psychology in Practice*, 24 (3): 225–36.

Giddens, A. (1976) *New Rules of Sociological Method: A Positive Critique of Interpretive Sociology*. London: Hutchins.

Golding, K.S. (2008) *Nurturing Attachments: Supporting Children who are Adopted or Fostered*. London: Jessica Kingsley.

Gollwitzer, P.M., Heckhausen, H. and Steller, B. (1990) 'Deliberative vs. implemental mind-sets: cognitive tuning toward congruous thoughts and information', *Journal of Personality and Social Psychology*, 59: 1119–27.

Goode, W. (1960) 'Encroachment, charlatanism and the emerging professions: psychology, sociology and medicine', *American Sociological Review*, 25: 194–209.

Gordon, G. and Whitchurch, C. (eds) (2010) *Academic and Professional Identities in Higher Education: The Challenge of a Diversifying Workforce*. New York: Routledge.

Gosling, D. (2009) 'Educational development in the UK: a complex and contradictory reality', *International Journal for Academic Development*, 14: 5–18.

Gummesson, E. (1991) 'Marketing orientation revisited: the crucial role of the part-time marketer', *European Journal of Marketing*, 225 (2): 60–75.

Gunn, R. and Hills, S. (2008) 'The impact of league tables on university application rates', *Higher Education Quarterly*, 62: 273–96.

Guy, A., Thomas, R., Stephenson, S. and Loewenthal, D. (2011) *NICE Under Scrutiny: The Impact of the National Institute for Health and Clinical Excellence Guidelines on the Provision of Psychotherapy in the UK*. London: United Kingdom Council for Psychotherapy.

Hackley, C. (2000) 'Silent running: tacit, discursive and psychological aspects of management in a top UK advertising agency', *British Journal of Management*, 11 (3): 239–54.

Hackley, C. (2003a) '"We are all customers now": rhetorical strategy and ideological control in marketing management texts', *Journal of Management Studies*, 40 (5): 1325–52.

Hackley, C. (2003b) 'Account planning: current agency perspectives on an advertising enigma', *Journal of Advertising Research*, 43 (2): 235–46.

Hackley, C. (2007) 'Marketing psychology and the hidden persuaders', *The Psychologist* 20 (8): 488–90. Retrieved 30 May 2012 from: www.thepsychologist.org.uk/archive/archive_home.cfm/volumeID_20-editionID_150-ArticleID_1228-getfile_getPDF/thepsychologist%5C0807hack.pdf

Hackley, C. (2009) *Marketing: A Critical Introduction.* London: Sage.

Hackley, C. (2010a) *Advertising and Promotion: An Integrated Marketing Communications Approach* (2nd edn). London: Sage.

Hackley, C. (2010b) 'Theorizing advertising: managerial, scientific and cultural approaches', in P. MacLaran, M. Saren, B. Stern and M. Tadajewski (eds), *The Sage Handbook of Marketing Theory*. London: Sage. pp. 89–107.

Hackley, C. and Kover, A. (2007) 'The trouble with creatives: negotiating creative identity in advertising agencies', *International Journal of Advertising*, 26 (1): 63–78.

Hagstrom, H.P., Fry, M.K.,Cramblet, L.D and Tanner, K. (2007) 'Educational psychologists as scientist-practitioners: an expansion of the meaning of a scientist practitioner', *American Behavioural Scientist*, 50: 797–808.

Halsey, A.H. and Trow, M.A. (1971) *The British Academics.* London: Faber & Faber.

Hammersley, D. (2003) 'Training and professional development in Counselling Psychology', in R. Woolfe, W. Dryden and S. Strawbridge (eds), *Handbook of Counselling Psychology* (2nd edn). London: Sage.

Handy, C. (1984) *The Future of Work.* London: Blackwell.

Hanin, Y.L. (2000) *Emotions in Sport.* Champaign, IL: Human Kinetics.

Hanin, Y.L. and Stambulova, N.B. (2002) 'Metaphoric description of performance states: an application of the IZOF model', *The Sport Psychologist*, 16 (4): 396–415.

Hardman, D. (2009) *Judgment and Decision Making: Psychological Perspectives.* Oxford: Blackwell.

Harper, D. (2004) 'Introducing social constructionist psychology into clinical psychology training', in G. Larner and D. Paré (eds), *Collaborative Practice in Psychology and Therapy*. New York: Haworth Press.

Harre, R., Moghaddam, F., Cairnie, T., Rothbart, D. and Sabat, S. (2009) 'Recent advance in positioning theory', *Theory and Psychology*, 19 (1): 5–31.

Hart, C. (2002) *Doing a Literature Review: Releasing the Social Science Research Imagination.* London: Sage.

Hartley, J. and Branthwaite, A. (eds) (1989) *The Applied Psychologist* (2nd edn). Buckingham: Open University Press.

Hartwig, S.G. (2002) 'Surveying psychologists' public image with drawings of a "typical" psychologist', *South Pacific Journal of Psychology*, 14: 69–75. Retrieved 30 May 2012 from: spjp.massey.ac.nz/issues/2002-v14/v14-hartwig.pdf

Hatcher, R. (2008) 'Psychological skills in working with offenders', in G.H. Davies, C. Hollin and R. Bull (eds), *Forensic Psychology*. Chichester: John Wiley and Sons. pp. 294–322.

Hatton, C., Gray, I. and Whittaker, A. (2000) 'Improving selection of clinical psychologists: the clearing house research project', *Clinical Psychology Forum*, 136: 35–8.

Hauser, M. (2006) *Moral Minds: How Nature Designed our Universal Sense of Right and Wrong.* London: Little, Brown.

Haward, L.R.C. (1981) *Forensic Psychology.* London: Batsford.

Hearnshaw, L.S. (1964) *A Short History of British Psychology 1840–1940*. London: Methuen.

Hefferon, K. and Boniwell, I. (2011) *Positive Psychology: Theory, Research and Applications*. Maidenhead: McGraw-Hill.

Help Age International (2010) *A Study of Humanitarian Financing for Older People*. London: Help Age International.

Hirschman, E.C. (1986) 'Humanistic inquiry in consumer research: philosophy, method and criteria', *Journal of Marketing Research*, 23: 237–49.

Hirschman, E.C. and Holbrook, M.B. (1982) 'Hedonic consumption: emerging concepts, methods and propositions', *Journal of Marketing*, 46: 92–101.

HM Government (1989) *The Children Act*. London: HMSO.

Hobfall, S.E., Watson, P., Bell, C.C., Bryant, R.A., Brymer, M.J., Friedman, M.J., Friedman, M., Gersons, B.P., de Jong, J.T, Layne, C.M., Maguen, S., Neria, Y., Norwood, A.E., Pynoos, R.S., Reissman, D., Ruzek, J.I., Shalev, A.Y., Solomon, Z., Steinberg, A.M. and Ursano, R.J. (2007) 'Five essential elements of immediate and mid-term mass trauma intervention: empirical evidence', *Psychiatry*, 70 (4): 283–315.

Hodgins, S. (1997) 'An overview of research on the prediction of dangerousness', *Nordic Journal of Psychiatry*, 51 (Suppl. 39): 33–8.

Hodkinson, P. and Issit, M. (eds) (1995) *The Challenges of Competence: Professionalism through Policies for Vocational Training in England and Wales*. London: Cassell.

Hoffman, B.M., Papas, R.K., Chatkoff, D.K. and Kerns, R.D. (2007) 'Meta-analysis of psychological interventions for chronic low back pain', *Health Psychology*, 26 (1): 1–9.

Holbrook, M.B. and Hirschman, E.C. (1982) 'The experiential aspects of consumption: consumer fantasies, feelings and fun', *Journal of Consumer Research*, 9 (September): 132–40.

Holmes, G. (2003) 'An audit: do the people I see get better?', *Clinical Psychology*, 24: 47–50.

Holttum, S. and Goble, L. (2006) 'Factors influencing levels of research activity in clinical psychologists: a new model', *Clinical Psychology and Psychotherapy*, 13: 339–51.

Home Office (1992) *Memorandum of Good Practice on Video Recorded Interviews with Child Witnesses for Criminal Procedures*. London: HMSO.

Home Office (2002) *Achieving Best Evidence in Criminal Proceedings: Guidance for Vulnerable or Intimidated Witnesses, including Children*. London: HMSO.

Home Office (2007) *Achieving Best Evidence in Criminal Proceedings: Guidance on Interviewing Victims and Witnesses, and using Special Measures*. London: HMSO.

Horton, I. (2012) 'Integration and its problems', in C. Feltham and I. Horton (eds), *The Sage Handbook of Counselling and Psychotherapy* (3rd edn). London: Sage.

Hoshmand, L.T. and Polkinghorne, D.E. (1992) 'Redefining the science–practice relationship and professional training', *American Psychologist*, 47: 55–66.

Howard, S. and Bauer, M. (2001) 'Psychology in the press 1988–1999', *The Psychologist*, 14: 632–6.

Hoyningen-Huene, D. von (1992) 'The distinctive nature of Fachhochschulen', *Metropolitan Universities*, 2: 4–13.

HPC (Health Professions Council) (2009) *Standards of Proficiency: Practitioner Psychologists*. London: HPC.

Huisman, J. (2007) 'Editorial: the anatomy of autonomy', *Higher Education Policy*, 20 (3): 219–21.

Humanitarian Emergency Response Review (HERR) (2011) *Humanitarian Emergency Response Review (Chair: Paddy Ashdown)*. London: HERR. Retrieved 29 May 2012 from: www.dfid.gov.uk/Documents/publications1/HERR.pdf

Hutton, J. (2011) 'Patients or people? The Local Authority as an employer of health psychologists', *Health Psychology Update*, 20 (1): 24–8.

Hyland, T. (1994) *Competence, Education and NVQs: dissenting perspectives*. London: Cassell.

Innocence Project (2011) from http://www.innocenceproject.org

Inter-Agency Standing Committee (IASC) (2007) *IASC Guidelines on Mental Health and Psychosocial Support in Emergency Settings*. Geneva: IASC.

International Task Force on Assessment Center Guidelines (2009) 'Guidelines and ethical considerations for Assessment Center Operations', *International Journal of Selection and Assessment*, 17: 243–53.

iPED Research Network (2009) *Academic Futures: Inquiries into Higher Education and Pedagogy*. Newcastle upon Tyne: Cambridge Scholars Publishing.

Jansari, A. (2005) 'Cognitive neuropsychology', in N. Braisby (ed.), *Cognitive Psychology: A Methods Companion*. Oxford: Oxford University Press.

Jansari, A., Davis, K., McGibbon, T., Firminger, S. and Kapur, N. (2010) 'When "long-term memory" no longer means "forever": analysis of accelerated long-term forgetting in a patient with temporal lobe epilepsy', *Neuropsychologia*, 48: 1707–15.

Jeffery, R.W., Drewnowski, A., Epstein, L.H., Stunkard, A.J., Wilson, G.T., Wing, R.R. and Hill, D.R. (2000) 'Long-term maintenance of weight loss: current status', *Health Psychology*, 19 (Suppl. 1): 5–16.

Jenkins, A., Breen, R. and Lindsay, R. (2003) *Reshaping Teaching in Higher Education: Linking Teaching with Research*. London: Kogan Page/SEDA.

Jenkins, S. (1995) *Accountable to None: The Tory Nationalisation of Britain*. London: Hamish Hamilton.

John, C. (2010) 'Virtual and real conversations with people who experieneced the QCoP', *Counselling Psychology Review*, 25 (3): 59–65.

John, I. (1998) 'The scientist-practitioner model: a critical examination', *Australian Psychologist*, 33: 24–30.

Johnson, E.J. and Goldstein, D. (2003) 'Medicine: Do defaults save lives?', *Science*, 302: 1338–9.

Johnstone, L. (2001) *Users and Abusers of Psychiatry* (2nd edn). London: Routledge.

Johnstone, L. and Dallos, R. (2006) *Formulation in Psychology and Psychotherapy*. Hove: Routledge.

Jones, A. (1998) 'What's the bloody point? More thoughts on fraudulent identity', *Clinical Psychology Forum*, 112: 3–9.

Kagan, C., Burton, M., Duckett, P., Lawthom, R. and Sidiquee, A. (2011a) *Critical Community Psychology*. Chichester: Wiley-Blackwell.

Kagan, C., Duggan, K., Richards, M. and Siddiquee, A. (2011b) 'Community psychology', in P.R. Martin, F.M. Cheung, M.C. Knowles, M. Kyrios, L. Littlefield, J.B. Overmier and J.M. Prieto (eds), *The IAAP Handbook of Applied Psychology*. Chichester: Wiley-Blackwell.

Kaplan, A. (1964) *The Conduct of Enquiry*. San Francisco, CA: Chandler.

Kazdin, A.E. (2006) 'Arbitrary metrics: implications for identifying evidence-based treatments', *American Psychologist*, 61: 42–9.

Kebbell, M., Hurren, E. and Mazerolle P. (2006) 'Sex offenders' perceptions of police interviewing: implications for improving interviewing effectiveness', *Canadian Journal of Police and Security Services*, 4: 28–36.

Kelly, B. Woolfson, L. and Boyle, J. (2008) *Frameworks for Practice in Educational Psychology*. London: Jessica Kingsley.

Kelly, C. and Gersch, I.S. (2000) 'How newly trained psychologists see the profession developing: a crystal ball gaze towards the Year 2010', *Division of Educational and Child Psychology Newsletter – British Psychological Society*, 94: 10–19.

Kelly, P. and Moloney, P. (2013) 'Psychological therapies', in J. Cromby, D. Harper and P. Reavey, *Psychology, Mental Health and Distress*. Basingstoke: Palgrave Macmillan.

Kennedy, J.E. (1924) *Reason Why Advertising, Plus Intensive Advertising*. Chicago, IL: TWI Press, Inc.

Kennedy, P. (2008) *Coping Effectively with Spinal Cord Injuries: A Therapist Guide*. Treatments that Work Series. Oxford: Oxford University Press.

Kennedy, P. and Llewelyn, S. (2001) 'Does the future belong to the scientist-practitioner?', *The Psychologist*, 14: 74–8.

Kerlinger, F. (1970) *Foundations of Behavioural Research*. New York: Holt, Rinehart and Winston.

Kinderman, P. (2005) 'The applied psychology revolution', *The Psychologist*, 18: 744–6.

Kivinen, O. and Nurmi, J. (2010) 'Different but equal? Assessing European dual HE systems', *Higher Education*, 60: 369–93.

Kline, P. (1998) *The New Psychometrics*. London: Routledge.

Knight, J. (2007) *Instructional Coaching: A Partnership Approach to Improving Instruction*. Thousand Oaks, CA: Corwin Press.

Knutson, B., Rick, S., Wimmer, S.G., Prelec, D. and Loewenstein, G. (2007) 'Neural predictors of purchases', *Neuron*, 53 (1): 147–56.

Kolb, D.A., Rubin, I.M. and McIntyre, J.M. (1974) *Organizational Psychology: An Experiential Approach*. Upper Saddle River, NJ: Prentice-Hall.

Kotler, P. and Levy, S. (1969) 'Broadening the concept of marketing', *Journal of Marketing*, 33: 10–15.

Kugelmann, R. (2003) 'Pain as symptom, pain as sign', *Health*, 7 (1): 29–50.

Kuncel, N.R., Ones, D.S. and Sackett, P.R. (2010) 'Individual differences as predictors of work, educational and broad life outcomes', *Personality and Individual Differences*, 49: 331–8.

Kutchins, H. and Kirk, S.A. (1997) *Making us Crazy: DSM: The Psychiatric Bible and the Creation of Mental Disorders*. New York: Free Press.

Kwiatkowski, R. and Duncan, D.C. (2006) 'UK occupational/organisational psychology, applied science and applied humanism: some further thoughts on what we have forgotten', *Journal of Occupational and Organizational Psychology*, 79: 217–24.

Kwiatkowski, R., Duncan, D.C. and Shimmin, S. (2006) 'What have we forgotten and why?', *Journal of Occupational and Organizational Psychology*, 79: 183–201.

Lambert, R. (2003) *Lambert Review of Business–University Collaboration*. London: HM Treasury.

Laming, W. (2003) *The Victoria Climbié Inquiry Report*. London: HMSO.

Lane, D.A. and Corrie, S. (eds) (2006) *The Modern Scientist-Practitioner: A Guide to Practice in Psychology*. Hove: Psychology Press.

Larner, G. (2001) 'The critical-practitioner model in therapy', *Australian Psychologist*, 36: 36–43.

Law, H.C. (2002) 'Coaching Psychology Interest Group – an introduction', *The Occupational Psychologist*, 47: 31–2.

Law, H.C., Ireland, S. and Hussain, Z. (2007) *Psychology of Coaching, Mentoring and Learning*. Chichester: John Wiley.

Layard. R. (2006) 'The case for psychological treatment centres', *British Medical Journal*, 332: 1030–2.

Lazarus, R.S. (2003) 'Does the positive psychology movement have legs?', *Psychological Inquiry*, 14 (2): 93–109.

Leaning, J. (2008) 'Human security and conflict', in M. Green (ed.), *Risking Human Security: Attachment and Public Life*. London: Karnac. pp. 125–49.

Learmonth, M. (2006) 'NICE Guidelines on Depression: a full digest for Arts Therapists', *Insider Art*, May. Retrieved 11 May 2011 from: www.insiderart.org.uk/UserFiles/File/The%20NICE%20Guidelines%20on%20Depression,%20an%20analysis%20from%20an%20art%20therapy%20perspective.pdf

Lechuga, V.M. (2006) *The Changing Landscape of the Academic Profession: The Culture of Faculty at For-Profit Colleges and Universities*. London: Routledge.

Lederach, J.P. (2001) 'Civil society and reconciliation', in C. Crocker, F. Osler Hampson and P. Aall (eds), *Turbulent Peace: The Challenges of Managing International Conflict*. Washington, DC: United States Institute of Peace Press. pp. 841–54.

LeDoux, J. (1998) *The Emotional Brain*. New York: Weidenfeld & Nicolson.

Leisyte, L., Enders, J. and de Boer, H. (2009) 'The balance between teaching and research in Dutch and English universities in the context of university governance reforms', *Higher Education*, 58: 619–35.

Lerner, B. and Locke, E. (1995) 'The effects of goal setting, self-efficacy, competition, and personal traits on the performance of an endurance task', *Journal of Sport and Exercise Psychology*, 2: 138–52.

Levy, S. (1959) 'Symbols for sale', *Harvard Business Review*, 37: 117–24.

Liddle., I. and Macmillan, S. (2010) 'Evaluating the FRIENDS programme in a Scottish setting', *Educational Psychology in Practice*, 26 (1): 53–68.

Lilienfeld, S.O. (2012) Public skepticism of psychology: why many people perceive the study of human behavior as unscientific', *American Psychologist*, 67: 111–29.

Lincoln, N.B., Willis, D., Philips, S.A., Juby, L.C. and Berman, P. (1997) 'Comparison of rehabilitation practice on hospital wards for stroke patients', *Stroke*, 28: 543–9.

Lincoln, Y. and Guba, E. (1985) *Naturalistic Inquiry*. Beverly Hills, CA: Sage.

Lindow, V. (2001) 'Survivor research', in C. Newnes, G. Holmes and C. Dunn (eds), *This is Madness Too: Critical Perspectives on Mental Health Services*. Ross-on-Wye: PCCS books.

Llewelyn, S. and Cuthbertson, A. (2009) 'Leadeship, teamwork and consultancy in clinical psychology', in H. Beinart, P. Kennedy and S. Llewelyn (eds), *Clinical Psychology in Practice*. Oxford: Wiley-Blackwell.

Locke, E.A. and Latham, G.P. (1990) *A Theory of Goal Setting and Task Performance*. Englewood Cliffs, NJ: Prentice Hall.

Lokman, P., Gabriel, Y. and Nicolson, P. (2011) 'Hospital doctors' anxieties at work', *International Journal of Organizational Analysis*, 19 (1): 29–48.

Long, C.G. and Hollin, C.R. (1997) 'The scientist-practitioner model in clinical psychology: a critique', *Clinical Psychology and Psychotherapy*, 4: 75–83.

Longmore, R.J. and Worrell, M. (2007) 'Do we need to challenge thoughts in cognitive behavior therapy?', *Clinical Psychology Review*, 27: 173–87.

Luft, J. and Ingham, H. (1955) 'The Johari window, a graphic model of interpersonal awareness', in *Proceedings of the Western Training Laboratory in Group Development*. Los Angeles: UCLA.

Lykken, D. and Tellegen, A. (1996) 'Happiness is a stochastic phenomenon', *Psychological Science*, 7 (3): 186–9.

MacKay, T. (2008) 'Can psychology change the world?', *The Psychologist*, 21: 928–31.

Macrodimitris, S.D. and Endler, N.S. (2001) 'Coping, control, and adjustment in type 2 diabetes', *Health Psychology*, 20 (3): 208–16.

Management Advisory Service (MAS) (1989) *Review of Clinical Psychology Services, Activities and Possible Models*. Cheltenham: MAS.

Marks, D.F. (1996) 'Health psychology in context', *Journal of Health Psychology*, 1 (1): 7–21.

Marks, D.F. (2002a) *Perspectives on Evidence-Based Practice*. London: National Institute for Health and Clinical Excellence. Retrieved 30 May 2012 from: www.nice.org.uk/aboutnice/whoweare/aboutthehda/evidencebase/publichealthevidencesteeringgroupproceedings/perspectives_on_evidence_based_practice.jsp

Marks, D.F. (2002b) *The Health Psychology Reader*. London: Sage.

Marks, D.F. (2009) 'How should psychology interventions be reported?', *Journal of Health Psychology*, 44: 475–89.

Marks, D.F., Murray, M.P., Evans, B., Willig, C., Woodall, C. and Sykes, C.M. (2005) *Health Psychology: Theory, Research and Practice* (2nd edn). London: Sage.

Martinson, R. (1974) 'What works? Questions and answers about prison reform', *Public Interest*, 10: 22–54.

Maruna, S. (2011) 'Why do they hate us? Making peace between prisoners and psychology', *International Journal of Offender Therapy and Comparative Criminology*, 55: 671–5.

Maruna, S. and Mann, R.E. (2006) 'A fundamental attribution error? Rethinking cognitive distortions', *Legal and Criminological Psychology*, 11: 155–77.

Matarazzo, J.D. (1980) 'Behavioural health and behavioural medicine: frontiers for a new health psychology', *American Psychologist*, 35: 807–17.

Maudsley Debates, The (2002) http://tinyurl.com/3ceo3oj. Accessed 27 August 2011.

Maxwell, N. (2007) *From Knowledge to Wisdom: A Revolution for Science and the Humanities*. London: Pentire.

McIntyre, L. (2006) *Dark Ages: The Case for a Science of Human Behavior*. Cambridge, MA: MIT Press.

McKay, L. (2005) 'How can humanitarian work be stressful?', in *The Headington Institute Online Training Module: Understanding and Coping with Traumatic Stress*. Pasadena, CA: Headington Institute. Retrieved from: http://www.headington-institute.org./Default.aspx?tabid=1786

McKay, L. (2010) *Spirituality and Humanitarian Work: Maintaining Your Vitality. Online Training Module Published by the Headington Institute*. Pasadena, CA: Headington Institute. Retrieved 30 May 2012 from: http://www.headington-institute.org/Default.aspx?tabid=2909

McKenna, P. and Todd, D. (1997) 'Longitudinal utilization of mental health services: a timeline method, nine retrospective accounts, and a preliminary conceptualization', *Psychotherapy Research*, 7: 383–95.

McLeod, J. (2003) *An Introduction to Counselling* (3rd edn). Milton Keynes: Open University Press.

McLeod, J. (2009) *An Introduction to Counselling* (4th edn). Milton Keynes: Open University Press.

McLeod, J. (2010) *Case Study Research in Counselling and Psychotherapy*. London: Sage.

McLeod, J. (2011) 'The role of qualitative methods in outcome research', in *Qualitative Research in Counselling and Psychotherapy*. London: Sage. pp. 161–80.

McLeod, C., O'Donohoe, S. and Townley, B. (2009) 'The elephant in the room? Class and creative careers in British advertising agencies', *Human Relations*, 62 (7): 1011–39.

McMahon, M. and Patton, W. (1995) 'Development of a systems theory of career development', *Australian Journal of Career Development*, 4 (2): 15–20.

McNamara, E. (2000) *Positive Pupil Management and Motivation: A Secondary Teacher's Guide*. London: Davild Fulton.

Medawar, P. (1972) *The Hope of Progress*. London: Methuen.

Megginson, D. and Clutterbuck, D. (1995) *Techniques for Coaching and Mentoring*. Oxford: Elsevier Butterworth-Heinemann.

MHChoice (2007) www.mhchoice.csip.org.uk/psychological therapies/iapt commisioned_pathfinder_sites.html

Michelsen, S. (2010) 'Humboldt meets Bologna', *Higher Education Policy*, 23: 151–72.

Michie, S. and West, M.A. (2004) 'Managing people and performance: an evidence-based framework applied to health service organizations', *International Journal of Management Reviews*, 5–6 (2): 91–111.

Midlands Psychology Group (2010) 'Welcome to NICEworld', *Clinical Psychology Forum*, 212: 52–6.

Milewa, T. (2006) 'Health technology adoption and the politics of governance in the UK', *Social Science and Medicine*, 63: 3102–12.

Milewa, T. and Barry, C. (2005) 'Health policy and the politics of evidence', *Social Policy and Administration*, 39: 498–512.

Miller, G.A. (1969) 'Psychology as a means of promoting human welfare', *American Psychologist*, 24: 1063–75.

Mills, J.S. (1874) *A System of Logic*. New York: Harper.

Mills, K.I. (2009) 'Getting beyond the couch: how does the general public view the science of psychology?', *APA Monitor on Psychology*, 40 (3): 38.

Milne, D. (1999) 'Editorial: Important differences between the "scientist-practitioner" and the "evidence-based practitioner"', *Clinical Psychology Forum*, 133: 5–9.

Milne, D. and Paxton, R. (1998) 'A psychological reanalysis of the scientist-practitioner model', *Clinical Psychology and Psychotherapy*, 5: 216–30.

Milne, D., Britton, P. and Wilkinson, I. (1990) 'The scientist-practitioner in practice', *Clinical Psychology Forum*, 30: 27–30.

Milne, D., Keegan, D., Paxton, R. and Seth, K. (2000) 'Is the practice of psychological therapists evidence-based?', *International Journal of Health Care Quality Assurance*, 13: 8–14.

Misra, G. (1993) 'Psychology from a constructionist perspective: an interview with Kenneth J. Gergen', *New Ideas in Psychology*, 11: 399–414.

Moncrieff, J. (2013) 'Psychiatric medication', in J. Cromby, D. Harper and P. Reavey (eds), *Psychology, Mental Health and Distress*. Basingstoke: Palgrave Macmillan.

Moscovici, S. (1984) 'The phenomenon of social representations', in R.M. Farr and S. Moscovici (eds), *Social Representations*. Cambridge: Cambridge University Press. pp. 3–70.

Moscovici, S. and Faucheux, C. (1972) 'Social influence, conformity bias and the study of active minorities', in L. Berkowitz (ed.), *Advances in Experimental Social Psychology, Volume 6*. New York: Academic Press. pp. 149–202.

Mount, M.K. and Barrick, M.R. (1998) 'Five reasons why the "Big Five" article has been cited', *Personnel Psychology*, 51: 849–57.

Mowbray, D. (2010) 'Finding clinical psychology (again)', *Mowbray Occasional Paper*, 3 (6): 1–6.

Mulveen, R. and Hepworth, J. (2006) 'An interpretative phenomenological analysis of participation in a pro-anorexia internet site and its relationship with disordered eating', *Journal of Health Psychology*, 11 (2): 283–96.

Mulvey, M.R. (2006) 'Career guidance in England: retrospect and prospect', *British Journal of Guidance and Counselling*, 34 (1): 13–30.

Munley, P.H., Duncan, L.E., McDonnell, K.A., and Sauer, E.M. (2004) 'Counseling psychology in the United States of America', *Counselling Psychology Quarterly*, 17 (3): 247–71.

Munro, G.D. (2011) 'Falling on deaf ears', *The Psychologist*, 24: 178–81.

Munsterberg, H. (1908) *On the Witness Stand: Essays on Psychology and Crime*. New York: Clark Boardman.

Murray, M. (2000) 'Levels of narrative analysis in health psychology', *Journal of Health Psychology*, 5 (3): 337–47.

Murray, M. (2004) *Critical Health Psychology*. Basingstoke: Palgrave.

Murray, M. (2010) 'Health psychology in context', *The European Health Psychologist*, 12: 39–41.

Murray, M. and Chamberlain, K. (1999) *Qualitative Health Psychology: Theories and Methods*. London: Sage.

National Committee of Inquiry into Higher Education (NCIHE) (1997) *Higher Education in the Learning Society: The Report of the National Committee of Inquiry into Higher Education (the Dearing Report)*. London: HMSO.

NICE (National Institute For Health and Clinical Excellence) (2006) *Attention Deficit Hyperactivity Disorder (ADHD): Stakeholder Consultation Table.* London: NICE. Retrieved 11 May 2011 from: www.nice.org.uk/nicemedia/live/11632/34228/34228.pdf

Neisser, U. (1967) *Cognitive Psychology.* New York: Appleton-Century-Crofts.

Nelson-Jones, R. (1999) 'On becoming counselling psychology in the Society: establishing the Counselling Psychology Section', *Counselling Psychology Review*, 14 (3): 30–7.

Nerad, M. (2004) 'The PhD in the US: criticism, facts and remedies', *Higher Education Policy*, 17: 183–99.

Neumayer, E. and Plümper, T. (2007) 'The gendered nature of natural disasters: the impact of catastrophic events on the gender gap in life expectancy, 1981–2002', *Annals of the Association of American Geographers*, 97 (3): 551–66.

New Economics Foundation (2010) *The (un)Happy Planet Index (HPI).* London, UK: New Economics Foundation.

New Ways of Working in Mental Health (2007) *New Ways of Working for Applied Psychologists in Health and Social Care: The End of the Beginning.* London: Department of Health.

Newall, J.T., Wood, V.A., Hewer, R.L. and Tinson, D.J. (1997) 'Development of a neurological rehabilitation environment: an observational study', *Clinical Rehabilitation*, 11: 146–55.

Nichols, K., Cormack, M. and Walsh, S. (1992) 'Preventative personal support: a challenge for training courses', *Clinical Psychology Forum*, 45: 29–31.

Nicolson, P. (2003a) 'Health psychology', in R. Bayne and I. Horton (eds), *Applied Psychology.* London: Sage. pp. 219–221.

Nicolson, P. (2003b) 'Reflexivity, "bias" and the in-depth interview: developing shared meanings', in L. Finlay and B. Gough (eds), *Reflexivity: A Practical Guide for Researchers in Health and Social Sciences.* Oxford: Blackwell. pp. 133–45.

Nicolson, P. (2010) *Domestic Violence and Psychology: A Critical Perspective.* London: Taylor and Francis.

Nicolson, P. and Anderson, P. (2000) 'The patient's burden: physical and psychological effects of acute exacerbations of chronic bronchitis', *Journal of Antimicrobial Chemotherapy*, 45 (Suppl. 2): 25–32.

Nicolson, P. and Anderson, P. (2001) 'The psychosocial impact of spasticity-related problems for people with multiple sclerosis: a focus group study', *Journal of Health Psychology*, 6 (5): 551–67.

Nicolson, P. and Anderson, P. (2003) 'Quality of life, distress and self-esteem: a focus group study of people with chronic bronchitis', *British Journal of Health Psychology*, 8: 251–70.

Nicolson, P., Kopp, Z., Chapple, C.R. and Kelleher, C. (2008) 'It's just the worry about not being able to control it! A qualitative study of living with overactive bladder', *British Journal of Health Psychology*, 13 (2): 343–59.

Nicolson, P., Rowland, E., Lokman, P., Fox, R., Gabriel, Y., Heffernan, K., Howorth, C., Ilan-Clarke, Y. and Smith, G. (2011) *Leadership and Better Patient Care: Managing in the NHS.* London: HMSO.

Niemeyer, G.J. and Diamond, A.K. (2001) 'The anticipated future of counselling psychology in the United States: a Delphi poll', *Counselling Psychology Quarterly*, 14 (1): 49–65.

Nithianantharajah, J. and Hannan, A.J. (2006) 'Enriched environments, experience-dependent plasticity and disorders of the nervous system', *Nature Reviews: Neuroscience*, 7: 697–709.

Noble, K.A. (1994) *Changing Doctoral Degrees: An International Perspective*. Buckingham: SRHE and Open University Press.

Norcross, J.C. and Goldfried, M.R. (eds) (2005) *Handbook of Psychotherapy Integration* (2nd edn). Oxford: Oxford University Press.

Norcross, J.C., Brust, A.M. and Dryden, W. (1992) 'British clinical psychologists: II. Survey findings and American comparisons', *Clinical Psychology Forum*, 40: 25–9.

Norcross, J.C., Karpiak, C.P. and Santoro, S.O. (2005) 'Clinical psychologists across the years: the Division of Clinical Psychology from 1960 to 2003', *Journal of Clinical Psychology*, 61: 1467–83.

Norman, D.A. (1988) *The Psychology of Everyday Things*. New York: Basic Books.

Nown, G. (1985) *The World's Worst Predictions*. London: Arrow Books.

Nybom, T. (2003) 'The Humboldt legacy: reflections on the past, present and future of the European university', *Higher Education Policy*, 16: 141–59.

O'Driscoll, P. (2010) *What are Counselling and Psychotherapy? BACP Information Sheet C2*. Lutterworth: BACP. Retrieved 30 May 2012 from: www.bacp.co.uk/admin/structure/files/repos/358_c2_what_are_counselling_and_psychotherapy.pdf

Oatley, K. (1992) *Best Laid Schemes: The Psychology of Emotions*. Cambridge: Cambridge University Press.

OfSted (2010) *A Statement is not Enough*. London: HMSO.

Ogden, J. (1991) *Health Psychology: A Textbook* (2nd Edition). Buckingham: Open University Press.

Orford, J. (2008) *Community Psychology: Challenges, Controversies And Emerging Consensus*. Chichester: Wiley.

Organisation for Economic Co-operation and Development (2004) *Career Guidance and Public Policy: Bridging the Gap*. Paris: OECD.

Organisation for Economic Co-operation and Development (2010) *Restoring Fiscal Stability and Lessons for the Public Sector*. Paris: OECD.

Orlans, V. and Van Scoyoc, S. (2009) *A Short Introduction to Counselling Psychology*. London: Sage.

Osborn, A. (1948) *Your Creative Power*. New York: Scribner.

Osipow, S.H. and Fitzgerald, L.F. (1996) *Theories of Career Development* (4th edn). Needham Heights, MA: Allyn & Bacon.

Packard, V. (1957/1984) *Hidden Persuaders*. New York: Washington Square Press.

Paley, G. and Shapiro, D.A. (2002) 'Lessons from psychotherapy research for psychological interventions for people with schizophrenia', *Psychology and Psychotherapy: Theory, Research and Practice*, 75: 5–17.

Palmer, S. and Cavenagh, M. (2012) 'Editorial: Coaching psychology coming of age in the 21st century', *International Coaching Psychology Review*, 7 (1): 4–5.

Palmer, S. and Whybrow, A. (eds) (2007) *Handbook of Coaching Psychology: A Guide for Practitioners.* London: Routledge.

Papworth, M. (2004) 'Getting on clinical psychology training courses: responses to frequently asked questions', *Clinical Psychology Forum*, 42: 32–6.

Papworth, M. (2007) 'Getting on clinical psychology training courses: responses to frequently asked questions (Part 2)', *Clinical Psychology Forum*, 177: 37–41.

Parker, J. (2008) 'Comparing research and teaching in university promotion criteria', *Higher Education Quarterly*, 62: 237–51.

Parkinson, C.N. (1958) *Parkinson's Law, or the Pursuit of Progress.* London: John Murray.

Pascarella, E. (2001) 'Identifying excellence in undergraduate education', *Change Magazine*, 33 (3): 18–23.

Passmore, J. (2008) 'Coaching assignments', *People and Organisation at Work*, Autumn: 1–2.

Passmore, J. (ed.) (2010) *Leadership Coaching: Working with Leaders to Develop Elite Performance.* London: Kogan Page.

Patel, N. (1999) *Getting the Evidence: Guidelines for Ethical Mental Health Research Involving Issues of 'Race', Ethnicity and Culture.* London: MIND/Transcultural Psychiatry Society.

Patton, W. and McMahon, M. (1999) *Career Development and Systems Theory: A New Relationship.* Pacific Grove, CA: Brooks/Cole.

Patton, W. and McMahon, M. (2006) *Career Development and Systems Theory: Connecting Theory and Practice* (2nd edn). Rotterdam: Sense Publishers.

Peltier, B. (2010) *The Psychology of Executive Coaching: Theory and Application* (2nd edn). London: Routledge.

Pembroke, L. (no date) *Politicising Self-Harm.* Retrieved 11 May 2011 from: http://www.soteria.freeuk.com/pembroke-jul.htm

Penn, P.R., Rose, F.D. and Johnson, D.A. (2009) 'Virtual enriched environments in the recovery from brain injury', *Developmental Neurorehabilitation*, 12 (1): 32–43.

Perkin, H.J. (1987) 'The academic profession in the United Kingdom', in B.B. Clark (ed.), *The Academic Profession.* Berkeley, CA: University of California Press.

Perkins, R. (2001) 'What constitutes success?', *British Journal of Psychiatry*, 179: 9–10.

Phillips, A., Hatton, C. and Gray, I. (2004) 'Factors predicting the short-listing and selection of trainee psychologists: a prospective national cohort study', *Clinical Psychology and Psychotherapy*, 11: 111–25.

Pilgrim, D. (2002) 'Psychiatric diagnosis: more questions than answers', *The Psychologist*, 13 (6): 302–5.

Pilgrim, D. and Treacher, A. (1992) *Clinical Psychology Observed.* London: Routledge.

Pluess, M., Boniwell, I., Hefferon, K. and Tunariu, A. (in preparation) 'Validation of SPARK Resilience Programme for secondary schools: quantitative and qualitative research findings'.

Potter, J. and Wetherell, M. (1987) *Discourse and Social Psychology: Beyond Attitudes and Behaviour.* London: Sage.

Preuss, L. (1998) 'On ethical theory in auditing', *Managerial Auditing Journal*, 13 (9): 500–8.

Prilleltensky, I. and Nelson, G. (2002) *Doing Psychology Critically: Making a Difference in Diverse Settings*. Basingstoke: Palgrave Macmillan.

Prochaska, J.O. and Norcross, J.C. (2009) *Systems of Psychotherapy: A Transtheoretical Analysis* (7th edn). Pacific Grove, CA: Brooks/Cole Pub Co.

Pugh, J. (2010) 'Cognitive behaviour therapy in schools: the role of educational psychology in the dissemination of empirically supported interventions', *Educational Psychology in Practice*, 26: 391–9.

Radford, J. (1994) 'Remote and ineffectual? The background to the profession of academic psychologist', *Psychology Teaching Review*, 3: 101–17.

Radford, J. (1995) 'The inadequacy of intelligence', in G. Kaufmann, T. Helstrup and K.H. Teigen (eds), *Problem Solving and Cognitive Processes*. Bergen: Fagbokforlaget Vigmostad and Bjorke AS.

Radford, J. (1997) 'Academic psychologists: parasites, priests, proletariat or professionals?', *Psychology Teaching Review*, 6: 170–80.

Radford, J. (2001) 'Doctor of what?', *Teaching in Higher Education*, 6: 257–59.

Radford, J. (2003a) 'The higher education context', in R. Bayne and I. Horton (eds), *Applied Psychology*. London: Sage.

Radford, J. (2003b) 'The professional academic', in R. Bayne and I. Horton (eds), *Applied Psychology*. London: Sage.

Radford, J. (2004) 'All for one and one for all?', *The Psychologist*, 17: 578–9.

Radford, J. (2008) 'Psychology in its place', *Psychology Teaching Review*, 14: 38–50.

Radford, J. (2010) 'A conspiracy against the laity?', *PsyPag Quarterly*, 77: 11–13.

Radford, J. (2011) 'Not a real doctor', *PsyPAG Quarterly*, 80: 4–7.

Radford, J. (2012) 'A response to Hartley: physician, heal thyself', *Psychology Teaching Review*, 18 (1): 35–42.

Radford, J. (in press) 'Physician, heal thyself: A reply to James Hartley', *Psychology Teaching Review*.

Radford, J. and Holdstock, L. (1995) 'Gender differences in higher education aims between computing and psychology students', *Research in Science and Technological Education*, 13: 163–76.

Radford, J. and Holdstock, L. (1996) 'Academic values rule', *New Academic*, 5: 10–11.

Radford, J. and Holdstock, L. (1997) 'Higher education: the views of parents of university students', *Journal of Further and Higher Education*, 20: 81–93.

Radford, J. and Holdstock, L. with Wu Rongxian (1999) 'Psychology as a subject, compared to other subjects: views of pre-university students', *Psychology Teaching Review*, 8: 26–36.

Radford, J. and Rose, D. (1989) *A Liberal Science: Psychology Education Past, Present and Future*. Milton Keynes: SRHE and Open University Press.

Radford, J., Raaheim, K., de Vries, P. and Williams, R. (1997) *Quantity and Quality in Higher Education*. London: Jessica Kingsley.

Rae, D. and Matlay, H. (2010) 'Enterprise education and university entrepreneurship', *Industry and Higher Education*, 23: 243–52.

Ravenette, A.T. (1999) *Personal Construct Theory in Educational Psychology: A Practitioner's View*. London: Whurr Publishers.

Reynierse, J. (2009) 'The case against type dynamics', *Journal of Psychological Type*, 69: 1–21.

Richards, D. and Suckling, R. (2010) 'Improving access to psychological therapies: Phase IV prospective cohort study', *British Journal of Clinical Psychology*, 48: 377–96.

Richards, G. (1987) 'Of what is history of psychology a history?', *British Journal of the History of Science*, 20: 201–11.

Richards, G. (1996) *Putting Psychology in its Place: An Introduction from a Critical Historical Perspective.* London: Routledge.

Rizzo, A., Schultheis, M., Kerns, K. and Mateer, C. (2004) 'Analysis of assets for virtual reality applications in neuropsychology', *Neuropsychological Rehabilitation*, 14 (1/2): 207–39.

Robbins Report (1963) *Great Britain: Committee in Higher Education: Report of the Committee.* London: HMSO.

Robertson, J. (2008) *Coaching Educational Leadership: Building Leadership Capacity through Partnership.* London: Sage.

Robertson, I.J., Baron, H., Gibbons, P., MacIver, R. and Nyfield, G. (2000) 'Conscientiousness and managerial performance', *Journal of Occupational and Organizational Psychology*, 73: 171–80.

Rogers, C.R. (2004) *On Becoming a Person.* London: Constable.

Rogers, E.S., Chamberlin, J., Ellison, M.L. and Crean, T. (1997) 'A consumer-constructed scale to measure empowerment among users of mental health services', *Psychiatric Services*, 48: 1042–7.

Rooke, D. and Torbert, W.R. (2005) 'Seven transformations of leadership', *Harvard Business Review*, 1 April.

Rose, F.D., Attree, E.A., Brooks, B.M. and Johnson, D.A. (1998) 'Virtual environments in brain damage rehabilitation: A rationale from basic neuroscience', in G. Riva, B.K. Wiederhold and E. Molinari (eds), *Virtual Environments in Clinical Psychology and Neuroscience: Methods and Techniques in Advanced Patient–Therapist Interaction.* Amsterdam: IOS Press. pp. 233–42.

Rose, D., Fleischmann, P., Wykes, T., Leese, M. and Bindman, J. (2003) 'Patients' perspectives on electroconvulsive therapy: systematic review', *British Medical Journal*, 326: 1363.

Rose, F.D., Brooks, B.M. and Rizzo, A.A. (2005) 'Virtual reality in brain damage rehabilitation: review', *Cyberpsychology and Behaviour*, 8 (3): 243–51.

Rose, D., Thornicroft, G. and Slade, M. (2006) 'Who decides what evidence is? Developing a multiple perspectives paradigm in mental health', *Acta Psychiatrica Scandinavica*, 113: 109–14.

Roth, A. and Fonagy, P. (2006) *What Works for Whom? A Critical Review of Psychotherapy Research* (2nd revised edn). New York: Guilford Press.

Roth, T. (1999) 'Evidence-based practice: is there a link between research and practice?', *Clinical Psychology Forum*, 133: 37–40.

Roth, T. and Leiper, R. (1995) 'Selecting for clinical training', *The Psychologist*, 8: 25–8.

Royal College of Psychiatrists (2011) *Schizophrenia* (leaflet). Retrieved 30 May 2012 from: http://www.rcpsych.ac.uk/mentalhealthinfo/problems/schizophrenia/schizophrenia.aspx

Roy-Chowdhury, S. (2003) 'Knowing the unknowable: what constitutes evidence in family therapy?', *Journal of Family Therapy*, 25: 64–85.

Rudkin, A. (2000) 'Having the courage to lack conviction', *Clinical Psychology Forum*, 141: 47–8.

Russo, N.F. and Denious, J.E. (2005) 'Controlling birth: science, politics, and public policy', *Journal of Social Issues*, 61 (1): 181–91.

Sackett, D.L., Rosenberg, W.M.C., Gray, J.A.M., Haynes, R.B. and Richardson, W.S. (1996) 'Evidence-based medicine: what it is and what it isn't', *British Medical Journal*, 312: 71–2.

Salter, B. and Tapper, T. (1994) *The State and Higher Education*. London: Woburn Press.

Sampson, E.E. (1993) 'Identity politics: challenges to psychology's understanding', *The American Psychologist*, 48: 1219–30.

Samuel, J. (2009) 'Intensive interaction for people with profound and complex learning disabilities', in H. Beinart, P. Kennedy and S. Llewelyn (eds), *Clinical Psychology in Practice*. Oxford: Wiley-Blackwell.

Sandelin, J. (2010) 'University–industry relationships: benefits and risks', *Industry and Higher Education*, 24: 55–62.

Save the Children (2005) *Psychosocial Care and Protection of Tsunami-Affected Children: Guiding Principles*. London: Save the Children. Retrieved 13 May, 2011 from: http://www.savethechildren.org.uk/en/54_5192.htm

Savickas, M.L. (1993) 'Career counseling in the postmodern era', *Journal of Cognitive Psychotherapy*, 7 (3): 205–15.

Savickas, M.L. (1995) 'Current theoretical issues in vocational psychology: convergence, divergence, and schism', in W.B. Walsh and S.H. Osipow (eds), *Handbook of Vocational Psychology: Theory, Research and Practice* (2nd edn). Mahwah, NJ: Lawrence Erlbaum Associates. pp. 1–34.

Savickas, M.L. (2002) 'Reinvigorating the study of careers', *Journal of Vocational Behavior*, 61 (3): 381–5.

Savickas, M.L. (2008) 'Helping people choose jobs: a history of the guidance profession', in J.A. Athanasou and R.V. Esbroeck (eds), *International Handbook of Career Guidance*. London: Springer Science + Business Media B.V. pp. 97–114.

Savickas, M.L., Nota, L., Rossier, J., Dauwalder, J.-P., Duarte, M.E., Guichard, J., Soresi, S., Van Esbroeck, R. and van Vianen, A.E.M. (2009) 'Life designing: a paradigm for career construction in the 21st century', *Journal of Vocational Behavior*, 75 (3): 239–50.

Scaife, J. (1995) *Training to Help: A Survival Guide*. Sheffield: Riding Press.

Schmidt, H.G., Cohen-Schotanus, J., van der Molen, H.T., Splinter, T.A.W., Bulte, J., Holdring, R. and van Rossum, M.J.M. (2010) 'Learning more by doing less: a "time for self-study" theory explaining curricular effects on graduation rates and study duration', *Higher Education*, 60: 287–300.

Schön, D.A. (1983) *The Reflective Practitioner: How Professionals Think in Action*. New York: Basic Books.

Schön, D.A. (1987) *Educating the Reflexive Practitioner*. San Francisco, CA: Jossey-Bass.

Schriewer, J. (2009) '"Rationalized myths" in European higher education: the construction of the Bologna model', *European Education*, 41: 31–51.

Schultheis, M.T. and Rizzo, A.A. (2001) 'The application of virtual reality technology in rehabilitation', *Rehabilitation Psychology*, 46: 296–311.

Scottish Government, The (2011) *Career Information, Advice and Guidance in Scotland: A Framework for Service Redesign and Improvement.* Edinburgh: The Scottish Government. Retrieved 30 May 2012 from: http://www.scotland.gov.uk/Publicat ions/2011/03/11110615/0

Scoville, W.B. and Milner, B. (1957) 'Loss of recent memory after bilateral hippocampal lesions', *Journal of Neurology, Neurosurgery & Psychiatry*, 20: 11–21.

Seligman, M.E.P. (1972) 'Learned helplessness', *Annual Review of Medicine*, 23: 407–12.

Seligman, M. (1998) *Learned Optimism: How to Change your Mind and your Life.* New York: Free Press.

Seligman, M. (2008) 'Positive health', *Applied Psychology*, 57: 3–18.

Seligman, M.E.P. (2011) *Flourish: A New Understanding of Happiness and Well-Being – and How to Achieve Them.* London: Nicholas Brealey Publishing.

Seligman, M.E.P. and Fowler, R. (2011) 'Comprehensive soldier fitness and the future of psychology', *American Psychologist*, 66: 82–6.

Seligman, M.P., Steen, T.A. and Peterson, C. (2005) 'Positive psychology progress: empirical validation of interventions', *American Psychologist*, 60: 410–21.

Shallice, T. and Warrington, E.K. (1970) 'Independent functioning of verbal memory stores: a neuropsychological study', *Quarterly Journal of Experimental Psychology*, 22: 261–73.

Shapiro, D.A. and Paley, G. (2002) 'Invited rejoinder: the continuing potential relevance of equivalence and allegiance to research on psychological treatment of psychosis', *Psychology and Psychotherapy: Theory, Research and Practice*, 75: 375–9.

Shapiro, M.B. (1961) 'A method of measuring psychological changes specific to the individual psychiatric patient', *British Journal of Medical Psychology*, 34: 151–5.

Sharmila, D. (2011) 'Doctors in distress', *The Lancet*, 377 (9764): 454–5.

Shattuck, M. (2008) 'The change from private to public governance of British higher education: its consequences for higher education policy making 1980–2006', *Higher Education Quarterly*, 62: 181–203.

Shearer-Underhill, C. and Marker, C. (2010) 'The use of the number needed to treat (NNT) in randomized clinical trials in psychological treatment', *Clinical Psychology: Science and Practice*, 17: 41–7.

Sheldon, K., Kashdan, T. and Steger, M. (2011) *Designing Positive Psychology: Taking Stock and Moving Forward.* New York: Oxford University Press.

Shinn, C.H. (1986) *Paying the Piper: The development of the University Grants Committee.* Lewes: Falmer Press.

Silver, H. (2007) *Tradition and Higher Education.* Winchester: Winchester University Press.

Simpson, J., Hemmings, R., Daiches, A. and Amor, C. (2010) 'Shortlisting from the clearing house application form: is it fit for purpose?', *Psychology Learning and Teaching*, 9 (2): 32–36.

Skills Commission, The (2008) *Inspiration and Aspiration – Realising our Potential in the 21st Century.* London: National Skills Forum.

Slater, J.J., Calleio Pérez, D.M. and Fain, S.M. (eds) (2008) *The War Against the Professions: The Impact of Politics and Economics on the Idea of a University*. Rotterdam: Sense Publishers.

Smail, D. (2005) *Power Interest and Psychology: Elements of a Social Materialist Understanding of Distress*. Ross-on-Wye: PCCS Books.

Smith, J.B. (1993) 'Teachers' grading styles: the languages of feeling and thinking', *Journal of Psychological Type*, 26: 37–41.

Smyth, J. (ed.) (1995) *Academic Work: The Changing Process in Higher Education*. Buckingham: SRHE and Open University Press.

Sphere Project, The (2011) *Humanitarian Charter and Minimum Response in Humanitarian Response.* Geneva: The Sphere Project, April 2011. Retrieved 30 May 2012 from: www.sphereproject.org/handbook/

Stedmon, J. and Dallos, R. (eds) (2009) *Reflective Practice in Psychotherapy and Counselling*. Maidenhead: Open University Press.

Stevens, A. (2011) 'Telling policy stories: an ethnographic study of the use of evidence in policy-making in the UK', *Journal of Social Policy*, 40: 237–56.

Stiglitz, J.E., Sen, A. and Fitoussi, J. (2009) *Report by the Commission on the Measurement of Economic Performance and Social Progress.* Retrieved 30 May 2012 from: www. stiglitz-sen-fitoussi.fr/documents/rapport_anglais.pdf

Stiles, D.A. and Stiles, W.B. (1989) 'Abuse of the drug metaphor in psychotherapy process-outcome research', *Clinical Psychology Review*, 9: 521–54.

Stobie, I., Boyle, J. and Woolfson, L. (2005) 'Solution-focussed approaches in the practice of UK educational psychologists: a study of the nature of their application and the evidence of their effectiveness', *School Psychology International*, 26 (1): 5–28.

Stockholm International Peace Research Institute (2011) *World Military Spending Reached $1.6 Trillion in 2010, Biggest Increase in South America, Fall in Europe according to new SIPRI data (11 April 2011)*. Stockholm: Stockholm International Peace Research Institute. Retrieved 16 August 2011 from: http://www.sipri.org/media/pressreleases/milex

Stolz, I., Hendel, D.D. and Horn, A.S. (2010) 'Ranking of rankings: benchmarking of twenty-five higher education ranking systems in Europe', *Higher Education*, 60: 507–28.

Stromquist, N.P. (ed.) (2007) *The Professsoriate in the Age of Globalization.* Rotterdam: Sense Publishers.

Summerfield, D. (1999) 'A critique of seven assumptions behind psychological trauma programmes in war-affected areas', *Social Science and Medicine*, 48: 1449–62.

Syer, J. and Connolly, C. (1998) *Sporting Body, Sporting Mind: An Athlete's Guide to Mental Training*. Simon and Schuster: London.

Szymanska, K. (2002) 'Trainee expectations in counselling psychology as compared to the reality of training experiences', *Counselling Psychology Review*, 17 (1): 22–7.

Taleb, N.N. (2007) *Fooled by Randomness.* London: Penguin.

Tan, S.J. and Halpern, D.F. (2006) 'Applying the science of psychology to a public that distrusts science', in S.I. Donaldson, D.E. Berger and K. Pezdek (eds), *Applied Psychology: New Frontiers and Rewarding Careers*. Mahwak, NJ: Lawrence Erlbaum Associates.

Tarrier, N., Haddock, G., Barrowclough, C. and Wykes, T. (2002) 'Invited commentary Paley and Shapiro: Are all psychological treatments for psychosis equal? The need for CBT in the treatment of psychosis and not for psychodynamic psychotherapy' *Psychology & Psychotherapy: Theory, Research & Practice*, 75: 365–74.

Thaler, R.H. and Sunstein, C.S. (2008) *Nudge: Improving Decisions about Health, Wealth, and Happiness*. New Haven: Yale University Press.

Thoma, V. and Henson, R.N. (2011) 'Object representations in ventral and dorsal visual streams: fMRI repetition effects depend on attention and part-whole configuration', *NeuroImage*, 57 (2): 513–25.

Thoma, V., Hummel, J.E. and Davidoff, J. (2004) 'Evidence for holistic representations of ignored images and analytic representations of attended images', *Journal of Experimental Psychology: Human Perception and Performance*, 30 (2): 257–67.

Thoma, V., Davidoff, J. and Hummel, J. (2007) 'Priming of plane-rotated objects depends on attention and view familiarity', *Visual Cognition*, 15 (2): 179–210.

Thorne, B. (1992) 'Psychotherapy and counselling: the quest for differences', *Counselling*, 3 (4): 244–8.

Tight, M. (2009) 'Are academic workloads increasing? The post-war survey evidence in the UK', *Higher Education Quarterly*, 64: 200–15.

Tolman, E.C. (1948) 'Cognitive maps in rats and men', *The Psychological Review*, 55 (4): 189–208.

Tonkin, M., Bull, R. and Santtila, P. (2011) 'The linking of burglary crimes using offender behavior: Testing research cross-nationally and exploring methodology', *Legal and Criminological Psychology*, 26 January (ePub ahead of print).

Towl, G. (2003) *Psychology in Prisons*. Oxford: Wiley-Blackwell.

Tuddenham, R. (1966) 'The nature and measurement of intelligence', in L. Postman (ed.), *Psychology in the Making*. New York: Alfred A. Knopf.

Tversky, A. and Kahneman, D. (1981) 'The framing of decisions and the psychology of choice', *Science*, 211: 453–8.

Tweed, R.G. and Lehman, D.R. (2002) 'Learning considered within a cultural context: Confucian and Socratic approaches', *American Psychologist*, 57: 89–99.

Tyrer, P., Duggan, C., Cooper, S., Crawford, M., Seivewright, H., Rutter, D., Maden, T., Byford, S. and Barrett, B. (2010) 'The successes and failures of the DSPD experiment: the assessment and management of severe personality disorder', *Medicine, Science and the Law*, 50: 95–9.

UK Commission for Employment and Skills (UKCES) (2010) *Ambition 2020: World Class Skills and Jobs for the UK*. Wath-upon-Dearne: UKCES. Retrieved 30 May 2012 from: www.ukces.org.uk/upload/pdf/UKCES_FullReport_USB_A2020.pdf

Usher, R. (2002) 'A diversity of doctorates: fitness for the knowledge economy?', *Higher Education Research and Development*, 21: 143–53.

Ussher, J.M. (2003) 'The ongoing silencing of women in families: an analysis and rethinking of premenstrual syndrome and therapy', *Journal of Family Therapy*, 25 (4): 388–405.

Ussher, J.M. and Nicolson, P. (eds) (1992) *Gender Issues in Clinical Psychology*. London: Routledge.

Ussher, J.M. and Perz, J. (2008) 'Empathy, egalitarianism and emotion work in the relational negotiation of PMS: the experience of women in lesbian relationships', *Feminism & Psychology*, 18 (1): 87–111.

Vanable, P.A., Ostrow, D.G., McKirnan, D.J., Taywaditep, K.J. and Hope, B.A. (2000) 'Impact of combination therapies on HIV risk perceptions and sexual risk among HIV-positive and HIV-negative gay and bisexual men', *Health Psychology*, 19 (2): 134–45.

Wallace, L. (2000) '"What did this course do for you?" The employability of master's graduates in health psychology', *Health Psychology Update*, 39: 4–10.

Walsh, D. and Bull, R. (2010) 'What really is effective in interviews with suspects? A study comparing interview skills against interview outcomes', *Legal and Criminological Psychology*, 15: 305–21.

Walsh, J.J. and McDermott, M.R. (2003) 'Health psychology', in R. Bayne and I. Horton (eds), *Applied Psychology*. London: Sage. pp. 79–93.

Walsh, S. and Cormack, M. (1994) '"Do as we say not as we do": personal, professional and organizational barriers to the receipt of support at work', *Clinical Psychology and Psychotherapy*, 1: 1101–10.

Walsh, S. and Scaife, J. (1998) 'Mechanisms for addressing personal and professional development in clinical training', *Clinical Psychology Forum*, 115: 21–4.

Wangenge-Ouma, G. and Langa, P.V. (2010) 'Universities and the mobilization of claims of excellence for competitive advantage', *Higher Education*, 59: 749–64.

Ward, T. (2010) 'Is offender rehabilitation a form of punishment?' *British Journal of Forensic Practice*, 12: 4–13.

Warnock, M. (1988) *A Common Policy for Education*. Oxford: Oxford University Press.

Warnock, M. (2010) *Dishonest to God: On Keeping Religion out of Politics*. London: Continuum.

Warren Piper, D. (1992) 'Are professors professional?', *Higher Education Quarterly*, 46: 145–156.

Warrington, E.K. and Taylor, A.M. (1978) 'Two categorical stages of object recognition', *Perception*, 7 (6): 695–705.

Watkins, J.M. and Mohr, B.J. (2001) *Appreciative Inquiry: Change at the Speed of Imagination*. San Francisco, CA: Jossey-Bass/Pfeiffer.

Watson, J. (1924) *Behaviorism*. Chicago: University of Chicago Press.

Welch, A. (ed.) (2005) *The Professoriate: Profile of a Profession*. Dordrecht: Springer.

Wessells, M. (2006) 'Negotiating the shrunken humanitarian space: Challenges and options', in G. Reyes and G. Jacobs (eds), *Handbook of International Disaster Psychology, Volume 1*. Westport, CT: Praeger. pp. 147–164.

Wessells, M. (2008) 'Do no harm: challenges in organizing psychosocial support to displaced people in emergency settings', *Refuge*, 25 (1): 6–14.

West, R., McNeill, A. and Raw, M. (2000) 'Smoking cessation guidelines for health professionals: an update', *Thorax*, 55 (12): 987–99.

Whitmore, J. (2002) *Coaching for Performance* (3rd edn). London: Brealey Publishing.

Wilkinson, R. and Pickett, K. (2009) *The Spirit Level: Why More Equal Societies Almost Always do Better*. London: Penguin.

Will, B., Galani, R., Kelche, C. and Rosenzweig, M.R. (2004) 'Recovery from brain injury in animals: relative efficacy of environmental enrichment, physical exercise or formal training (1990–2002)', *Progress in Neurobiology*, 72: 167–82.

Willig, C. (2000) 'A discourse-dynamic approach to the study of subjectivity in health psychology', *Theory & Psychology*, 10 (4): 547–70.

Wilson, B.A., Evans, J.J., Emslie H. and Malinek, V. (1997) 'Evaluation of NeuroPage: a new memory aid', *Journal of Neurology, Neurosurgery & Psychiatry*, 63: 113–5.

Wilson, R.A. (2008) *The Future of Work: What does Work Mean 2025 and Beyond?* London: DCSF/Futurelab. Retrieved 30 May 2012 from: http://www.beyondcurrent thorizons.org.uk/wp-content/uploads/bch_challenge_paper_work_wilson.pdf

Winter, D. (2010) 'Editorial for special issue: researcher allegiance in the psychological therapies', *European Journal of Psychotherapy & Counselling*, 12: 3–9.

Winter, H., Gaynor, G., Weiner, B., Tsalavoutas, S., Hawksley, J., Prescott, N., le Roux and Perella, F. (2011) 'Clinical psychology trainees: self-funded places for international trainees', *Clinical Psychology Forum*, 225: 6–7.

Winter, H., Gaynor, D., Weiner, B., Tsalavoutas, S., Hawksley, J. Prescott, N., leRoux, N. and Pirella, F. (in press) [Letter to the Editor] *Clinical Psychology Forum*.

Wolf, A. (1995) *Competence-Based Assessment*. Buckingham: Open University Press.

Woolfe, R. (1996) 'Counselling Psychology in Britain: past, present and future', *Counselling Psychology Review*, 11 (4): 7–18.

Woolfe, R. (2002) 'That is what gets results' (Letter to the Editor), *The Psychologist*, 15 (4): 168.

Woolfe, R., Strawbridge, S., Douglas, B. and Dryden, W. (2010) (eds) *Handbook of Counselling Psychology*. London: Sage.

Workman, L. (2011) 'The psychological transformer: interview with Kerry Chamberlain', *The Psychologist*, 24 (3): 190–1.

Young, R.A. and Collin, A. (2000) 'Introduction: framing the future of career', in A. Collin and R.A. Young (eds), *The Future of Career*. Cambridge: Cambridge University Press. pp. 1–17.

Zimbardo, P.G. (2004) 'Does psychology make a significant difference in our lives?', *American Psychologist*, 59: 339–51.

INDEX

References in *italics* are to figures and in **bold** are to tables.